D0139864

Ethical Issues
in the New
Reproductive
Technologies

Ethical Issues in the New Reproductive Technologies

Edited and with an introduction by

RICHARD T. HULL

State University of New York at Buffalo

Wadsworth Publishing Company
Belmont, California
A Division of Wadsworth, Inc.

Philosophy Editor: Kenneth King
Editorial Assistant: Michelle Palacio
Production: The Book Company
Print Buyer: Randy Hurst
Designer: Donna Davis
Copy Editor: Elizabeth Judd
Compositor: Typelink, Inc.
Cover: Vargas/Williams/Design

Printed in the United States of America

1 2 3 4 5 6 7 8 9 10—93 92 91 90

Library of Congress Cataloging in Publication Data

Ethical issues in the new reproductive technologies / edited and with an introduction
    by Richard T. Hull.
        p.   cm.
    Articles reprinted from various sources.
    Includes bibliographical references.
    ISBN 0-534-12558-1
    1. Human reproductive technology—Moral and ethical aspects.   I. Hull, Richard T.,
1936-   .
    [DNLM: 1. Ethics, Medical—collected works.   2. Fertilization in Vitro—collected
works.   3. Insemination, Artificial—collected works.   4. Reproduction Technics—collected
works.   WQ 205 E836]
RG133.5.E84   1989
176—dc20
DNLM/DLC   89-22643
for Library of Congress   CIP

ISBN 0-534-12558-1

This collection is dedicated to my late, great son, Geoff.

Contents

Preface

Works in biomedical ethics are usually one of two sorts; either they attempt to present a broad survey of a range of major theories, concepts, and issues as an introduction to the field of bioethics, or they attempt to develop one theory, concept, or issue in depth.

This work is of the latter sort: It presumes that the reader will have access to surveys of the conceptual theories and principles of ethics in application to a range of biomedical issues; it assumes some familiarity with the general terminology of bioethics; and it seeks to deepen the reader's understanding of a particular field of application and concern—that of the technology of reproduction. It lies squarely in the discipline of bioethics, because it is concerned with the application of biotechnology to problems of fertility and practices of childbearing. At the same time, it can be viewed as overlapping with the more general ethical concerns about having children that have come to characterize much of our social reflection on human institutions.

The field of reproductive technologies stretches beyond those explicitly covered in this work. The technologies of abortion and of contraception properly fall within the conceptual framework of reproductive technology, yet both have been omitted from consideration here, for various reasons. A number of excellent collections of works and monographs on the ethical and conceptual problems of abortion already exist. Moreover, abortion and contraception are technologies concerned with not having babies; this collection focuses on the technologies of having them, and the ethical issues that those technologies raise. Our concern here is first with the struggles of individuals who have unsuccessfully attempted to have children, with the professional ethical concerns and motivations of those who have sought to bring relief to their problems of infertility through the use of medical technology, and finally with the uses of the available technology, developed for medical purposes, to address the needs and wants of individuals not afflicted with biological problems of infertility.

This book is offered as a selection of the best and most recent thinking of individuals specializing in the ethical and legal problems involved in the new reproductive technologies. It aims, first, at providing factual information about those technologies and their scope and limitations. It also seeks to locate the varied uses of those technologies in the wider cultural contexts of our collective wisdom about human reproduction, broadly construed. It reflects interests as varied as those of the enthusiastic proponent of the new reproductive technologies, the feminist opposing the exploitation of women, the social critic worrying about erosion of the responsibilities of parenting, and the traditionalist concerned about the transformation of the fundamental moral character of the family. And finally, it seeks to stimulate appreciation of the complex and multitiered character of moral decision making as it is practiced by the individual, the medical professional, the affected member of the community, and the legislator or jurist who is charged with preserving, protecting, and applying justly the principles of the society.

My thanks are extended to LeRoy Walters, who provided valuable advice on an earlier prospectus for this work; to Morton Winston, who read a later proposal and made several excellent suggestions; and to Kenneth King, philosophy editor for Wadsworth Publishing Company, who demonstrated great patience and good sense in guiding this project to its completion.

My appreciation is extended as well to the publishers and authors of the essays and excerpts included herein for their kind permission to reprint their efforts.

Acknowledgments

Ethics Committee (1984-85) of the American Fertility Society. 1986. "The Constitutional Aspects of Procreative Liberty," in "Ethical Considerations of the New Reproductive Technologies." *Fertility and Sterility* 46(Sup.1):2S-6S. Reprinted with permission of the publishers from *Fertility and Sterility*.

Ethics Committee (1984-85) of the American Fertility Society. 1986. "The Moral Right to Reproduce and its Limitations," in "Ethical Considerations of the New Reproductive Technologies." *Fertility and Sterility* 46(Sup.1):21S-23S. Reprinted with permission of the publishers from *Fertility and Sterility*.

Congregation for the Doctrine of the Faith. Vatican translation. 1987. *Instruction on Respect for Human Life in Its Origin and on the Dignity of Procreation: Replies to Certain Questions of the Day* ("Foreword" and "Introduction" omitted). Boston: St. Paul Editions. Reprinted with permission of St. Paul Editions.

Ethics Committee (1986-87) of the American Fertility Society. 1988. "Ethical Consideration of the New Reproductive Technologies." *Fertility and Sterility* 49(Sup.2):2S-10S. Reprinted with permission of the publishers from *Fertility and Sterility*.

Corea, Gena. 1986. "The Subversive Sperm: 'A False Strain of Blood.'" From Gena Corea, *The Mother Machine: Reproductive Technologies from Artificial Insemination to Artificial Wombs*. New York: Harper & Row, pp. 34–48. Reprinted with permission of the author.

Smart, Carol. 1987. "'There is of course the distinction dictated by nature': Law and the Problem of Paternity." In Michelle Stanworth, ed., *Reproductive Technologies: Gender, Motherhood, and Medicine*. Minneapolis: University of Minnesota Press, pp. 98–117. Collection copyright © Michelle Stanworth 1987. Copyright © in each contribution held by authors 1987. Reprinted by permission of the University of Minnesota Press, Minneapolis.

Caplan, Arthur L. 1986. "The Ethics of In Vitro Fertilization." *Primary Care* 13(2):241-253. Reprinted with permission of W. B. Saunders Co. and the author.

Walters, LeRoy. 1987. "Test-Tube Babies: Ethical Considerations." *Clinics in Perinatology* 14(2):271-280. Reprinted with permission of W. B. Saunders Co. and the author.

Tiefel, Hans O. 1982. "Human In Vitro Fertilization: A Conservative View." *JAMA* 247:3235-3242. Copyright 1982 American Medical Association. Reprinted with permission of the author and the American Medical Association.

Zaner, Richard M. 1984. "A Criticism of Moral Conservatism's View of In Vitro Fertilization and Embryo Transfer." *Perspectives in Biology and Medicine* 27(2):201-212. Copyright 1984 by The University of Chicago. All rights reserved. Reprinted with permission of the author and The University of Chicago Press.

Robertson, John A. 1983. "Surrogate Mothers: The Case For and Against." *Hastings Center Report* 13(5):28-34. Reprinted with permission of the author and the publishers of the Hastings Center Report.

Wilentz, Hon. Robert N., Chief Justice, New Jersey Supreme Court. 1988. "In the Matter of Baby M, a Pseudonym for an Actual Person." *109 N.J.* 396, 421-474. Reprinted with permission of West Publishing Co.

Annas, George J. 1986. "The Baby Broker Boom." *Hastings Center Report* 16(3):30-32. Reprinted with permission of the author and publishers of the Hastings Center Report.

Andrews, Lori B. 1987. "The Aftermath of Baby M: Proposed State Laws on Surrogate Motherhood." *Hastings Center Report* 17(5):31-40. Reprinted with permission of the author and the publishers from Hastings Center Report.

Murray, Thomas H. 1987. "Moral Obligations to the Not-Yet-Born: The Fetus as Patient." *Clinics in Perinatology* 14(2):329-343. Reprinted with permission of W. B. Saunders Co. and the author.

Nelson, Lawrence J., and Nancy Milliken. 1988. "Compelled Medical Treatment of Pregnant Women: Life, Liberty and Law in Conflict." *JAMA* 259(7):1060-1066. Copyright 1988 American Medical Association. Reprinted with permission of the authors and the American Medical Association.

Bayles, Michael D. 1984. "Genetic Choice." From Michael D. Bayles, *Reproductive Ethics* (chap. 2), pp. 33-51. Englewood Cliffs, N.J.: Prentice-Hall. Copyright © 1984. Reprinted with permission of Prentice-Hall, Inc., Englewood Cliffs. N.J.

Mahowald, Mary B., Jerry Silver, and Robert A. Ratcheson. 1987. "The Ethical Options in Transplanting Fetal Tissue." *Hastings Center Report* 17(1):9-15. Reprinted with permission of the authors and publishers from the Hastings Center Report.

INTRODUCTION

Legal and Moral Claims About the Right to Assistance in Reproduction

REVIEW OF THE ISSUES

Perhaps one of the most general truisms of our time whose wisdom we still seek to embody in our social and medical ethics is that no action, development, or piece of technology has just one effect. Nowhere is the truth of that lesson more profound than in the burgeoning field of reproductive technology. Every new piece of technology, made for the specific purpose of addressing some clearly compelling medical need, has led to profound and controversial issues dimly apprehended, if at all, by its inventors.

Biomedical ethics as a discipline has repeatedly scrambled to comprehend the implications of these new powers even as those implications were being played out dramatically in the media and courts of law in this and other societies. The very pace of technological advance has denied philosophers their accustomed luxury of sedate and measured reflection, for bioethicists have quickly recognized that philosophy's traditional symbol of wisdom, the Owl of Minerva, if not chased from her perch, would spread her wings not even at dusk but only after nightfall. And so it has been with philosophy and the new reproductive technologies.

Most of us have experienced, in recent years, repeatedly having our attention riveted to ongoing published or broadcast reports of clashes in the courts between individuals locked in disputes over custody of children conceived under surrogacy agreements, of individuals seeking knowledge about a biological parent, of embryos orphaned while in a frozen state. These are only particularly dramatic public examples of the many more scenarios played out in the usually private contexts of individuals dealing with needs and desires about having children. And it is sobering to realize that as many as 2.4 million married couples experienced fertility problems in 1982 (Office of Technology Assessment, 1988), and many more will confront health problems of their children originating in genetic or maternal/paternal health factors during gestation. So our attention is not merely voyeuristic; we see in others' plights anticipations of our own fragile possibilities. And these anticipations irresistibly draw us into reflection on the possibilities of being confronted with such obstacles, and tempted by technology's ingenious and awesome ways around them.

A corollary of the truism that one cannot do just one thing is that there are virtually no significant actions that one can take today that affect only oneself. One may focus exclusively for a time on the hoped-for personal effects of an application of technology, but eventually one discovers results in oneself and others that were unimagined but are real, and sometimes troublesome. The care with which others regard us, coupled with a sometimes less myopic view of the probable results of what we do, may prompt them to seek to dissuade us from what we (think we) desire; and the fact that our actions have possible effects on their interests may lend their "interference" a self-protecting function.

Still others, charged by their groups or by society with safeguarding important institutions, may see in our contemplated courses of action trends that pose threats to those institutions; they may react with less than the full enthusiasm with which we individually embrace personal possibilities. Still others may side with us, in the service of yet other ideals, catching our personal excitement and reading it as a manifestation of the progress of human efforts to master, and not be mastered by, brute nature and personal misfortune.

We therefore encounter the phenomenon of fair-minded individuals disagreeing over moral matters. Appreciating the roots of those disagreements lies, in part, in realizing the kinds of considerations advanced by the types of moral reasoning, considered as theories; but it lies as well in grasping the role that a piece of argument plays, the interests in the service of which it is wielded. Perhaps only then can discussion, clarification, and appraisal of these issues be fully conducted.

I suggested earlier that there are at least four levels of moral argument about modern reproduction and its technologies at which we will find the authors of our selections engaged: the *personal level* of the patient—usually a couple, sometimes an individual, occasionally several; the *professional level* of the physician—frequently reflecting not only a differing view of the patient's needs than that of the patient but also a commitment to a tradition and its view of the proper role and use of the tools of medical technology; the *group level*—whether the group is religious, professional, philosophical, political—where individuals see their groups' interests in protecting and fostering a set of ideals intersecting in one way or another with both the interests of the patient and the potentials of the physician's technology; and the *level of government*, one of immense powers and checks of power, with its mandate to serve the just interests of all, impartially conceived and broadly construed.

At the personal level the deliberative attention is almost always focused on oneself or the closest ring of one's family, and an immediate problem: infertility, or the lack of a suitable mate, or one's economic needs or commitments to unfinished life projects. One is preoccupied with an inability to conceive, or one confronts the possibility of one's genetic heritage or behavior posing a threat to one's possible offspring. Here, the question is, What can and should I do? How can I maximize the chance of conception, or minimize the risk of damage to my offspring?

At this level we are generally not concerned with the impact our action may have on the national interest, not concerned even with the reaction that our overtures to a physician may provoke. Judging from the statistics, we may not even be primarily focused on conforming to the ideals of the various groups to which we belong. (A recent study indicated that the percentage of Roman Catholic women who obtain abortions is greater than that of non-Catholic women who do likewise.)

What ought to be done appears in first-level deliberation as that which factors optimally in the personal value hierarchy of the individual with the problem. The individual, in short, is engaging in egocentric reasoning. In this respect, infertility appears as an inability to engage in activity that is perceived by that individual as normal, natural, and necessary for his or her individual fulfillment. If it is a disability that may be treated or circumvented by application of medical science and technology, the individual will likely see it as a medical problem even if its origin is such a natural one as aging. Indeed, confronted with medicine as the sole keeper of powerful technology, one is going to be inclined to view as medical problems even desires and inconveniences imposed by one's adopted lifestyle.

Moral deliberation at the second level by physicians and other providers of health and medical care usually, but not always, also focuses on the individual's problem. A lack of shared commitment at the individual level occurs when the problem is not perceived by the physician as falling within the proper scope of medicine's traditional commitment to health. Consumers who see medical services and technology as ways of fulfilling what others perceive as their whims and wishes may find health-care professionals resistant to demands for services. A couple who wants to use the technology of amniocentesis and selective abortion to ensure a child of a particular sex, or a woman who wants to employ the technology of lavage and transfer of a preimplantation embryo to a surrogate gestational mother in order to avoid the professional disruption of pregnancy, might expect to encounter such resistance. But resistance may be encountered as well to requests for artificial insemination by a single woman, or one or both members of a lesbian couple, and so forth, because their problems do not strike the traditionally more conservative health-care provider as medical in character.

The health-care provider may also perceive the individual's problem as one of unwillingness to accept something inevitable, as unrealistic in pursuing functions that decline naturally for very good biological reasons, or as something that should have been anticipated before a prior step (such as surgical sterilization) was taken. A couple in their late forties or early fifties stand far greater risks of producing a child with one of the major birth defects; their single-minded pursuit of pregnancy at any cost may strike the physician as both insensitive to the risks to possible future children and naive about the effects of having such a child on their own psychological well-being. There is something remote about a statistical possibility with which one has no experience; the physician's experience in such possibilities-become-actualities looms vividly before the mind and may prompt discouragement of the incautious enthusiasm of the patient couple. At the same time, the couple who had a child and then opted for surgical sterilization, only to lose that child tragically, may appear to the physician to have the best of reasons for wanting their infertility treated by medicine, despite being of an age that poses risks to future offspring.

The third level of moral reasoning about these technologies is that of the groups or communities to which we give our membership and allegiance. Often, the influence of such a community's values is directly present in the individual, perhaps even in the health-care professional. It is certainly the case that the group, with a strong consensus concerning the permissibility or impermissibility of some technology, will seek to foster that consensus in its membership; on matters of great importance, continued membership in the group may be conditional upon adhering to the consensus. I suggest we view Vatican directives with respect to the impermissibility of artificial insemination, and the recommendation of the Ethics Committee of the American Fertility Society against the use of a gestational mother for a nonmedical reason, as similar in functioning to preserve a group consensus about a particular value.

If medicine were simply to leave up to each physician how, to whom, and for what reason to offer a particular technological service, something essential about medicine as an organized profession would be lost (see Jameton, 1984, chap. 2). Hence, medicine as a profession may seek to bolster the individual physician's adherence to an ideal, such as offering medical services only for the purpose of promoting or restoring health, through publication of its organizations' professional standards and ethics committees' directives, lobbying with state and federal legislatures and regulatory agencies, and even (in relatively rare cases) disciplining individual physicians who display patterns of unethical, unprofessional, or incompetent practices.

Finally, a level of moral reasoning and directive may occur at the various levels of government, from governors' and presidential commissions to legislative bodies, from regulatory agencies to the systems of civil and criminal courts. A major concern of government is the protection of the interests of its citizens against exploitation. An economically disadvantaged woman may agree to serve as a "surrogate mother" for another couple's child in exchange for payment, but find that the trauma of surrendering the child at birth is psychologically crippling to her and damaging to her natural children, who may come to wonder whether they, too, might be sold. This sort of possibility has prompted some states to outlaw surrogacy contracts.

Disputes over authority and responsibility for banked sperm or preembryos arise, and require regulation and adjudication. Situations not even anticipated in the initial agreement, such as responsibility for a child born via artificial insemination from a donor when the marriage ends in divorce, require the determination of the courts. Attempts to compel medical treatment on pregnant women collide with passionately held commitments to individual liberty in this society, raising constitutional issues that may ultimately be resolved only at the highest level of our court system.

Thus, reasoning about the ethical issues in reproductive technology is a complex, multifaceted, and multilevel process, requiring careful reflection on each technology and its possible uses as we seek both a social consensus and a personal or professional stance.

An Office of Technology Assessment (OTA) report in May 1988 indicates that Americans spend about $1 billion annually on medical care to combat infertility (defined as a couple's failure to conceive after a year of unprotected intercourse). About 20 percent of the cases of infertility result from sexually transmitted diseases, such as gonorrhea, chlamydia, and so forth, and are preventable with "safe sex" techniques. The most widely successful and common methods of treatment are "low-tech" measures, such as medical treatment, surgery, ovulation induction, and artificial insemination. "High-tech" methods, such as in vitro fertilization and gamete intrafallopian transfer, involve reproduction without intercourse (as does artificial insemination), but are considerably more expensive. Still other practices involve social arrangements that involve what has been called preconception adoption contracts, the misnamed "surrogate mother," and other strategies permitting a couple's biological child to be gestated in another woman's womb.

Despite the variety of low- and high-tech possibilities that currently exist, OTA reports that as many as half the infertile couples seeking treatment are ultimately unsuccessful. Nonetheless, reproductive technology offers for many couples the only possibility of rearing normal children, since the combination of the ready accessibility of abortion on demand and long waiting lists for normal, adoptive children, together with standard age limitations for adoptive parents and delays in starting families, alert many infertile couples to their problem well into the childbearing years. Thus, infertile couples and their social networks of families and friends represent a potent political force that may be expected to press for increased accessibility of many techniques currently not covered by medical insurance and thus unavailable to couples without substantial disposable income.

PREVIEW OF THE SELECTIONS

The 1984–85 Ethics Committee of the American Fertility Society, a professional medical society composed mostly of physicians with a sprinkling of ethicists, lawyers, and religious leaders, issued a lengthy report titled "Ethical Considerations of the New Reproductive Technologies." In the two sections of that report reproduced here, the Committee takes up the questions of legal and moral reproductive rights and responsibilities, observing that the legal right to reproduce is virtually unlimited in the United States (even in unmarried individuals). The Committee argues that the legal right to reproduce should extend to noncoital, assisted means of reproduction, but only as a negative liberty right of noninterference by the state, not as a positive legal claim or welfare right to financial assistance by the state in obtaining access to reproductive technology.

On the other hand, the Committee concludes that the moral right to reproduce may be limited by a variety of considerations having to do with predictable or possible harms to offspring. Finally, there may be a moral claim against society by the infertile couple of limited means for help in obtaining reproductive assistance, depending on whether society accepts the obligation to provide an adequate level of health care for every citizen and on whether inability to reproduce is viewed as an "unhealthy" condition.

Shortly after the Committee's deliberations were published, the Vatican published a pamphlet addressing a variety of current issues in reproductive ethics. In the portions of that pamphlet included here, the Church condemns all reproductive technologies except those that seek to restore the damaged or diseased reproductive system to normalcy and that involve the mechanisms of coital reproduction by a married couple without the direct intervention of any third party. Thus, not only are surrogacy and in vitro fertilization (IVF) ruled out, but so are gamete intrafallopian transfer (GIFT), artificial insemination from a donor (AID), and even artificial insemination from the husband (AIH).

But the Church statement went beyond its apparent aim of offering moral instruction to Catholic congregations. In the section on "Moral and Civil Law" it advocates legislative prohibition of AIH, IVF, donation of gametes, surrogacy, and of the use of aborted fetuses for research purposes.

The publication of this pamphlet prompted the 1986–87 Ethics Committee of the American Fertility Society to review the Vatican's document. The Ethics Committee located its differences and reasserted its position on a number of issues. The Committee's full response is included in its entirety, including its response to the Vatican's proposed criminalization of reproductive technology.

Works Cited

1. Jameton, Andrew. *Nursing Practice: The Ethical Issues*. Englewood Cliffs, N.J.: Prentice-Hall, 1984.
2. Office of Technology Assessment, U.S. Congress. *Infertility: Medical and Social Choices*. Washington, D.C.: U.S. Government Printing Office, 1988.

The Constitutional Aspects of Procreative Liberty

ETHICS COMMITTEE OF THE AMERICAN FERTILITY SOCIETY*

Currently, there is little direct regulation of in vitro fertilization (IVF) and donor-assisted reproduction in the United States, although it is likely that further regulation will occur. Regulation of noncoital reproduction raises questions of the constitutional power of the state in intervening with procreative choice. This chapter addresses the constitutional status of that choice and its application to IVF and donor-assisted reproduction.

Procreative Liberty and the Right to Procreate

In discussions of procreative liberty, actions designed to avoid procreation and actions designed to bring it about must be distinguished. In the United States, a constitutional right *not to procreate* has been clearly established by a series of Supreme Court decisions involving contraception and abortion. The burdens of unwanted pregnancy and child rearing are deemed so substantial that any competent person—married, single, adult, minor—may choose to abort until the time of viability and use contraceptives to avoid pregnancy.[1]

The right *to procreate*—to do those things that will lead to biologic descendants—is also of great significance to persons, but it has not received explicit legal recognition because the state has never attempted to restrict married couples from having children when and how they can.[2] Without attempts at state regulation, the need or occasion to define the limits of a married couple's right to procreate has not arisen.

---

*Ed. note: Members of the 1984–85 Committee included Lori B. Andrews, J.D., Celso-Ramon Garcia, M.D., Clifford Grobstein, Ph.D., Gary D. Hodgen, Ph.D., Howard W. Jones, Jr., M.D., Richard J. McCormick, S.J., Richard Marrs, M.D., C. Alvin Paulsen, M.D., John Robertson, J.D., Edward E. Wallach, M.D., LeRoy Walters, Ph.D.

Noncoital conception and donor-assisted reproduction raise questions that require a more precise definition of a constitutional right to procreate. Although there are few precedents directly on the point, there is good reason to expect the courts to recognize a constitutional right to procreate by noncoital and donor-assisted means. Such a right will not prevent regulation, but it will protect individual procreative choice unless there is a compelling need for state intervention.

The Argument for a Constitutional Right to Procreate

Most persons would consider the right to reproduce to be a fundamental human right. Indeed, several international declarations of human rights speak about the right of "men and women of full age . . . to marry and found a family" (United Nations, 1978).[3] However, these declarations have not been ratified by the United States and therefore have no legal effect.

Moreover, there have been few cases brought to the United States Supreme Court that test the question directly. Aside from laws involuntarily sterilizing mentally retarded persons and laws on fornication and cohabitation that attempt to confine reproduction to marriage, there have been few attempts by the state to stop people from reproducing.[4] However, on several occasions, the Supreme Court has indicated strong support for procreative liberty, particularly of married persons. Although these cases have not involved state attempts to prevent married couples from reproducing, they do suggest that the Court would recognize such a right if it were ever faced with a direct limitation on a married couple's desire to reproduce by sexual intercourse.

The language in these cases is broad and presumably would extend to both coital and noncoital reproduction, even if the latter were not contemplated at the time. In *Skinner v Oklahoma*, the Court struck down a mandatory sterilization law for habitual criminals because it interfered with marriage and procreation, which are among "the basic rights of man."[5] In *Meyer v Nebraska*, the Court stated that constitutional liberty includes "the right of an individual to marry, establish a home and bring up children."[6] In *Stanley v Illinois*, the Court observed that "the rights to conceive and raise one's children have been deemed 'essential,' 'basic civil rights of man,' and 'rights far more precious than property rights.'"[7] Another case recognized that "freedom of personal choice in matters of marriage and family life" is one of the liberties protected by the due process clause of the Fourteenth Amendment.[8] Finally, Justice Brennan, in *Eisenstadt v Baird*, stated: "If the right of privacy means anything, it is the right of the individual, married or single, to be free of unwarranted governmental intrusion into matters so fundamentally affecting a person as the decision whether to bear or beget a child."[9]

Because these statements do not arise in cases in which the state has tried to prevent married persons from procreating, much less from reproducing by noncoital or donor-assisted means, they are not precedents that are binding in later cases. However, they do strongly suggest that the Supreme Court would recognize some right to reproduce, at least for married persons. For example, it is likely that laws limiting a married couple's right to have children when and as they choose by sexual intercourse (such as mandatory sterilization, conception, or abortion laws) would be struck down as a violation of the fundamental right to procreate.*

The argument for the right to reproduce coitally is clearest in the case of married persons but can also be made for unmarried persons. Although most of the Supreme Court dicta cited above apply explicitly to married persons, a strong argument can be made that unmarried persons also have a right to reproduce coitally.[10] Unmarried persons also have needs or desires to have and rear biologic descendants and may be as competent parents as married couples.† They may not be able or willing to marry to satisfy this desire. Indeed, banning coital or noncoital conception by single persons seems inconsistent because an unmarried person cannot be forced to use contraception, abort, or relinquish the rearing of an illegitimate child.‡

Although the argument for the right of unmarried persons to reproduce coitally persuades many persons, it is not clear that this argument would be accepted by the Supreme Court. The single person's right to use contraception and to continue a pregnancy does not necessarily entail a right to conceive in the first place.§ The Supreme Court has not yet held that fornication laws violate an unmarried person's right of privacy. Given the tradition of reproduction within marriage and the importance of the family,* the Court is more likely to recognize a married couple's right to reproduce than to recognize the right of unmarried persons to reproduce.

---

*Severe overpopulation might constitute the compelling interest necessary to uphold interference with reproduction by sexual intercourse, as might the situation in which a couple knowingly and avoidably conceives and brings to term a severely handicapped child, then passes to others the cost and burdens of rearing that child.

†Single parenthood is especially difficult for poor, young, single mothers who are unemployed or lack skills. But even they and older, more financially secure single persons may be competent rearers of children.

‡A single woman may have a right to go to term once she has conceived, because she cannot be forced to have an abortion. But this right may be based on a right of bodily integrity, rather than on a right to reproduce. Similarly, a single woman who has given birth cannot be forced to relinquish a child just because she is single. But in this case, it would be a heavy intrusion to separate mother and child on the basis of moral disapproval of her unmarried status. Also, a single person may have access to contraceptives in order to avoid the burdens of reproduction. Thus, recognition of a right not to procreate does not necessarily mean that fornication laws are also unconstitutional.

§The distinction is admittedly strained. In one case, the state is forcing one type of burden on the woman; in the second case, another type of burden altogether. But difference in type of burden seems less important than the significance or magnitude of the burden. On this score, there appears to be no morally recognizable difference.

*The importance of family tradition is evident in Justice Powell's opinion in *Moore v City of East Cleveland*, 431 US 494 (1977), in which a zoning ordinance preventing a grandmother from living with grandchildren was struck down on the basis of a substantive due process right to live with one's lineal descendants. Surely the right of a married couple to have children is a stronger candidate for fundamental right status than is a grandmother's right to live with grandchildren.

The lack of explicit constitutional protection, however, does not mean that it is unlawful or unethical for physicians to treat infertility in single persons or otherwise to assist their reproduction. State and federal law do not now prohibit noncoital reproduction by unmarried persons. Thus, physicians are legally free to assist single persons in reproduction.

Inclusion of Noncoital and Donor-Assisted Reproduction Within the Right to Reproduce

The Supreme Court statements supporting a couple's right to marry and found a family generally assume that reproduction will occur only as a result of sexual intercourse, because the statements were made before IVF and widespread use of donor sperm occurred. However, the couple's interest in reproducing is the same, no matter how reproduction occurs. The values and interests underlying a right of coital reproduction strongly suggest a married couple's right to noncoital reproduction as well and, arguably, to have the assistance of donors and surrogates, as needed.*

Coital reproduction is legally protected not for the coitus but for what the coitus makes possible: it enables the couple to unite egg and sperm in order to acquire the possibility of rearing a child of their own genes and gestation.† The use of noncoital techniques, such as IVF or artificial insemination (AIH), to unite egg and husband's sperm, necessitated by the couple's infertility, should then also be protected.

The married couple's right to reproduce should thus extend to noncoital means of conception, which include the wide range of choices made possible by developments in IVF. The couple would then have the right to create, store, and have transferred to them extracorporeal preembryos created by their egg and sperm. They would have the right to determine whether their gametes would be used for reproduction and determine the disposition of preembryos created with their gametes,‡ which would include a right to donate preembryos to other couples. Indeed, the right might also be

---

*This view was recognized for IVF between a married couple in Flannery (1979). A specific analysis of this view as applied to collaborative reproduction with donors appears in Robertson (1986 a).

†A traditional Catholic view is that the unitive and the procreative should be combined in one act, thus making the separation of sex and reproduction, either to procure pleasure or to procure offspring, wrong. See McCormick (1982) for a description of this view. The law does not, and is unlikely to, reflect this view.

‡In this sense, married couples may be said to "own" their gametes and resulting preembryos. However, their right of "ownership" might be constitutionally limited by laws limiting preembryo research and discard, as long as significant procreative interests of the couple are not infringed.

found to extend to posthumous reproduction, which might occur with stored sperm or preembryos after the death of a spouse.*

A strong legal argument can also be made that a married couple's procreative liberty would include the right to enlist the assistance of a third-party donor or surrogate to provide the gametes or uterine function necessary for the couple to beget, bear, or otherwise acquire for rearing a child genetically related to one of the partners. Although not as directly entailed as the right of noncoital conception, the logic and values behind protecting marital procreation suggest that the need for assistance of a third-party collaborator should be similarly treated. The donor is essential if the couple are to rear a child who has a gametic or gestational connection to them.† Because the couple would be free, if fertile, to reproduce as often as they wanted to, they should be free to procreate with the help of gamete donors or the uterus of another party.

If this argument is accepted, couples attempting to reproduce would have the right to engage in a wide range of activities involving donors and extracorporeal preembryos. They would have the right to contract with others for the provision of gametes or preembryos, with the contract settling the parties' rearing rights and duties toward resulting offspring.‡ A contractual approach would also extend to contracts with surrogates for them to gestate the couple's preembryo and to return it to them for rearing. Strictly analyzed, the logic of marital procreative liberty would require the state to enforce such contracts and would allow fees to be paid to donors for the various services provided.§ States might then regulate the circumstances under which parties would enter into reproductive contracts, but they could not ban such transactions altogether.

In short, the interests and values supporting the right to reproduce by sexual intercourse apply equally to noncoital activities involving the extracorporeal preembryo.

---

*However, the couple's right to reproduce might not include doing everything possible with extracorporeal preembryos and preembryo or gamete storage. Questions concerning the ability to transfer stored gametes and preembryos to others or to manipulate the genes of future offspring may or may not be included within the couple's procreative liberty. This will depend on the social practices and meanings that evolve as these technologies become available and the full range of their risks and benefits becomes known (Robertson, 1983; see footnote * on p. 11).

†With donor egg or sperm, the wife will be bearing, and the couple rearing, the genetic child of one partner. When they contribute an embryo to another couple, they are reproducing by providing the genes for another's child. If they receive an embryo donation, they are reproducing in the sense of gestating and rearing children, the usual result of coital reproduction. In the case of surrogates, the couple will be rearing a child with genes of one or both partners.

‡The contractual right reflects the growing importance of contract in the marital relation (Weitzman, 1974; Shultz, 1982). Recognition of the right asserted here raises certain questions: Why would contracts of adoption made before conception, or after conception but before birth, not be valid? Why should parties not be free, after birth of the child, to make private contracts for adoption directly with women who want to relinquish their children? It may be that the law of adoption needs to be rethought in view of the reproductive rights of married couples to contract with donors and surrogates.

§See Flannery (1979) and Robertson (1986 a).

Although the case is strongest for a couple's right to reproduce noncoitally, a strong argument can also be made for their right to enlist the aid of gamete donors and surrogates. Both methods enable a couple to rear a child who is the biologic descendant of, or who has been gestated by, one of them. Unmarried persons would also have the right to reproduce through extracorporeal fertilization and donor assistance if their right to coital reproduction were recognized.*

Limits on the Right of Noncoital Reproduction

If the logic of procreative rights is strictly analyzed by the courts, the procreative rights of married couples would extend to noncoital activities that are essential for them to reproduce. Constitutional rights, however, are not absolute, and restrictions might be imposed when necessary to serve important state interests. The question is whether noncoital and donor-assisted techniques pose harm to state interests sufficient to justify restriction of the procreative choices involving them.

Noncoital and donor-assisted reproduction raise a variety of concerns, from duties to extracorporeal preembryos to concern for the welfare of offspring, the family, and donors and surrogates. There are also more general societal concerns about dehumanizing or reifying reproduction through excessive technologizing and commercialization.

Although these are valid concerns that will influence individual choice, they may not be a constitutionally sufficient basis for preventing couples from using these techniques when the need for any particular restriction is scrutinized. Preembryo freezing and donation or contracts with gamete donors and surrogates may not risk sufficient tangible harm to the parties or the offspring to warrant state interference with the constitutional right to procreate.†

Existing laws that appear to limit noncoital reproduction by married persons are constitutionally dubious and may well be struck down if challenged in the courts. Fetal and preembryo research laws that appear to restrict a married couple's control of preembryos for reproduction are most vulnerable to attack. Also, existing legal presumptions about who is the rearing father or mother in situations of donor ga-

---

*Refusal to enforce a reproductive contract or to ban payments would amount to an interference with procreative liberty because it would prevent couples from acquiring the donor or surrogate assistance needed to acquire a child genetically or gestationally related to themselves. If the courts analyze the issue correctly, refusal to enforce, or bans on, such contracts will be constitutional only to prevent a tangible harm and not merely to register societal disapproval of such uses of reproductive capacity. A right to contract enforcement is satisfied by awards of damages from donors and surrogates and would not necessarily require specific performance of the contract (Robertson, 1986 a).

†See Flannery (1979) and Robertson (1986 a).

metes and surrogacy may also fall when the full implications of marital procreative liberty are recognized.*

Two kinds of state restrictions, however, are constitutionally permissible. One would be laws that prevent the couple, donors, and surrogates from maintaining anonymity if the offspring's welfare required disclosure.† A second restriction would be regulations designed to assure free, informed entry into donor and surrogate transactions in order to protect the autonomy of the parties.†

Intangible religious, moral, or societal concerns about the nature of reproduction, family, the reproductive roles of women, and the power of science would not ordinarily justify interference with procreative liberty. Such deeply held religious or moral views about reproductive relations are of immense importance to individuals and to society, for these views represent value choices that constitute individual and societal moral commitment. However, moral, religious, or symbolic concerns that do not have direct, tangible effects on others are not sufficient constitutional grounds for interfering with fundamental rights of persons with different views.‡

Views of the rightness or wrongness of particular means of conception might properly animate individual and institutional choices to avoid, seek, or provide such services. Neither physicians nor institutions in the private sector are obligated to provide noncoital or extracorporeal reproductive services of any particular kind. Nor are persons obligated to use their reproductive capacity to assist the reproduction of others. The state is not constitutionally obligated to fund such services any more than it is obligated to fund abortions.§ But there is a limit to direct state interference with noncoital reproductive choice.

The constitutional status of procreative liberty illustrates the recurring dilemma of fundamental rights in a society of limited governmental powers. Recognition of procreative rights is essential in the constitutional scheme; yet, it permits activities that may run counter to the values that a majority hold and may even lead to a transformation of those values. Even so, the community may not legally prevent the exercise of those rights other than by persuasion, even if an impact on its value structure occurs.

---

*Artificial insemination laws may mean that the husband of a surrogate who has been artificially inseminated is the legal father. There are also presumptions that the birthing mother is the rearing mother (Robertson, 1986).

†See Flannery (1979) and Robertson (1986 a).

‡There is no way to understand *Griswold v Connecticut, Roe v Wade, Eisenstadt v Baird*, and similar cases than as standing for the proposition that symbolic or moral evaluation of conduct alone does not justify interference with fundamental rights. The community's power to enforce or impose morality stops at the threshold of another person's fundamental rights.

§Because procreative liberty (like most constitutional rights) is a negative, not a positive, right, it obligates the state to refrain from interferences with reproductive arrangements among consenting adults and physicians. The state is not obligated to fund these activities or allow them in state institutions, any more than it is obligated to fund abortions or contraception. (*Harris v McCrae*, 448 US 297 [1980]; *Maher v Roe*, 432 US 464 [1977]; *Poelker v Doe*, 432 US 519 [1977].)

Currently, it appears that the constitutional status of procreative liberty requires that the legal system leave noncoital and donor-assisted reproduction largely to the moral decision of the physicians, patients, and institutions involved.

The Moral Right to Reproduce and Its Limitations

According to Article 16.1 of the United Nations Declaration of Human Rights, "Men and women of full age, without any limitation due to race, nationality or religion, have the right to marry and found a family" (United Nations, 1978). The goal of this chapter is to explore the scope and possible limits of the moral right to "found a family."

Moral philosophers generally distinguish two types of rights: negative (liberty) rights and positive (welfare) rights. Applied to the question of procreation, a liberty right would encompass the moral freedom to reproduce, or to assist others in reproducing, without violating any countervailing moral obligations. A welfare right to reproduce would morally entitle one to be assisted by another party (or other parties) in achieving the goal of reproduction.

The Liberty Right to Reproduce

The thesis of this section is that the *moral* right to freedom in reproductive decisions may be limited, whereas the *legal* liberty right is virtually unlimited in current United States constitutional law. Because discussions of moral rights usually postdate and frequently borrow from discussions of legal rights, this section begins with a discussion of legal rights.

The United States Supreme Court has reviewed the liberty right to reproduce primarily in two contexts: the proposed sterilization of a criminal or of a mentally retarded person and access to contraceptive measures. In a line of important decisions between 1942 and 1977, the Supreme Court clearly affirmed the right of couples to use contraceptives to avoid pregnancy and indicated its strong support for procreative liberty, particularly the procreative liberty of married persons. Presumably, this sphere of procreative liberty would be broad enough to include a couple's freedom to employ a newly available technique for assisting in reproduction (Flannery, 1979).

However, our moral obligations are sometimes more stringent than our legal obligations. Reciprocally, our moral rights may be narrower in their scope than our legal rights. In addition, ethical standards, unlike legal rules, are generally not enforced by the coercive power of the state. Thus, a greater role may be given to moral suasion or moral counseling.

The ethical question "What are appropriate limitations on the moral right to reproduce?" can also be formulated as follows: "Under what circumstances does one have a moral obligation to refrain from reproducing or from assisting others in reproducing?" In the Committee's view, these questions should be considered by everyone who is considering reproduction, whether by conventional or by technically assisted means. If one remembers that the ethical sphere is one for thoughtful discussion or counseling, rather than for coercion, then these questions can be considered calmly, without fear of government intrusion.

Parents

From an ethical standpoint, at least six grounds can be envisioned on the basis of which one might have a moral duty not to reproduce, that is, on the basis of which one's liberty right to reproduce might be ethically constrained. The last three of these grounds remain controversial.

Transmission of Disease to Offspring   Past discussions of this constraint on the moral right to reproduce have centered on the transmission of genetic or chromosomal abnormalities to one's offspring (Hoering, 1976). One ethicist has even sought to develop an "ethic of genetic duty" (Ramsey, 1970). According to this view, couples whose members both carry a serious genetic defect have a moral obligation to refrain from producing children who have a high risk of being afflicted with the defect. In more recent times, men and women afflicted with Acquired Immune Deficiency Syndrome or seropositive for antibody to the HTLV-III/LAV virus have faced the moral question of whether they should bear or beget children and thereby place the children at risk of contracting this devastating disease.

Unwillingness to Provide Proper Prenatal Care   Some congenital defects are caused by the voluntary behavior of the parents. Fetal-alcohol syndrome is one example of a teratogenic effect caused by maternal behavior. Similarly, a husband's exposure of his wife to toxic chemicals or sexually transmitted disease could be deleterious both to her and to the fetus that she is carrying. Unless a couple is prepared to "be good to the baby before it is born," the couple ought not, from a moral point of view, conceive a child.

Inability to Rear Children   Constitutional law emphasizes the liberty of couples to make decisions about bearing or begetting children. However, a positive decision to bear or beget, unlike a decision to employ contraceptives, normally carries with it an obligation not only to bear or beget but also to rear a child to adulthood. Therefore, it can be argued that a person who is not in a position to take on the responsibilities of providing food, clothing, shelter, education, and health care for a child ought not, from an ethical standpoint, bear or beget a child (O'Neill, 1979).

Psychologic Harm to Offspring   Some critics of technologically assisted modes of reproduction—particularly those involving third parties—contend that these modes could produce psychologic damage to children who later discover the circumstances of their conception. Like the data on the psychologic effects of adoption, the data on the potential harm to children are currently inconclusive. Such harm therefore remains speculative.

Overpopulation   It can be argued that when the population of a region or nation already places a serious strain on available resources, that fact of life may place a constraint on the liberty right to reproduce (Bayles, 1979). One thinks, for example, of China with its perceived need to limit population growth and of several African countries that are experiencing severe food shortages. However, this possible ground for limiting the moral right to reproduce does not seem to apply in the context of the United States at present.

Nonmarriage   It can also be argued that single persons or homosexual couples ought not to bring children into the world. This view holds that it is helpful for children to have role models of both genders. Also, two parents are better able than one to cope with the demands of child rearing. However, changing patterns of family life, particularly with respect to divorce and adoption, have called the traditional presumption into question. Other things being equal, the Committee regards the setting of heterosexual marriage as the most appropriate context for the rearing of children. But because other factors are often not equal, the Committee is unwilling to view nonmarriage as a *general* constraint on the liberty right to reproduce.

The common thread running through these six possible constraints on the moral right to reproduce is a concern about *harm*, particularly harm to the child, but also harm to the public good. In light of the foregoing discussion, it seems reasonable to say that couples have a liberty right to reproduce, limited by ethical constraints. This right is a moral right that exists independently of statutory, constitutional, or case law. The moral right to reproduce would seem to encompass the freedom to resort to newly developed means for assisting reproduction.

The Committee would include within the moral right to reproduce the freedom to enlist the services of third parties in cases in which one or both members of the couple are physically incapable of reproducing by themselves.

Donors

Two of the above six constraints also apply to prospective donors whose assistance in reproduction may be requested.

Transmission of Disease to Offspring   The freedom to serve as a provider of gametes or as a surrogate mother or carrier—either with or without remuneration—should be constrained by the moral duty not to transmit genetic or infectious disease. For this reason, prospective gamete donors or surrogates have a moral obligation to disclose familial genetic problems and to cooperate in appropriate screening programs.

Unwillingness to Provide Proper Prenatal Care   The freedom to serve as a surrogate mother should be constrained by the moral duty to adopt a healthy lifestyle for the sake of the fetus that one is carrying on behalf of an adopting couple. This constraint may require special emphasis because the surrogate knows that she will not bear long-term responsibility for rearing the child that she is carrying.

The Welfare Right to Assistance in Reproduction

The majority of persons seeking to reproduce need to lodge no moral claims against third parties in order to initiate a pregnancy. However, a substantial minority of couples, perhaps 1 in 14 in the United States (Mosher, 1982), need assistance from third parties if they are to reproduce at all or if they are to reduce the probability of transmitting a serious disease to their offspring. In addition, some single persons desire to reproduce. Couples or single persons in this position might conceivably assert moral welfare rights against three distinct types of moral agents: (a) health professionals, (b) gamete providers or surrogates, and (c) society at large.

Health Professionals

In this case, a single person or a couple would claim, as a moral entitlement, the assistance of health professionals in overcoming infertility problems or possible disease-transmission problems. There are health professionals who have expertise in the alleviation of such problems. However, it is not clear that any particular health professional—or health professionals as a group—has a moral obligation to provide such service to infertile couples, unless a satisfactory mutual agreement to enter into a professional-patient relationship can be worked out. Any other view on this question would seem to violate the liberty rights of health providers.

Gamete Providers or Surrogates

A given couple may need the assistance of a sperm or an egg provider (often called a "donor") or of a surrogate mother if the couple is to have a child who is in some sense the couple's own. However, it is again not clear that any particular person has a moral obligation to provide assistance to a particular couple or to infertile couples generally.

Particular persons may, at their discretion, agree to come to the aid of such couples, but such assistance is likely to be either a benevolent gift or the sale of a product or service, not the fulfillment of a strict moral obligation.

Society as a Whole

Perhaps the most difficult question in this chapter is whether infertile couples have any special moral welfare rights against the larger society in their quest to overcome involuntary infertility or other reproductive difficulties. The correlative question, phrased in terms of obligations, is this: "Does the larger society have any special moral obligations to infertile couples?"

If one accepts the notion that society as a whole ought to provide volunteer subjects for nontherapeutic research or whole blood for transfusion or organs for transplantation, then one might accept the notion that society as a whole ought to encourage its members to provide gametes for couples who are physically incapable of producing functional gametes. In fact, Great Britain and France seem to be moving toward voluntary nonprofit systems for fulfilling this perceived obligation (Great Britain, 1984). This general obligation of society would, of course, not apply to any member of the society who is conscientiously opposed to gamete donation. Also, it seems unlikely that such a system would be adequate for surrogate motherhood arrangements.

Society may have a moral obligation to provide, either directly or indirectly, access to health services for the treatment of infertility. One approach to the resolution of this problem is that taken in the United States by the President's Commission for the Study of Ethical Problems in Medicine and Biomedical and Behavioral Research. In its report entitled *Securing Access to Health Care* (1983), the Commission argued that society has an ethical obligation to provide an adequate level of health care to every citizen. If this general obligation is accepted as binding, the specific question in the case of noncoital reproduction becomes this: "Are techniques of assisted reproduction for infertile couples included within the notion of 'an adequate level of health care'?" This is surely a controversial question, one that will need to be addressed through surveys of public opinion and an open, democratic policy-making process. At least one state, Maryland, has implicitly answered this question in the affirmative by requiring private health insurance plans written in the state to include in vitro fertilization as a covered service on the same basis as other infertility services.[1]

Notes

1. *Griswold v Connecticut*, 381 US 479 (1965); *Roe v Wade*, 410 US 113 (1973); *Planned Parenthood v Danforth*, 482 US 52 (1976); *Bellotti v Baird*, 443 US 622 (1979); *City of Akron v Akron Reproductive Center*, 103 S Ct 2481 (1983)

2. *Dandridge v Williams*, 397 US 471 (1970) (Indirect restrictions, such as limits on welfare benefits, are not considered restrictions on procreative choice.)

[1]Maryland General Assembly: SB 793. Insurance—In Vitro Fertilization. Laws, ch. 237 (1985).

3. For similarly worded statements, see *The International Covenant of Civil and Political Rights*, Art. 23, 1976; *European Convention on Human Rights*, Art. 12, 1953

4. *Buck v Bell*, 274 US 200 (1927) (Upholding the state's right in certain circumstances to sterilize mentally retarded persons involuntarily.)

5. 316 US 535, 541 (1942)

6. 262 US 390, 399 (1923)

7. 405 US 645, 651 (1972)

8. 414 US 632, 639–640 (1974)

9. 405 US 438, 453 (1972)

10. *Eisenstadt v Baird*, 405 US 438, 653 (1972); *Carey v Population Services*, 431 US 678 (1977)

References

1. Bayles, M. "Limits to a right to procreate." In *Having Children: Philosophical and Legal Reflections on Parenthood*. Ed. by O. O'Neill and W. Ruddick. New York: Oxford University Press, 1979, p. 13.

2. Flannery, D. M., Weisman, C. D., Lipsett, C. R., and Braverman, A. N. "Test tube babies: legal issues raised by in vitro fertilization. *Georgetown Law Journal* 67: 1295, 1979.

3. Great Britain: Dept. of Health and Social Security. *Report of the Committee of Inquiry into Human Fertilisation and Embryology*. Ed. by M. Warnock. London, Her Majesty's Stationery Office, 1984, pp. 27, 63.

4. Hoering, B. "Genetics and responsible parenthood." *Social Thought* 2:7, 1976.

5. McCormick, R. A. "Notes on moral theology." *Theological Studies* 45:96, 1984.

6. Mosher, W. D., Pratt, W. F. "Reproductive impairments among married couples: United States." In *Vital Health Statistics*, ser. 23. Washington, D.C.: National Center for Health Statistics, 1982, pp. 13, 32.

7. O'Neill, O. "Begetting, bearing and rearing." In *Having Children: Philosophical and Legal Reflections on Parenthood*. Ed. by O. O'Neill and W. Ruddick. New York: Oxford University Press, 1979, p. 13.

8. Ramsey, P. "Moral and religious implications of genetic control." In *Fabricated Man: The Ethics of Genetic Control*. New Haven: Yale University Press, 1970, pp. 30, 57.

9. Robertson, J. "Procreative liberty and the control of conception, pregnancy and childbirth." *Virginia Law Review* 69:405, 1983.

10. Robertson, J. "Extracorporial embroyos and the abortion debate." *Journal of Contemporary Health Law Policy* 2:53, 1986.

11. Robertson, J. "Embryos, families and procreative liberty." *Southern California Law Review* 59(5):(July), 1986a.

12. Shultz, M. "Contractual ordering of marriage: a new model for state policy." *California Law Review* 70:211, 1982.

13. United Nations. *Universal Declaration of Human Rights*, Art. 16(1). New York: United Nations, 1978.

Instruction on Respect for Human Life in Its Origin and on the Dignity of Procreation

CONGREGATION FOR THE DOCTRINE OF THE FAITH

Replies to Certain Questions of the Day

I
Respect for
Human Embryos

Careful reflection on this teaching of the Magisterium and on the evidence of reason enables us to respond to the numerous moral problems posed by technical interventions upon the human being in the first phases of his life and upon the processes of his conception.

1. What Respect Is Due to the Human Embryo, Taking into Account His Nature and Identity?

The human being must be respected—as a person—from the very first instant of his existence.

The implementation of procedures of artificial fertilization has made possible various interventions upon embryos and human fetuses. The aims pursued are of various kinds: diagnostic and therapeutic, scientific and commercial. From all of this, serious problems arise. Can one speak of a right to experimentation upon human embryos for the purpose of scientific research? What norms or laws should be worked out with regard to this matter? The response to these problems presupposes a detailed reflection on the nature and specific identity—the word "status" is used—of the human embryo itself.

At the Second Vatican Council, the Church for her part presented once again to modern man her constant and certain doctrine according to which: "Life, once conceived, must be protected with the utmost care; abortion and infanticide are abominable crimes.[1] More recently, the *Charter of the Rights of the Family*, published by the Holy See, confirmed that "Human life must be absolutely respected and protected from the moment of conception."[2]

This Congregation is aware of the current debates concerning the beginning of human life, concerning the individuality of the human being and concerning the identity of the human person. The Congregation recalls the teachings found in the *Declaration on Procured Abortion*: "From the time that the ovum is fertilized, a new life is begun which is neither that of the father nor of the mother; it is rather the life of a new human being with his own growth. It would never be made human if it were not human already. To this perpetual evidence . . . modern genetic science brings valuable confirmation. It has demonstrated that, from the first instant, the program is fixed as to what this living being will be: a man, this individual-man with his characteristic aspects already well determined. Right from fertilization is begun the adventure of a human life, and each of its great capacities requires time . . . to find its place and to be in a position to act."[3] This teaching remains valid and is further confirmed, if confirmation were needed, by recent findings of human biological science which recognize that in the zygote* resulting from fertilization the biological identity of a new human individual is already constituted.

Certainly no experimental datum can be in itself sufficient to bring us to the recognition of a spiritual soul; nevertheless, the conclusions of science regarding the human embryo provide a valuable indication for discerning by the use of reason a personal presence at the moment of this first appearance of a human life: how could a human individual not be a human person? The Magisterium has not expressly committed itself to an affirmation of a philosophical nature, but it constantly reaffirms the moral condemnation of any kind of procured abortion. This teaching has not been changed and is unchangeable.[4]

Thus the fruit of human generation, from the first moment of its existence, that is to say from the moment the zygote has formed, demands the unconditional respect that is morally due to the human being in his bodily and spiritual totality. The human being is to be respected and treated as a person from the moment of conception; and therefore from that same moment his rights as a person must be recognized, among which in the first place is the inviolable right of every innocent human being to life.

This doctrinal reminder provides the fundamental criterion for the solution of the various problems posed by the development of the biomedical sciences in this field: since the embryo must be treated as a person, it must also be defended in its integrity, tended and cared for, to the extent possible, in the same way as any other human being as far as medical assistance is concerned.

2. Is Prenatal Diagnosis Morally Licit?

If prenatal diagnosis respects the life and integrity of the embryo and the human fetus and is directed towards its safeguarding or healing as an individual, then the answer is affirmative.

---

*The zygote is the cell produced when the nuclei of the two gametes have fused.

For prenatal diagnosis makes it possible to know the condition of the embryo and of the fetus when still in the mother's womb. It permits, or makes it possible to anticipate earlier and more effectively, certain therapeutic, medical or surgical procedures.

Such diagnosis is permissible, with the consent of the parents after they have been adequately informed, if the methods employed safeguard the life and integrity of the embryo and the mother, without subjecting them to disproportionate risks.[5] But this diagnosis is gravely opposed to the moral law when it is done with the thought of possibly inducing an abortion, depending upon the results: a diagnosis which shows the existence of a malformation or a hereditary illness must not be the equivalent of a death-sentence. Thus a woman would be committing a gravely illicit act if she were to request such a diagnosis with the deliberate intention of having an abortion should the results confirm the existence of a malformation or abnormality. The spouse or relatives or anyone else would similarly be acting in a manner contrary to the moral law if they were to counsel or impose such a diagnostic procedure on the expectant mother with the same intention of possibly proceeding to an abortion. So too the specialist would be guilty of illicit collaboration if, in conducting the diagnosis and in communicating its results, he were deliberately to contribute to establishing or favoring a link between prenatal diagnosis and abortion.

In conclusion, any directive or program of the civil and health authorities or of scientific organizations which in any way were to favor a link between prenatal diagnosis and abortion, or which were to go as far as directly to induce expectant mothers to submit to prenatal diagnosis planned for the purpose of eliminating fetuses which are affected by malformations or which are carriers of hereditary illness, is to be condemned as a violation of the unborn child's right to life and as an abuse of the prior rights and duties of the spouses.

3. Are Therapeutic Procedures Carried Out on the Human Embryo Licit?

As with all medical interventions on patients, *one must uphold as licit procedures carried out on the human embryo which respect the life and integrity of the embryo and do not involve disproportionate risks for it but are directed towards its healing, the improvement of its condition of health, or its individual survival.*

Whatever the type of medical, surgical or other therapy, the free and informed consent of the parents is required, according to the deontological rules followed in the case of children. The application of this moral principle may call for delicate and particular precautions in the case of embryonic or fetal life.

The legitimacy and criteria of such procedures have been clearly stated by Pope John Paul II: "A strictly therapeutic intervention whose explicit objective is the healing of various maladies such as those stemming from chromosomal defects will, in principle, be considered desirable, provided it is directed to the true promotion of the personal well-being of the individual without doing harm to his integrity or worsening his conditions of life. Such an intervention would indeed fall within the logic of the Christian moral tradition."[6]

4. How Is One Morally To Evaluate Research and Experimentation* on Human Embryos and Fetuses?

Medical research must refrain from operations on live embryos, unless there is a moral certainty of not causing harm to the life or integrity of the unborn child and the mother, and on condition that the parents have given their free and informed consent to the procedure. It follows that all research, even when limited to the simple observation of the embryo, would become illicit were it to involve risk to the embryo's physical integrity or life by reason of the methods used or the effects induced.

As regards experimentation, and presupposing the general distinction between experimentation for purposes which are not directly therapeutic and experimentation which is clearly therapeutic for the subject himself, in the case in point one must also distinguish between experimentation carried out on embryos which are still alive and experimentation carried out on embryos which are dead. *If the embryos are living, whether viable or not, they must be respected just like any other human person; experimentation on embryos which is not directly therapeutic is illicit.*[7]

No objective, even though noble in itself, such as a foreseeable advantage to science, to other human beings or to society, can in any way justify experimentation on living human embryos or fetuses, whether viable or not, either inside or outside the mother's womb. The informed consent ordinarily required for clinical experimentation on adults cannot be granted by the parents, who may not freely dispose of the physical integrity or life of the unborn child. Moreover, experimentation on embryos and fetuses always involves risk, and indeed in most cases it involves the certain expectation of harm to their physical integrity or even their death.

To use human embryos or fetuses as the object or instrument of experimentation constitutes a crime against their dignity as human beings having a right to the same respect that is due to the child already born and to every human person.

The *Charter of the Rights of the Family* published by the Holy See affirms: "Respect for the dignity of the human being excludes all experimental manipulation or exploitation of the human embryo."[8] The practice of keeping human embryos alive *in vivo* or *in vitro* for experimental or commercial purposes is totally opposed to human dignity.

In the case of experimentation that is clearly therapeutic, namely, when it is a matter of experimental forms of therapy used for the benefit of the embryo itself in a final attempt to save its life, and in the absence of other reliable forms of therapy, recourse to drugs or procedures not yet fully tested can be licit.[9]

---

*Since the terms "research" and "experimentation" are often used equivalently and ambiguously, it is deemed necessary to specify the exact meaning given them in this document.

1) By *research* is meant any inductive-deductive process which aims at promoting the systematic observation of a given phenomenon in the human field or at verifying a hypothesis arising from previous observations.

2) By *experimentation* is meant any research in which the human being (in the various stages of his existence: embryo, fetus, child or adult) represents the object through which or upon which one intends to verify the effect, at present unknown or not sufficiently known, of a given treatment (e.g., pharmacological, teratogenic, surgical, etc.).

The corpses of human embryos and fetuses, whether they have been deliberately aborted or not, must be respected just as the remains of other human beings. In particular, they cannot be subjected to mutilation or to autopsies if their death has not yet been verified and without the consent of the parents or of the mother. Furthermore, the moral requirements must be safeguarded, that there be no complicity in deliberate abortion and that the risk of scandal be avoided. Also, in the case of dead fetuses, as for the corpses of adult persons, all commercial trafficking must be considered illicit and should be prohibited.

5. How Is One Morally To Evaluate the Use for Research Purposes of Embryos Obtained by Fertilization In Vitro?

Human embryos obtained *in vitro* are human beings and subjects with rights: their dignity and right to life must be respected from the first moment of their existence. *It is immoral to produce human embryos destined to be exploited as disposable "biological material."*

In the usual practice of *in vitro* fertilization, not all of the embryos are transferred to the woman's body; some are destroyed. Just as the Church condemns induced abortion, so she also forbids acts against the life of these human beings. *It is a duty to condemn the particular gravity of the voluntary destruction of human embryos obtained* in vitro *for the sole purpose of research, either by means of artificial insemination or by means of "twin fission."* By acting in this way the researcher usurps the place of God; and, even though he may be unaware of this, he sets himself up as the master of the destiny of others inasmuch as he arbitrarily chooses whom he will allow to live and whom he will send to death, and kills defenseless human beings.

Methods of observation or experimentation which damage or impose grave and disproportionate risks upon embryos obtained *in vitro* are morally illicit for the same reasons. Every human being is to be respected for himself, and cannot be reduced in worth to a pure and simple instrument for the advantage of others. *It is therefore not in conformity with the moral law deliberately to expose to death human embryos obtained* in vitro. In consequence of the fact that they have been produced *in vitro*, those embryos which are not transferred into the body of the mother and are called "spare" are exposed to an absurd fate, with no possibility of their being offered safe means of survival which can be licitly pursued.

6. What Judgment Should Be Made on Other Procedures of Manipulating Embryos Connected with the "Techniques of Human Reproduction"?

Techniques of fertilization *in vitro* can open the way to other forms of biological and genetic manipulation of human embryos, such as attempts or plans for fertilization between human and animal gametes and the gestation of human embryos in the uterus of animals, or the hypothesis or project of constructing artificial uteruses for the human embryo. *These procedures are contrary to the human dignity proper to the embryo, and at the same time they are contrary to the right of every person to be conceived and to be born within marriage and from marriage.*[10] *Also, attempts or hypotheses for obtaining a human being without any connection with sexuality through "twin fission," cloning or parthenogenesis are to be considered contrary to the moral law, since they are in opposition to the dignity both of human procreation and of the conjugal union.*

The freezing of embryos, even when carried out in order to preserve the life of an embryo—cryopreservation—*constitutes an offense against the respect due to human beings* by exposing them to grave risks of death or harm to their physical integrity, and depriving them, at least temporarily, of maternal shelter and gestation, thus placing them in a situation in which further offenses and manipulation are possible.

Certain attempts to influence chromosomic or genetic inheritance are not therapeutic but are aimed at producing human beings selected according to sex or other predetermined qualities. These manipulations are contrary to the personal dignity of the human being and his or her integrity and identity. Therefore, in no way can they be justified on the grounds of possible beneficial consequences for future humanity.[11] Every person must be respected for himself: in this consists the dignity and right of every human being from his or her beginning.

II
Interventions Upon Human Procreation

By "artificial procreation" or "artificial fertilization" are understood here the different technical procedures directed towards obtaining a human conception in a manner other than the sexual union of man and woman. This instruction deals with fertilization of an ovum in a test tube (*in vitro* fertilization) and artificial insemination through transfer into the woman's genital tracts of previously collected sperm.

A preliminary point for the moral evaluation of such technical procedures is constituted by the consideration of the circumstances and consequences which those procedures involve in relation to the respect due the human embryo. Development of the practice of *in vitro* fertilization has required innumerable fertilizations and destructions of human embryos. Even today, the usual practice presupposes a hyper-ovulation on the part of the woman: a number of ova are withdrawn, fertilized and then cultivated *in vitro* for some days. Usually not all are transferred into the genital tracts of the woman; some embryos, generally called "spare," are destroyed or frozen. On occasion, some of the implanted embryos are sacrificed for various eugenic, economic or psychological reasons. Such deliberate destruction of human beings or their utilization for different purposes to the detriment of their integrity and life is contrary to the doctrine on procured abortion already recalled.

The connection between *in vitro* fertilization and the voluntary destruction of human embryos occurs too often. This is significant: through these procedures, with apparently contrary purposes, life and death are subjected to the decision of man, who thus sets himself up as the giver of life and death by decree. This dynamic of violence and domination may remain unnoticed by those very individuals who, in wishing to utilize this procedure, become subject to it themselves. The facts recorded and the cold logic which links them must be taken into consideration for a moral judgment on IVF and ET (*in vitro* vertilization and embryo transfer): the abortion-mentality which has made this procedure possible thus leads, whether one wants it or not, to man's domination over the life and death of his fellow human beings and can lead to a system of radical eugenics.

Nevertheless, such abuses do not exempt one from a further and thorough ethical study of the techniques of artificial procreation considered in themselves, abstracting as far as possible from the destruction of embryos produced *in vitro*.

The present instruction will therefore take into consideration in the first place the problems posed by heterologous artificial fertilization (II, 1–3),* and subsequently those linked with homologous artificial fertilization (II, 4–6).†

Before formulating an ethical judgment on each of these procedures, the principles and values which determine the moral evaluation of each of them will be considered.

A
Heterologous Artificial Fertilization

1. Why Must Human Procreation Take Place in Marriage?

Every human being is always to be accepted as a gift and blessing of God. However, from the moral point of view a truly responsible procreation vis-à-vis the unborn child must be the fruit of marriage.

For human procreation has specific characteristics by virtue of the personal dignity of the parents and of the children: the procreation of a new person, whereby the man and the woman collaborate with the power of the Creator, must be the fruit and the sign of the mutual self-giving of the spouses, of their love and of their fidelity.[12] *The fidelity of the spouses in the unity of marriage involves reciprocal respect of their right to become a father and a mother only through each other.*

The child has the right to be conceived, carried in the womb, brought into the world and brought up within marriage: it is through the secure and recognized rela-

---

*By the term *heterologous artificial fertilization* or *procreation*, the instruction means techniques used to obtain a human conception artificially by the use of gametes coming from at least one donor other than the spouses who are joined in marriage. Such techniques can be of two types:
a) *Heterologous IVF and ET*: the technique used to obtain a human conception through the meeting *in vitro* of gametes taken from at least one donor other than the two spouses joined in marriage.
b) *Heterologous artificial insemination*: the technique used to obtain a human conception through the transfer into the genital tracts of the woman of the sperm previously collected from a donor other than the husband.

†By *artificial homologous fertilization* or *procreation*, the instruction means the technique used to obtain a human conception using the gametes of the two spouses joined in marriage. Homologous artificial fertilization can be carried out by two different methods:
a) *Homologous IVF and ET*: the technique used to obtain a human conception through the meeting *in vitro* of the gametes of the spouses joined in marriage.
b) *Homologous artificial insemination*: the technique used to obtain a human conception through the transfer into the genital tracts of a married woman of the sperm previously collected from her husband.

tionship to his own parents that the child can discover his own identity and achieve his own proper human development.

The parents find in their child a confirmation and completion of their reciprocal self-giving: the child is the living image of their love, the permanent sign of their conjugal union, the living and indissoluble concrete expression of their paternity and maternity.[13]

By reason of the vocation and social responsibilities of the person, the good of the children and of the parents contributes to the good of civil society; the vitality and stability of society require that children come into the world within a family and that the family be firmly based on marriage.

The tradition of the Church and anthropological reflection recognize in marriage and in its indissoluble unity the only setting worthy of truly responsible procreation.

2. Does Heterologous Artificial Fertilization Conform to the Dignity of the Couple and to the Truth of Marriage?

Through IVF and ET and heterologous artificial insemination, human conception is achieved through the fusion of gametes of at least one donor other than the spouses who are united in marriage. *Heterologous artificial fertilization is contrary to the unity of marriage, to the dignity of the spouses, to the vocation proper to parents, and to the child's right to be conceived and brought into the world in marriage and from marriage.*[14]

Respect for the unity of marriage and for conjugal fidelity demands that the child be conceived in marriage; the bond existing between husband and wife accords the spouses, in an objective and inalienable manner, the exclusive right to become father and mother solely through each other.[15] Recourse to the gametes of a third person, in order to have sperm or ovum available, constitutes a violation of the reciprocal commitment of the spouses and a grave lack in regard to that essential property of marriage which is its unity.

Heterologous artificial fertilization violates the rights of the child; it deprives him of his filial relationship with his parental origins and can hinder the maturing of his personal identity. Furthermore, it offends the common vocation of the spouses who are called to fatherhood and motherhood: it objectively deprives conjugal fruitfulness of its unity and integrity; it brings about and manifests a rupture between genetic parenthood, gestational parenthood and responsibility for upbringing. Such damage to the personal relationships within the family has repercussions on civil society: what threatens the unity and stability of the family is a source of dissension, disorder and injustice in the whole of social life.

These reasons lead to a negative moral judgment concerning heterologous artificial fertilization: consequently fertilization of a married woman with the sperm of a donor different from her husband and fertilization with the husband's sperm of an ovum not coming from his wife are morally illicit. Furthermore, the artificial fertilization of a woman who is unmarried or a widow, whoever the donor may be, cannot be morally justified.

The desire to have a child and the love between spouses who long to obviate a sterility which cannot be overcome in any other way constitute understandable motivations; but subjectively good intentions do not render heterologous artificial fertilization conformable to the objective and inalienable properties of marriage or respectful of the rights of the child and of the spouses.

3. Is "Surrogate"* Motherhood Morally Licit?

No, for the same reasons which lead one to reject heterologous artificial fertilization: for it is contrary to the unity of marriage and to the dignity of the procreation of the human person.

Surrogate motherhood represents an objective failure to meet the obligations of maternal love, of conjugal fidelity and of responsible motherhood; it offends the dignity and the right of the child to be conceived, carried in the womb, brought into the world and brought up by his own parents; it sets up, to the detriment of families, a division between the physical, psychological and moral elements which constitute those families.

B
Homologous Artificial Fertilization

Since heterologous artificial fertilization has been declared unacceptable, the question arises of how to evaluate morally the process of homologous artificial fertilization: IVF and ET and artificial insemination between husband and wife. First a question of principle must be clarified.

4. From the Moral Point of View What Connection Is Required Between Procreation and the Conjugal Act?

a) The Church's teaching on marriage and human procreation affirms the "inseparable connection, willed by God and unable to be broken by man on his own initiative, between the two meanings of the conjugal act: the unitive meaning and the procreative meaning. Indeed, by its intimate structure, the conjugal act, while most closely uniting husband and wife, makes them capable of the generation of new lives, according to laws inscribed in the very being of man and of woman."[16] This principle, which is based upon the nature of marriage and the intimate connection of the goods of marriage, has well-known consequences on the level of responsible fatherhood and motherhood. "By safeguarding both these essential aspects, the unitive and the procreative, the conjugal act pre-

---

*By "surrogate mother" the instruction means:

a) The woman who carries in pregnancy an embryo implanted in her uterus and who is genetically a stranger to the embryo because it has been obtained through the union of the gametes of "donors." She carries the pregnancy with a pledge to surrender the baby once it is born to the party who commissioned or made the agreement for the pregnancy.

b) The woman who carries in pregnancy an embryo to whose procreation she has contributed the donation of her own ovum, fertilized through insemination with the sperm of a man other than her husband. She carries the pregnancy with the pledge to surrender the child once it is born to the party who commissioned or made the agreement for the pregnancy.

serves in its fullness the sense of true mutual love and its ordination toward man's exalted vocation to parenthood."[17]

The same doctrine concerning the link between the meanings of the conjugal act and between the goods of marriage throws light on the moral problem of homologous artificial fertilization, since "it is never permitted to separate these different aspects to such a degree as positively to exclude either the procreative intention or the conjugal relation."[18]

Contraception deliberately deprives the conjugal act of its openness to procreation and in this way brings about a voluntary dissociation of the ends of marriage. Homologous artificial fertilization, in seeking a procreation which is not the fruit of a specific act of conjugal union, objectively effects an analogous separation between the goods and the meanings of marriage.

Thus, *fertilization is licitly sought when it is the result of a "conjugal act which is per se suitable for the generation of children to which marriage is ordered by its nature and by which the spouses become one flesh."*[19] *But from the moral point of view procreation is deprived of its proper perfection when it is not desired as the fruit of the conjugal act, that is to say of the specific act of the spouses' union.*

b) The moral value of the intimate link between the goods of marriage and between the meanings of the conjugal act is based upon the unity of the human being, a unity involving body and spiritual soul.[20] Spouses mutually express their personal love in the "language of the body," which clearly involves both "spousal meanings" and parental ones.[21] The conjugal act by which the couple mutually express their self-gift at the same time expresses openness to the gift of life. It is an act that is inseparably corporal and spiritual. It is in their bodies and through their bodies that the spouses consummate their marriage and are able to become father and mother. In order to respect the language of their bodies and their natural generosity, the conjugal union must take place with respect for its openness to procreation; and the procreation of a person must be the fruit and the result of married love. The origin of the human being thus follows from a procreation that is "linked to the union, not only biological but also spiritual, of the parents, made one by the bond of marriage."[22] Fertilization achieved outside the bodies of the couple remains by this very fact deprived of the meanings and the values which are expressed in the language of the body and in the union of human persons.

c) Only respect for the link between the meanings of the conjugal act and respect for the unity of the human being make possible procreation in conformity with the dignity of the person. In his unique and unrepeatable origin, the child must be respected and recognized as equal in personal dignity to those who give him life. The human person must be accepted in his parents' act of union and love; the generation of a child must therefore be the fruit of that mutual giving[23] which is realized in the conjugal act wherein the spouses cooperate as servants and not as masters in the work of the Creator who is Love.[24]

In reality, the origin of a human person is the result of an act of giving. The one conceived must be the fruit of his parents' love. He cannot be desired or conceived as the product of an intervention of medical or biological techniques; that would be equivalent to reducing him to an object of scientific technology. No one may subject the coming of a child into the world to conditions of technical efficiency which are to be evaluated according to standards of control and dominion.

The moral relevance of the link between the meanings of the conjugal act and between the goods of marriage, as well as the unity of the human being and the dignity of his origin, demand that the procreation of a human person be brought about as the fruit of the conjugal act specific to the love between spouses. The link between procreation and the conjugal act is thus shown to be of great importance on the anthropological and moral planes, and it throws light on the positions of the Magisterium with regard to homologous artificial fertilization.

5. Is Homologous *In Vitro* Fertilization Morally Licit?

The answer to this question is strictly dependent on the principles just mentioned. Certainly one cannot ignore the legitimate aspirations of sterile couples. For some, recourse to homologous IVF and ET appears to be the only way of fulfilling their sincere desire for a child. The question is asked whether the totality of conjugal life in such situations is not sufficient to ensure the dignity proper to human procreation. It is acknowledged that IVF and ET certainly cannot supply for the absence of sexual relations[25] and cannot be preferred to the specific acts of conjugal union, given the risks involved for the child and the difficulties of the procedure. But it is asked whether, when there is no other way of overcoming the sterility which is a source of suffering, homologous *in vitro* fertilization may not constitute an aid, if not a form of therapy, whereby its moral licitness could be admitted.

The desire for a child—or at the very least an openness to the transmission of life—is a necessary prerequisite from the moral point of view for responsible human procreation. But this good intention is not sufficient for making a positive moral evaluation of *in vitro* fertilization between spouses. The process of IVF and ET must be judged in itself and cannot borrow its definitive moral quality from the totality of conjugal life of which it becomes part nor from the conjugal acts which may precede or follow it.[26]

It has already been recalled that, in the circumstances in which it is regularly practiced, IVF and ET involves the destruction of human beings, which is something contrary to the doctrine on the illicitness of abortion previously mentioned.[27] But even in a situation in which every precaution were taken to avoid the death of human embryos, homologous IVF and ET dissociates from the conjugal act the actions which are directed to human fertilization. For this reason the very nature of homologous IVF and ET also must be taken into account, even abstracting from the link with procured abortion.

Homologous IVF and ET is brought about outside the bodies of the couple through actions of third parties whose competence and technical activity determine the success of the procedure. Such fertilization entrusts the life and identity of the embryo into the power of doctors and biologists and establishes the domination of technology over the origin and destiny of the human person. Such a relationship of domination is in itself contrary to the dignity and equality that must be common to parents and children.

Conception *in vitro* is the result of the technical action which presides over fertilization. *Such fertilization is neither in fact achieved nor positively willed as the expression and fruit of a specific act of the conjugal union. In homologous IVF and ET, therefore, even if it is considered in the context of* de facto *existing sexual relations, the generation of the human person is objectively deprived of its proper perfection: namely, that of being the result and fruit of a conjugal act* in which the spouses can become "cooperators with God for giving life to a new person."[28]

These reasons enable us to understand why the act of conjugal love is considered in the teaching of the Church as the only setting worthy of human procreation. For the same reasons the so-called "simple case," i.e., a homologous IVF and ET procedure that is free of any compromise with the abortive practice of destroying embryos and with masturbation, remains a technique which is morally illicit because it deprives human procreation of the dignity which is proper and connatural to it.

Certainly, homologous IVF and ET fertilization is not marked by all that ethical negativity found in extra-conjugal procreation; the family and marriage continue to constitute the setting for the birth and upbringing of the children. Nevertheless, in conformity with the traditional doctrine relating to the goods of marriage and the dignity of the person, *the Church remains opposed from the moral point of view to homologous* in vitro *fertilization. Such fertilization is in itself illicit and in opposition to the dignity of procreation and of the conjugal union, even when everything is done to avoid the death of the human embryo*.

Although the manner in which human conception is achieved with IVF and ET cannot be approved, every child which comes into the world must in any case be accepted as a living gift of the divine Goodness and must be brought up with love.

6. How Is Homologous Artificial Insemination To Be Evaluated from the Moral Point of View?

Homologous artificial insemination within marriage cannot be admitted except for those cases in which the technical means is not a substitute for the conjugal act but serves to facilitate and to help so that the act attains its natural purpose.

The teaching of the Magisterium on this point has already been stated.[29] This teaching is not just an expression of particular historical circumstances but is based on the Church's doctrine concerning the connection between the conjugal union and procreation and on a consideration of the personal nature of the conjugal act and of human procreation. "In its natural structure, the conjugal act is a personal action, a simultaneous and immediate cooperation on the part of the husband and wife, which by the very nature of the agents and the proper nature of the act is the expression of the mutual gift which, according to the words of Scripture, brings about union 'in one flesh.'"[30] Thus moral conscience "does not necessarily proscribe the use of certain artificial means destined solely either to the facilitating of the natural act or to ensuring that the natural act normally performed achieves its proper end."[31] If the technical means facilitates the conjugal act or helps it to reach its natural objectives, it can be morally acceptable. If, on the other hand, the procedure were to replace the conjugal act, it is morally illicit.

Artificial insemination as a substitute for the conjugal act is prohibited by reason of the voluntarily achieved dissociation of the two meanings of the conjugal act. Masturbation, through which the sperm is normally obtained, is another sign of this dissociation: even when it is done for the purpose of procreation, the act remains deprived of its unitive meaning: "It lacks the sexual relationship called for by the moral order, namely the relationship which realizes 'the full sense of mutual self-giving and human procreation in the context of true love.'"[32]

7. What Moral Criterion Can Be Proposed with Regard to Medical Intervention in Human Procreation?

The medical act must be evaluated not only with reference to its technical dimension but also and above all in relation to its goal, which is the good of persons and their bodily and psychological health. The moral criteria for medical intervention in procreation are deduced from the dignity of human persons, of their sexuality and of their origin.

Medicine which seeks to be ordered to the integral good of the person must respect the specifically human values of sexuality.[33] *The doctor is at the service of persons and of human procreation. He does not have the authority to dispose of them or to decide their fate.* "A medical intervention respects the dignity of persons when it seeks to assist the conjugal act either in order to facilitate its performance or in order to enable it to achieve its objective once it has been normally performed."[34]

On the other hand, it sometimes happens that a medical procedure technologically replaces the conjugal act in order to obtain a procreation which is neither its result nor its fruit. In this case the medical act is not, as it should be, at the service of conjugal union but rather appropriates to itself the procreative function and thus contradicts the dignity and the inalienable rights of the spouses and of the child to be born.

The humanization of medicine, which is insisted upon today by everyone, requires respect for the integral dignity of the human person first of all in the act and at the moment in which the spouses transmit life to a new person. It is only logical therefore to address an urgent appeal to Catholic doctors and scientists that they bear exemplary witness to the respect due to the human embryo and to the dignity of procreation. The medical and nursing staff of Catholic hospitals and clinics are in a special way urged to do justice to the moral obligations which they have assumed, frequently also as part of their contract. Those who are in charge of Catholic hospitals and clinics and who are often religious will take special care to safeguard and promote a diligent observance of the moral norms recalled in the present instruction.

8. The Suffering Caused by Infertility in Marriage

The suffering of spouses who cannot have children or who are afraid of bringing a handicapped child into the world is a suffering that everyone must understand and properly evaluate.

On the part of the spouses, the desire for a child is natural: it expresses the vocation to fatherhood and motherhood inscribed in conjugal love. This desire can be even stronger if the couple is affected by sterility which appears incurable. Nevertheless, marriage does not confer upon the spouses the right to have a child, but only the right to perform those natural acts which are *per se* ordered to procreation.[35]

A true and proper right to a child would be contrary to the child's dignity and nature. The child is not an object to which one has a right, nor can he be considered as an object of ownership: rather, a child is a gift, "the supreme gift"[36] and the most gratuitous gift of marriage, and is a living testimony of the mutual giving of his parents. For this reason, the child has the right, as already mentioned, to be the fruit of the specific act of the conjugal love of his parents; and he also has the right to be respected as a person from the moment of his conception.

Nevertheless, whatever its causes or prognosis, sterility is certainly a difficult trial. The community of believers is called to shed light upon and support the suffering of those who are unable to fulfill their legitimate aspiration to motherhood and fatherhood. Spouses who find themselves in this sad situation are called to find in it an opportunity for sharing in a particular way in the Lord's cross, the source of spiritual fruitfulness. Sterile couples must not forget that "even when procreation is not possible, conjugal life does not for this reason lose its value. Physical sterility in fact can be for spouses the occasion for other important services in the life of the human person, for example, adoption, various forms of educational work, and assistance to other families and to poor or handicapped children."[37]

Many researchers are engaged in the fight against sterility. While fully safeguarding the dignity of human procreation, some have achieved results which previously seemed unattainable. Scientists therefore are to be encouraged to continue their research with the aim of preventing the causes of sterility and of being able to remedy them so that sterile couples will be able to procreate in full respect for their own personal dignity and that of the child to be born.

Moral and Civil Law: The Values and Moral Obligations that Civil Legislation Must Respect and Sanction in this Matter

The inviolable right to life of every innocent human individual and the rights of the family and of the institution of marriage constitute fundamental moral values, because they concern the natural condition and integral vocation of the human person; at the same time they are constitutive elements of civil society and its order.

For this reason the new technological possibilities which have opened up in the field of biomedicine require the intervention of the political authorities and of the legislator, since an uncontrolled application of such techniques could lead to unforeseeable and damaging consequences for civil society. Recourse to the conscience of each individual and to the self-regulation of researchers cannot be sufficient for ensuring respect for personal rights and public order. If the legislator responsible for the common good were not watchful, he could be deprived of his prerogatives by researchers claiming to govern humanity in the name of the biological discoveries and the alleged "improvement" processes which they would draw from those discoveries. "Eugenism" and forms of discrimination between human beings could come to be legitimized: this would constitute an act of violence and a serious offense to the equality, dignity and fundamental rights of the human person.

The intervention of the public authority must be inspired by the rational principles which regulate the relationships between civil law and moral law. The task of the civil law is to ensure the common good of people through the recognition of and the defense of fundamental rights and through the promotion of peace and of public morality.[38] In no sphere of life can the civil law take the place of conscience or dictate norms concerning things which are outside its competence. It must sometimes tolerate, for the sake of public order, things which it cannot forbid without a greater evil resulting. However, the inalienable rights of the person must be recognized and respected by civil society and the political authority. These human rights depend neither on single individuals nor on parents; nor do they represent a concession made by society and the state: they pertain to human nature and are inherent in the person by virtue of the creative act from which the person took his or her origin.

Among such fundamental rights one should mention in this regard: a) every human being's right to life and physical integrity from the moment of conception until death; b) the rights of the family and of marriage as an institution and, in this area, the child's right to be conceived, brought into the world and brought up by his parents. To each of these two themes it is necessary here to give some further consideration.

In various states certain laws have authorized the direct suppression of innocents: the moment a positive law deprives a category of human beings of the protection which civil legislation must accord them, the state is denying the equality of all before the law. When the state does not place its power at the service of the rights of each citizen, and in particular of the more vulnerable, the very foundations of a state based on law are undermined. The political authority consequently cannot give approval to the calling of human beings into existence through procedures which would expose them to those very grave risks noted previously. The possible recognition by positive law and the political authorities of techniques of artificial transmission of life and the experimentation connected with it would widen the breach already opened by the legalization of abortion.

As a consequence of the respect and protection which must be ensured for the unborn child from the moment of his conception, the law must provide appropriate penal sanctions for every deliberate violation of the child's rights. The law cannot tolerate—indeed it must expressly forbid—that human beings, even at the embryonic stage, should be treated as objects of experimentation, be mutilated or destroyed with the excuse that they are superfluous or incapable of developing normally.

The political authority is bound to guarantee to the institution of the family, upon which society is based, the juridical protection to which it has a right. From the very fact that it is at the service of people, the political authority must also be at the service of the family. Civil law cannot grant approval to techniques of artificial procreation which, for the benefit of third parties (doctors, biologists, economic or governmental powers), take away what is a right inherent in the relationship between spouses; and, therefore, civil law cannot legalize the donation of gametes between persons who are not legitimately united in marriage.

Legislation must also prohibit, by virtue of the support which is due to the family, embryo banks, *post mortem* insemination and "surrogate motherhood."

It is part of the duty of the public authority to ensure that the civil law is regulated according to the fundamental norms of the moral law in matters concerning human rights, human life and the institution of the family. Politicians must commit themselves, through their interventions upon public opinion, to securing in society the widest possible consensus on such essential points and to consolidating this consensus wherever it risks being weakened or is in danger of collapse.

In many countries, the legalization of abortion and juridical tolerance of unmarried couples makes it more difficult to secure respect for the fundamental rights recalled by this instruction. It is to be hoped that states will not become responsible for aggravating these socially damaging situations of injustice. It is rather to be hoped that nations and states will realize all the cultural, ideological and political implications connected with the techniques of artificial procreation and will find the wisdom and courage necessary for issuing laws which are more just and more respectful of human life and the institution of the family.

The civil legislation of many states confers an undue legitimation upon certain practices in the eyes of many today; it is seen to be incapable of guaranteeing that morality which is in conformity with the natural exigencies of the human person and with the "unwritten laws" etched by the Creator upon the human heart. All men of good will must commit themselves, particularly within their professional field and in the exercise of their civil rights, to ensuring the reform of morally unacceptable civil laws and the correction of illicit practices. In addition, "conscientious objection" vis-à-vis such laws must be supported and recognized. A movement of passive resistance to the legitimation of practices contrary to human life and dignity is beginning to make an ever sharper impression upon the moral conscience of many, especially among specialists in the biomedical sciences.

Conclusion

The spread of technologies of intervention in the processes of human procreation raises very serious moral problems in relation to the respect due to the human being from the moment of conception, to the dignity of the person, of his or her sexuality, and of the transmission of life.

With this instruction the Congregation for the Doctrine of the Faith, in fulfilling its responsibility to promote and defend the Church's teaching in so serious a matter, addresses a new and heartfelt invitation to all those who, by reason of their role and their commitment, can exercise a positive influence and ensure that, in the family and in society, due respect is accorded to life and love. It addresses this invitation to those responsible for the formation of consciences and of public opinion, to scientists and medical professionals, to jurists and politicians. It hopes that all will understand the incompatibility between recognition of the dignity of the human person and contempt for life and love, between faith in the living God and the claim to decide arbitrarily the origin and fate of a human being.

In particular, the Congregation for the Doctrine of the Faith addresses an invitation with confidence and encouragement to theologians, and above all to moralists, that they study more deeply and make ever more accessible to the faithful the contents of the teaching of the Church's Magisterium in the light of a valid anthropology in the matter of sexuality and marriage and in the context of the necessary interdisciplinary approach. Thus they will make it possible to understand ever more clearly the reasons for and the validity of this teaching. By defending man against the excesses of his own power, the Church of God reminds him of the reasons for his true nobility; only in this way can the possibility of living and loving with that dignity and liberty which derive from respect for the truth be ensured for the men and women of tomorrow. The precise indications which are offered in the present instruction, therefore, are not meant to halt the effort of reflection but rather to give it a renewed impulse in unrenounceable fidelity to the teaching of the Church.

In the light of the truth about the gift of human life and in the light of the moral principles which flow from that truth, everyone is invited to act in the area of responsibility proper to each and, like the good Samaritan, to recognize as a neighbor even the littlest among the children of men (cf. Lk. 10:29–37). Here Christ's words find a new and particular echo: "What you do to one of the least of my brethren, you do unto me" (Mt. 25:40).

During an audience granted to the undersigned Prefect after the plenary session of the Congregation for the Doctrine of the Faith, the Supreme Pontiff, John Paul II, approved this instruction and ordered it to be published.

Given at Rome, from the Congregation for the Doctrine of the Faith, February 22, 1987, the Feast of the Chair of St. Peter, the Apostle.

JOSEPH CARDINAL RATZINGER
Prefect

✠ ALBERTO BOVONE
Titular Archbishop of Caesarea in Numidia
Secretary

Notes

1. Pastoral Constitution *Gaudium et spes*, no. 51.

2. Holy See, *Charter of the Rights of the Family*, no. 4: *L'Osservatore Romano*, November 25, 1983.

3. Sacred Congregation for the Doctrine of the Faith, *Declaration on Procured Abortion*, nos. 12–13: *AAS* 66 (1974), 738.

4. Cf. Pope Paul VI, *Discourse to participants in the Twenty-third National Congress of Italian Catholic Jurists*, December 9, 1972: *AAS* 64 (1972), 777.

5. The obligation to avoid disproportionate risks involves an authentic respect for human beings and the uprightness of therapeutic intentions. It implies that the doctor "above all . . . must carefully evaluate the possible negative consequences which the necessary use of a particular exploratory technique may have upon the unborn child and avoid recourse to diagnostic procedures which do not offer sufficient guarantees of their honest purpose and substantial harmlessness. And if, as

often happens in human choices, a degree of risk must be undertaken, he will take care to assure that it is justified by a truly urgent need for the diagnosis and by the importance of the results that can be achieved by it for the benefit of the unborn child himself" (Pope John Paul II, *Discourse to Participants in the Pro-life Movement Congress*, December 3, 1982: *Insegnamenti di Giovanni Paolo II*, V, 3 [1982] 1512). This clarification concerning "proportionate risk" is also to be kept in mind in the following sections of the present instruction, whenever this term appears.

6. Pope John Paul II, *Discourse to the participants in the 35th General Assembly of the World Medical Association*, October 29, 1983: *AAS* 76 (1984), 392.

7. Cf. Pope John Paul II, *Address to a Meeting of the Pontifical Academy of Sciences*, October 23, 1982: *AAS* 75 (1983), 37: "I condemn, in the most explicit and formal way, experimental manipulations of the human embryo, since the human being, from conception to death, cannot be exploited for any purpose whatsoever."

8. Holy See, *Charter of the Rights of the Family*, no. 4b: *L'Osservatore Romano*, November 25, 1983.

9. Cf. Pope John Paul II, *Address to the Participants in the Convention of the Pro-Life Movement*, December 3, 1982: *Insegnamenti di Giovanni Paolo II*, V, 3 (1982), 1511: "Any form of experimentation on the fetus that may damage its integrity or worsen its condition is unacceptable, except in the case of a final effort to save it from death." Sacred Congregation for the Doctrine of the Faith, *Declaration on Euthanasia*, no. 4: *AAS* 72 (1980), 550: "In the absence of other sufficient remedies, it is permitted, with the patient's consent, to have recourse to the means provided by the most advanced medical techniques, even if these means are still at the experimental stage and are not without a certain risk."

10. No one, before coming into existence, can claim a subjective right to begin to exist; nevertheless, it is legitimate to affirm the right of the child to have a fully human origin through conception in conformity with the personal nature of the human being. Life is a gift that must be bestowed in a manner worthy both of the subject receiving it and of the subjects transmitting it. This statement is to be borne in mind also for what will be explained concerning artificial human procreation.

11. Cf. Pope John Paul II, *Discourse to those taking part in the 35th General Assembly of the World Medical Association*, October 29, 1983: *AAS* 76 (1984), 391.

12. Cf. Pastoral Constitution on the Church in the Modern World, *Gaudium et spes*, no. 50.

13. Cf. Pope John Paul II, Apostolic Exhortation *Familiaris consortio*, no. 14: *AAS* 74 (1982), 96.

14. Cf. Pope Pius XII, *Discourse to those taking part in the 4th International Congress of Catholic Doctors*, September 29, 1949: *AAS* 41 (1949), 559. According to the plan of the Creator, "A man leaves his father and his mother and cleaves to his wife, and they become one flesh" (Gn. 2:24). The unity of marriage, bound to the order of creation, is a truth accessible to natural reason. The Church's Tradition and Magisterium frequently make reference to the book of Genesis, both directly and through the passages of the New Testament that refer to it: Mt. 19:4–6; Mk. 10:5–8; Eph. 5:31. Cf. Athenagoras, *Legatio por christianis*, 33: *PG* 6, 965–967; St. Chrysostom, *In Matthaeum homiliae*, LXII, 19, 1: *PG* 58, 597; St. Leo the Great, *Epist. ad Rusticum*, 4; *PL* 54, 1204; Innocent III, *Epist. Gaudemus in Domino: DS* 778; Council of Lyons II, *IV Session: DS* 860; Council of Trent, *XXIV Session: DS* 1798, 1802; Pope Leo XIII, Encyclical *Arcanum Divinae Sapientiae: AAS* 12 (1879/80), 388–391; Pope Pius XI, Encyclical *Casti connubii: AAS* 22 (1930), 546–547; Second Vatican Council, *Gaudium et spes*, no. 48; Pope John Paul II, Apostolic Exhortation *Familiaris consortio*, no. 19: *AAS* 74 (1982), 101–102; *Code of Canon Law*, Can. 1056.

15. Cf. Pope Pius XII, *Discourse to those taking part in the 4th International Congress of Catholic Doctors*, September 29, 1949: *AAS* 41 (1949), 560; *Discourse to those taking part in the Congress of the Italian Catholic Union of Midwives*, October 29, 1951: *AAS* 43 (1951), 850; *Code of Canon Law*, Can. 1134.

16. Pope Paul VI, Encyclical Letter *Humanae vitae*, no. 12: *AAS* 60 (1968), 488–489.

17. *Loc. cit., ibid.*, no. 489.

18. Pope Pius XII, *Discourse to those taking part in the Second Naples World Congress on Fertility and Human Sterility*, May 19, 1956: *AAS* 48 (1956), 470.

19. *Code of Canon Law*, Can. 1061. According to this Canon, the conjugal act is that by which the marriage is consummated if the couple "have performed (it) between themselves in a human manner."

20. Cf. Pastoral Constitution *Gaudium et spes*, no. 14.

21. Cf. Pope John Paul II, *General Audience on January 16, 1980: Insegnamenti di Giovanni Paolo II*, III, 1 (1980), 148–152.

22. Pope John Paul II, *Discourse to those taking part in the 35th General Assembly of the World Medical Association*, October 29, 1983: *AAS* 76 (1984), 393.

23. Cf. Pastoral Constitution *Gaudium et spes*, no. 51.

24. Cf. Pastoral Constitution *Gaudium et spes*, no. 50.

25. Cf. Pope Pius XII, *Discourse to those taking part in the 4th International Congress of Catholic Doctors*, September 29, 1949: *AAS* 41 (1949), 560: "It would be erroneous . . . to think that the possibility of resorting to this means (artificial fertilization) might render valid a marriage between persons unable to contract it because of the *impedimentum inpotentiae*."

26. A similar question was dealt with by Pope Paul VI, Encyclical *Humanae vitae*, no. 14: *AAS* 60 (1968), 490–491.

27. Cf. *supra*: I, 1ff.

28. Pope John Paul II, Apostolic Exhortation *Familiaris consortio*, no. 14: *AAS* 74 (1982), 96.

29. Cf. *Response of the Holy Office*, March 17, 1897: *DS* 3323; Pope Pius XII, *Discourse to those taking part in the 4th International Congress of Catholic Doctors*, September 29, 1949: *AAS* 41 (1949), 560; *Discourse to the Italian Catholic Union of Midwives*, October 29, 1951: *AAS* 43 (1951), 850; *Discourse to those taking part in the Second Naples World Congress on Fertility and Human Sterility*, May 19, 1956: *AAS* 48 (1956), 471–473; *Discourse to those taking part in the 7th International Congress of the International Society of Hematology*, September 12, 1958: *AAS* 50 (1958), 733; Pope John XXIII, Encyclical *Mater et magistra*, III: *AAS* 53 (1961), 447.

30. Pope Pius XII, *Discourse to the Italian Catholic Union of Midwives*, October 29, 1951: *AAS* 43 (1951), 850.

31. Pope Pius XII, *Discourse to those taking part in the 4th International Congress of Catholic Doctors*, September 29, 1949: *AAS* 41 (1949), 560.

32. Sacred Congregation for the Doctrine of the Faith, *Declaration on Certain Questions Concerning Sexual Ethics*, no. 9: *AAS* 68 (1976), 86, which quotes the Pastoral Constitution *Gaudium et spes*, no. 51. Cf. *Decree of the Holy Office*, August 2, 1929: *AAS* 21 (1929), 490; Pope Pius XII, *Discourse to those taking part in the 26th Congress of the Italian Society of Urology*, October 8, 1953: *AAS* 45 (1953), 678.

33. Cf. Pope John XXIII, Encyclical *Mater et magistra*, III: *AAS* 53 (1961), 447.

34. Cf. Pope Pius XII, *Discourse to those taking part in the 4th International Congress of Catholic Doctors*, September 29, 1949: *AAS* 41 (1949), 560.

35. Cf. Pope Pius XII, *Discourse to those taking part in the Second Naples World Congress on Fertility and Human Sterility*, May 19, 1956: *AAS* 48 (1956), 471–473.

36. Pastoral Constitution *Gaudium et spes*, no. 50.

37. Pope John Paul II, Apostolic Exhortation *Familiaris consortio*, no. 14: *AAS* 74 (1982), 97.

38. Cf. Declaration *Dignitatis humanae*, no. 7.

Ethical Considerations of the New Reproductive Technologies

ETHICS COMMITTEE OF THE AMERICAN FERTILITY SOCIETY*

Foreword

In September 1986, The American Fertility Society issued a report, *Ethical Considerations of the New Reproductive Technologies*, Fertil Steril 46:[Suppl 1], 1986) setting forth the then-held ethical position of the Society on the various new reproductive technologies. In 1987, the Congregation for the Doctrine of the Faith issued the *Instruction on the Respect for Human Life in its Origin and on the Dignity of Procreation*.

Because of the conflicting conclusions of the two documents, the present Ethics Committee (1986–87) of The American Fertility Society was convened and considered the Fertility Society guidelines in the light of the *Instruction*. The succeeding document represents the deliberations of the 1986–87 Ethics Committee. These deliberations were approved by the Board of Directors of The American Fertility Society at its meeting in September 1987.

Introduction

The Vatican's *Instruction on Respect for Human Life* is a further addition to the international discussion of the new reproductive technologies. This discussion began in the early 1970s. It has led in the 1980s to a profusion of views, articles, and committee statements on the value dimensions of medically assisted reproduction and research involving early human pre-embryos. Professional societies, governmental committees, and religious bodies have been participants in the ongoing international study and debate. The Vatican *Instruction* is, without doubt, a significant contribution to the discussion.

In its conclusion, the *Instruction* clearly anticipates that its readers will be stimulated to re-evaluate their own moral assessment of the new reproductive technolo-

*Ed. note: Members of the 1986–87 Committee included Lori B. Andrews, J.D., Celso-Ramon Garcia, M.D., Gary D. Hodgen, Ph.D., Howard W. Jones, Jr., M.D., Richard J. McCormick, S.J., Richard Marrs, M.D., C. Alvin Paulsen, M.D., John Robertson, J.D., Edward E. Wallach, M.D., LeRoy Walters, Ph.D.

gies. "The precise indications which are offered in the present *Instruction* . . . are not meant to halt the effort of reflection, but rather to give it a renewed impulse. . . ." This brief document by the Ethics Committee (1986–87) of The American Fertility Society is part of that "effort of reflection" and is put forward to further additional exploration.

There is much in the *Instruction* with which people of good will, whether they are adherents of religious bodies or not, can identify. For example, the *Instruction* places safeguarding "the values and rights of the human person" at the center of its concern. In fact, the good of the human person, considered as an integral unity of body and mind, becomes the fundamental ethical criterion for judging all acts, policies, and technologies. The Ethics Committee (1985–86) of The American Fertility Society adopted a similar view in its September 1986 report when it asserted, "There is a more general ethical criterion which these appeals illuminate and to which they point. That criterion is *the human person integrally and adequately considered. Integrally and adequately* refers to the sum of dimensions of the person that constitute human well being: bodily health; intellectual and spiritual well being, which includes the freedom to form one's own convictions on important moral and religious questions; and social well being in all its forms: familial, economic, political, international, and religious."

The *Instruction* also acknowledges the potentially constructive role that science and medicine can play in helping to achieve the good of human beings. "Applied biology and medicine work together for the integral good of human life when they come to the aid of a person stricken by illness and infirmity and when they respect his or her dignity as a creature of God." However, the *Instruction* notes that some applications of technology can be demeaning to human beings. It therefore asserts that "what is technically possible is not, for that very reason, morally admissible."

On two other important points, the *Instruction* delineates a carefully nuanced approach. First, the document cautions against a blanket rejection of newer technical possibilities simply on the grounds of their artificiality: "Artificial interventions in procreation and the origin of human life . . . are not to be rejected on the grounds that they are artificial." Second, the *Instruction* clearly expresses sympathy for the suffering experienced by "spouses who cannot have children or who are afraid of bringing a handicapped child into the world." It encourages researchers to continue their effort to discover and overcome the causes of infertility. The *Instruction* also recognizes the value of the religious community's sympathetic support for the involuntarily infertile.

While acknowledging the value of such positive contributions of the *Instruction*, the Committee finds areas about which it has questions or disagreements with the document. The following discussion, which focuses on major issues, is divided into five sections:

I. Homologous Artificial Insemination and In Vitro Fertilization

II. The Use of Heterologous Gametes

III. Biomedical Research and Respect for the Pre-Embryo

IV. The Role of Law in Regulating Reproductive Technologies

V. Summary and Conclusions.

SECTION ONE
Homologous Artificial Insemination and In Vitro Fertilization

The *Instruction* rejects homologous artificial insemination and in vitro fertilization on grounds that they involve a separation between "the goods and meanings of marriage," that is, the unitive and the procreative. The separation of these two dimensions means that procreation thus achieved is "deprived of its proper perfection" and is therefore "not in conformity with the dignity of the person." The child must be conceived through an act of love and, indeed, of sexual intercourse.

It is this conclusion of the *Instruction* that the Committee finds problematic. In its own statement, the Committee had unanimously found that artificial insemination by the husband and in vitro fertilization are "ethically acceptable" in principle. The Committee therefore offers the following reflection on the analysis and conclusion of the *Instruction*.

First, the Committee agrees with the *Instruction* that "the one conceived must be the fruit of his parents' love," but it cannot understand how the conclusion is drawn that this love must, in all circumstances, mean sexual intercourse.

Second, the Committee wonders how separating the unitive and procreative in an *individual act*, "whether to prevent or achieve pregnancy," involves separation of the goods *of marriage*. What happens to the goods and meaning of marriage would seem to involve *the relationship*, not necessarily the individual act. Further, the Committee finds no radical separation of the unitive and procreative in these procedures, because it sees such interventions not as a replacement of sexual intimacy, but as its logical and technical extension—a view strongly supported by those who have experienced such interventions.

Third, the Committee would question whether an action "deprived of its proper perfection" is necessarily morally wrong. Many human actions, occurring as they do amid situations of deprivation, imperfection, and conflict, are not ideal and in that sense are "deprived of their proper perfection." Such actions, however, are not always morally wrong. The Committee believes that the *Instruction*, in its laudable effort to avoid mechanizing marriage and procreation, has too easily accepted natural procedures as morally normative.

Finally, the Committee notes the very broad ecumenical and scientific consensus with regard to assisted reproduction in the so-called "simple case" (between husband and wife). No major national committee or other religious body has rejected such intervention, given appropriate conditions of safety and respect for the pre-embryo. The Committee believes that such consensus reflects *basic known human experience and intuition* about the morally appropriate and inappropriate. The *Instruction* seems to take no account of this consensus, but to rely exclusively on previous ecclesiastical pronouncements.

SECTION TWO
The Use of
Heterologous Gametes

Although the introduction of a third party with the use of heterologous gametes may pose a problem for some, it is undeniable that it can provide a child to the infertile couple under certain circumstances. In specific instances, the use of heterologous gametes may protect the offspring, for example, when a serious genetic disease would be conveyed by the gametes of one of the parents. For these reasons, in their September 1986 statement, a majority of the Committee found the use of heterologous gametes to be ethically acceptable when medically indicated.

Donation customarily is viewed as a charitable act, as in the giving of a gift, giving of love, donation of an organ, or giving of life. As the *Instruction* indicates, "In reality the origin of a human person is the result of an act of giving." The donation of a gamete to an infertile couple can, in the Committee's view, also be an act of generosity.

As an alternative to childbearing with conjugal gametes, in the view of a significant number of people, the principle of using heterologous gametes presents a justifiable relaxation of unity between the genetic and gestational components of procreation and therefore does not constitute a violation of the unity of marriage. Since medical practice is directed toward the relief of suffering and illness, physicians do not discriminate between the suffering and illness associated with infertility and that attendant upon any other disease process. With regard to the use of heterologous gametes, the physician assists the couple without dominating the process.

While the *Instruction* suggests damage by heterologous artificial insemination to personal family relations, as well as to the offspring and its repercussion on civil society, the lengthy experience with heterologous insemination challenges this conclusion. Considerable supportive consensus reflects this concept, and there are no data to support the assertion of any deleterious effects, on the family or society, associated with the use of heterologous gametes. It seems likely that continuing improvement in knowledge and practices associated with the use of donated eggs and sperm will serve to strengthen the safety of and moral support for procedures involving heterologous gametes.

SECTION THREE
Biomedical Research
and Respect for
the Pre-embryo

Centuries of international debate on when a human life begins persist even to the present and are at the root of pluralism of the fundamental precepts affecting learned opinions about the relative value of human pre-embryos versus extant persons. It may be worthy of reiteration that the Committee finds real and significant moral values in the human pre-embryo from the time of fertilization onward in development, but the degree and nature of respect and moral value accorded to the human pre-embryo or fetus rises continuously until birth. Thus, proximity to birth is a principal factor in apportioning greater moral value upon developing human life.

The *Instruction* sets forth, without providing a rational basis, that "from the first moment of its existence until birth . . . no moral distinction is considered between zygotes, pre-embryos, embryos or fetuses." Although our knowledge of biologic processes that accompany human fertilization and subsequent embryonic development remains limited, it is growing. Certain scientific inferences on early human differentiation and development are warranted alongside viewpoints derived from substantive theological grounds. For example: (1) technically, because fertilization is a process, not an event, and the genome of the new generation is not segregated and surrounded by a nuclear envelope until the 2-cell stage, the early human zygote (before the 2-cell stage) would elude prohibitions aimed at postfertilization stages of development, such as those named in the *Instruction*, and (2) it remains fundamentally inconsistent to assign the status of human *individual* to the human zygote or early pre-embryo when compelling biologic evidence demonstrates that individuation, even in a primitive biologic sense, is not yet established. Thus, homologous (identical) twins may result from spontaneous cleavage of the pre-embryo at some point after fertilization but prior to the completion of implantation. Furthermore, during very early development, an embryo is not clearly established and awaits the differentiation between the trophoblast and the embryoblast. The Committee notes that although the *Instruction* preliminarily addresses biologic evidence on early human development, these data ultimately are put aside in favor of a predetermined position (revelation) that is not persuasive.

At numerous points in the *Instruction*, a strong bias against technology is evident, despite an initial claim that biomedical science is acceptable and consistent with appropriate moral behavior. The *Instruction* indirectly suggests that the motives of physicians, scientists, and others responding to the suffering of infertile couples and their wish to establish families are of questionable moral derivation. A case in point is the statement that "no biologist or doctor can reasonably claim by virtue of a scientific competence to be able to decide on people's origin and destiny." Indeed, no group has a special competence to decide these matters. Accordingly, physicians and scientists have sought a wider spectrum of opinion for ethical guidance. This is achieved broadly by the 1985–86 Committee's previously reported *Ethical Considerations*, and more narrowly by recommendations that human pre-embryo experimentations not be undertaken until properly constituted Institutional Review Boards have approved or rejected the proposed study. Even with approval, strict limitations have been specified.

The present Committee finds it unfortunate that the *Instruction* colors the good intention of biomedical research by choosing words and expressions that attach moral irresponsibility to persons and institutions seeking to provide new medical services to infertile couples, despite the statement that human service is an obligatory moral behavior. Moreover, certain statements are offered to indicate that human pre-embryos are wantonly destroyed with some frequency, either on frivolous or casual grounds. In addition, the *Instruction* states: "Cryopreservation constitutes an offense against the respect for human beings by exposing them to great risks of death or horror. . . ." Nowhere is there mention of the fact that cryopreservation preserves life and avoids, in many instances, the hazards to mother and offspring of multiple pregnancy.

The Committee regrets this remarkable and one-sided characterization, especially when such extensive efforts have been undertaken by physicians and scientists, in connection with theologians, ethicists, and lawyers, to define appropriate positions on the new reproductive technologies.

Finally, to associate the issues pertinent to infertility treatment by new reproductive technologies with the extant divisiveness of abortion and contraception seems unreasonable to the Committee. Instead, the single issue here is the attainment of a wanted pregnancy.

SECTION FOUR
The Role of Law in Regulating Reproductive Technologies

The *Instruction* applies past papal teaching to the issue of medically assigned reproduction and concludes that noncoital reproductive technologies are morally illicit. In this respect, the document may be persuasive to adherents of the Catholic faith in their own personal decisions about whether to participate in medically assisted reproduction as patient, health care provider, donor, or surrogate.

However, the *Instruction* does not stop at an attempt to provide a religious framework for decisions about reproductive technologies. The *Instruction* urges lawmakers to codify, in a set of laws, the conclusions of this religious framework. In doing so, the *Instruction* overlooks the difficulties involved in formulating public policies on private familial matters, like reproduction, and disputed ethical questions, like the moral status of early human embryos, especially in democratic, pluralistic societies. Although reproductive technologies provide technical means to facilitate procreation without coitus, there is dispute about the nature of the risks that these technologies pose for individuals, families, and society, and about whether a prohibitory law, rather than, for example, moral suasion, is the most appropriate means to deal with each risk.

The *Instruction* calls for the "reform of morally unacceptable civil laws for the correction of illicit practices" regarding reproductive technologies. The *Instruction* also advocates making it a crime to engage in (1) artificial insemination with one's husband's sperm, (2) in vitro fertilization, (3) research on the conceptus (except that which is therapeutic to the potential child and not disproportionately risky), and (4) donor or surrogate aid in reproduction. Under this approach, a couple and a doctor could be prosecuted if they attempted to overcome the husband's infertility by inseminating the wife with his sperm or by using in vitro fertilization.

To many people in the United States, even those with serious moral reservations about reproductive technologies, the idea of subjecting a couple to prosecution for trying to become parents in this fashion would be unacceptable. Moreover, such an approach would likely conflict with the protection of the United States Constitution.

The *Instruction* justifies its legislative recommendations on the grounds that they further fundamental values: the recognition of the conceptus as a human being from the moment of fertilization and the limitation of childbearing to a conjugal act within marriage. However, the constitutional legal framework in the United States highlights a different set of fundamental values. For the Vatican statement to be an adequate basis for statutory enactment, it must frame its arguments according to the generally accepted view of what is fundamental. Even though it is possible that some states might ban reproductive technologies based on the Vatican *Instruction*, such laws most likely would not be upheld as constitutional based on the reasoning of the *Instruction* alone.

There is a well-defined legal test that legislation must meet, if it interferes with an individual's or couple's right to privacy, a right that encompasses the seeking of medical aid in achieving or preventing procreation. There must be a compelling need for such a law, and a law must meet that need in the least restrictive manner possible.

At the heart of the conflict between the Vatican's approach to public policy and the constitutional approach is the difference in what is considered to be of fundamental value. The Constitution protects the right to privacy as fundamental. This right encompasses a right to autonomy in procreative decisions. Because of the importance of the biologic and social experiences that bearing and rearing a child entails, reproductive technologies potentially provide the only means by which one or both of the potential rearing parents would be able to create his or her genetic or gestational child. Consequently, decisions to use these technologies are likely to be protected by the constitutional right to privacy. As a result, particular reproductive technologies can be banned only if they present compelling risks that can only be satisfactorily met by outright prohibition. These risks must be imminent and substantial. They might be risks to the adult participant in a given reproductive technology or to the prospective child or to society. The Vatican *Instruction* alludes to certain risks but does not support them sufficiently to meet the constitutional test. For example, it states that heterologous artificial insemination by "threatening the unity and stability of the family is a source of dissension, disorder, and injustice in the whole social life." Without citing specific evidence for such assertions, the *Instruction* does not provide the grounds for legally upholding the legislative position that it advocates in the context of the United States.

Moreover, the *Instruction* lacks adequate discussion of the role that law should play in the enforcement of moral values. It overlooks the fact that there is not a consensus in the wider society about many of the issues under scrutiny. For example, there are divergent views on what moral and legal protection ought to be accorded to a pre-embryo or whether heterologous artificial reproduction threatens the institution of the family. In addition, the *Instruction* truncates the possibility for full social discussion or attempts to achieve a consensus around these issues by calling immediately for a legal ban on the new reproductive technologies.

SECTION FIVE
Summary and Conclusions

In September 1986, The American Fertility Society issued a report, *Ethical Considerations of the New Reproductive Technologies*, setting forth the then-held ethical position of the Society on the various new reproductive technologies. In 1987, the Congregation for the Doctrine of the Faith issued the *Instruction on the Respect for Human Life and Its Origin and on the Dignity of Procreation*. While both documents state that very similar moral criteria were used to derive ethical positions with respect to various reproductive procedures, the conclusions as to the ethical acceptability of the various procedures differ sharply in the two documents.

The question can be raised about the procedure used by the Congregation of the Faith to derive its conclusions from the stated premises. Thus, while stating that "the individual integrally and adequately considered" is to be the basis of the moral judgment, the fact is that most conclusions are based on and referenced to past Catholic statements.

While the difference in conclusion from similar premises may be troubling to society, it can be especially paralyzing to four groups: (1) those who face problems that might be solved by one or another of the new reproductive technologies; (2) those who are involved in applying them; (3) those who are responsible for institutional policies where such techniques may be applied; and (4) those who are in a position to influence public policy in a legislative or regulatory way.

Because of the conflicting conclusions of the two documents, the present Ethics Committee (1986–87) of The American Fertility Society was convened and considered these guidelines in the light of the *Instruction*.

For reasons set forth previously, the Committee reaffirmed the finding of the 1985–86 Committee that basic in vitro fertilization with homologous gametes is ethically acceptable.

The Committee reaffirmed the finding that the use of heterologous gametes is also ethically acceptable, provided that various precautions and guidelines are observed, as outlined in its previous report.

The Committee recognized and re-evaluated the long-debated and very complex issue of the moral status of the gamete, zygote, pre-embryo, embryo, and fetus. The reasons for believing that progressive degrees of respect are due with progressive development were set forth here and in the previous document. The Committee reaffirmed the position that experimentation on the pre-embryo in conformity with the policies and guidelines, as previously expressed, can be ethically justifiable and, indeed, necessary, if the human condition is to be improved.

The Committee was especially concerned lest the pluralistic nature of society be overlooked. It recognized that societal judgments about the reproductive technologies have changed and continue to change, necessitating a continuing dialogue to assure that these changes are reflected in current and future practices. For this reason, the Committee views with alarm the call for legislation based on doctrines not adequately supported by human experience or scientific data.

The Committee welcomes and encourages continued re-evaluation of the changing societal and moral issues and views involved in the ever-evolving new reproductive technologies.

□□□■

CHAPTER 1

Artificial Insemination

CASES FOR PRELIMINARY DISCUSSION

Case 1.1

A woman in her early thirties made an appointment with a fertility clinic counselor concerning the fact that she and her husband were childless after a number of years of trying. During the meeting, the woman disclosed that her husband was sterile and had insisted that they use his father's semen for artificial insemination. Her father-in-law, who was quite wealthy, had indicated that he would not recognize a child who was artificially produced as his legitimate heir unless the couple agreed to use his semen. While the woman admired her father-in-law and did not object to the procedure since the insemination would be artificial, she had some reservations. Nevertheless, she asked if the counselor could give her a go-ahead for the procedure.

—Adapted from "Artificial Insemination from a Father-in-Law," in *Case Studies in Medical Ethics*, by Robert M. Veatch (Cambridge, Mass.: Harvard University Press, 1976).

Case 1.2

"The facts in this proceeding are briefly stated. During the marriage the child was born of consensual AID. The husband was listed as the father on the birth certificate. Later the couple separated and the separation was followed by a divorce. Both the separation agreement and the divorce decree declare the child to be the 'daughter' and 'child' of the couple. The wife was granted support and the husband visitation rights. He has faithfully visited and performed all the support conditions of the decree. The wife later remarried and her new husband is petitioning to adopt the child. The first husband has refused his consent. Confronted with that legal impediment, the petitioner has suggested that the first husband's consent is not required since he is not the 'parent' of the child. . . ."

—From "In the Matter of the Adoption of Anonymous," 345 N.Y.S. 2d 430.

Case 1.3

A small-town physician is confronted with a starry-eyed couple one May morning, intent on a prenuptial physical prior to their June wedding, which has already been announced. A nagging doubt in the back of his mind prompts the physician to check his records, where he discovers to his consternation that they are half-brother and sister, each sired by the same anonymous sperm donor in AID arrangements with their parents nearly two decades previously. Grimly, he steels himself for an unpleasant interview in which he must tell them that the laws of the state prohibit their marriage.

Case 1.4

A 32-year-old lesbian lawyer requests that her gynecologist artificially inseminate her so that she can have a child. As she indicates to the physician, she is a successful attorney and, even as a single parent, can provide at least as much support and care as occurs with many working couples. In addition, there are many single-parent families headed by women. She would hope to raise the child, whether male or female, with an openness to being either heterosexual or homosexual. The physician is hesitant, in part because the woman is unmarried and would be raising the child alone, and in part because of her committed homosexual lifestyle.

—From Baruch A. Brody and H. Tristram Engelhardt, Jr., *Bioethics: Readings and Case Studies* (Englewood Cliffs, N.J.: Prentice-Hall, 1987).

REVIEW OF THE ISSUES

Men who experience diminished fertility do so for a number of causes: cryptorchidism involving undescended testes, varicocele, sports and other injuries, diseases producing high fever or damage to reproductive structures, licit drugs taken to deal with conditions such as high blood pressure, smoking and excessive alcohol consumption, illicit drugs, surgery for testicular cancer or strangulated vas deferens, irreversible surgical sterilization, exposure to radiation or toxic substances, spinal cord injuries, and natural aging.

Diminished fertility can often be successfully dealt with through medical treatment and surgery and even through alteration of clothing styles or the use of practices or devices designed to lower the temperature of the testes. However, infertility may well persist despite such measures; couples then turn to fertility specialists seeking technical assistance in achieving pregnancy.

Perhaps the oldest technique of reproductive technology is artificial insemination, or AI. AI permits semen to be collected from one or more ejaculations of a male who is chronically impotent or whose production of viable, active sperm in a given ejaculation falls below the numbers normally required to optimize the chances of fertilization. Batches of semen are then preserved through freezing, pooled, and introduced into the reproductive track of a woman at the time of ovulation. As a modern medical technique, it has been used for the better part of a quarter century to enable a husband to have children by his wife when normal coitus is impossible or when numbers of healthy, motile sperm are subcritical in number. The practice is widespread and relatively inexpensive: Some 172,000 American women underwent physician-induced artificial insemination in 1987, at an average cost of $953 each; slightly more than half these women have insurance coverage that on average pays 48 percent of the total cost.

Artificial insemination from the husband, or AIH, is possible as a home practice, using masturbation, a plastic bag, a refrigerator, a thermometer, and a syringe or baster, and there is no accurate record of how many couples have employed such practices on their own. However, the medically sanctioned form of AIH involves the intervention of the physician in the storage, pooling, and introduction of the husband's semen. Traditionalists, already dubious about the use of any artificial technique or device in reproductive activity (whether to prevent or encourage conception), have viewed the entry of the physician into the reproductive acts of husband and wife as a kind of adulterous intervention, or at least as a mechanization of the act of reproduction in a way that separates the natural spontaneity of an act of love from conception. (The charge of adultery is rather implausible since many physicians involved in this practice are themselves women.)

Despite such objections, AIH has become a widespread and commonly accepted practice, even among members of groups that officially disapprove. Some 35,000 children were born over a 12-month period in 1986–87, as a result of AIH performed by some 11,000 physicians. These live births represent 37.7 percent of the cases in which AI has been tried. More controversial, however, has been another application of the same techniques: artificial insemination of sperm from both husband and a donor.

Heterologous artificial insemination was originally introduced as an extention of AIH in cases where, even with the technique of artificial insemination, the husband's count of viable or motile sperm was inadequate to achieve a pregnancy. Semen taken from a donor is mixed with the sperm of the husband before artificial insemination. This technique originally permitted the husband to believe, because of the genuine possibility, that the offspring was his (although Redd Foxx expressed the problem here succinctly: "Momma's baby, Poppa's maybe"); the likelihood of such psychological—and social—certainty was enhanced by matching the donor to the husband for obvious characteristics such as hair and eye color and even blood type. (Now, the sophisticated new techniques of DNA analysis make these and other attempts to minimize doubts about paternity somewhat lame, since paternity can be definitively established.) However, heterologous AI has, in general, been supplanted by AID; the recent OTA reports do not mention heterologous AI as a practice.

The next obvious step was pure AID, using straight donor semen for cases where the infertility or impotence of the male partner was insurmountable, or where the male partner had a potential of transmitting a genetic disease, such as Huntington's chorea. And here the ascendancy of medical over private arrangements has proven to be more socially acceptable. Home-practice donor insemination almost always involves at least the woman knowing the identity of the biological father; many men willing to be donors are unwilling to place such a potent piece of information in the hands of someone who may, at a later date, find the desirability of revealing it to a child or some other individual to be greater than the inclination to keep the identity secret. Most, but not all, sperm banks and physicians practicing AID keep the donor's identity secret, although usually identifying records are kept that make it possible to connect information about a donor's genetic or infectious disease state with recipients of his semen.

It should be noted, however, that the various means of achieving AID can permit a close genetic relationship between the husband and the child who is the product of AID using semen from a male relative of the husband (such as a brother or even his father). There are thus cases on record where a man's wife has given birth to a child who is biologically his nephew or even his half-brother!

All the states that have dealt specifically with the rise of the practice of AID have statutorily decreed that any child born within wedlock is to be regarded presumptively as the issue of husband and wife, with the husband as responsible for the support of the child as if he were the biological father. This reflects the common medical practice of obtaining both husband and wife's consent when AID is to be performed.

AID carries with it some psychological risks. An infertile husband, confronted in a child with a daily reminder of his sterility (and perhaps impotence), may not succeed in stepping fully and wholesomely into the role of father. It is for this reason that couples seeking AID are evaluated psychologically as well as physiologically; where the chances for a rejection of the parental role or a worsening of the male's psychological state are significant, fertility clinics may disqualify the couple for AID.

In all but a very few such arrangements, the donor remains anonymous, known only to the physician or sperm bank personnel who have collected the sample. And frequently, donors have been attracted with the incentive of cash payment for their sperm. These two features, anonymity and cash transaction, have been the source of numerous complications and a troubling precedent. The complications will be mentioned here; the precedent will be introduced later in the discussion of surrogacy.

Such cases as that of the unwitting half-siblings seeking marital counseling, and the lack of knowledge of one's genetic family medical history, together with the typical curiosity about one's unknown biological parents, are the sorts of burdens carried by adopted childen; provided careful records have been kept, it may be possible, with the cooperation of the donor or surrendering parent, to determine their answers. But unlike adopted children, AID-conceived children are deliberately conceived in a manner that will confront them with such future questions. Adoption is undertaken under the test of the "best interests of the child doctrine," as an arrangement designed to rescue a child from an unfortunate and often tragic set of circumstances. AID-conceived children, however, are destined to grapple with such questions not as the unavoidable result of a society's efforts to protect their interests but as the unavoidable result of medicine's efforts to further the interests of their gestational/rearing parents. Thus, AID harbors moral complications more severe than those of simple adoption, placing the future individual at risk from the start for all of the problems of incompletely known parentage and close genetic connection to potential mates. The imposition of those burdens must be carefully weighed against the benefits to the infertile couple.

A corollary of these issues is that the individual donating semen may have a complex set of moral obligations to his several possible future children. Typically, financial responsibility for offspring produced with donated semen does not legally transfer with the genetic material. Still, one may arguably possess residual moral obligations to one's AID-sired offspring, at least to inform them of significant negatives in one's later health history. Some writers have speculated that the moral responsibility of the biological parent in AID and artificial inovulation from a donor remains fully that of a natural parent (Nelson and Nelson, 1989).

Seventy-eight percent of physicians sampled by the OTA reported testing for human immunosuppressive virus, or HIV; 74 percent require other diagnostic tests. Testing for HIV is tricky, because it is possible for semen to carry virus particles from a recent exposure of a male before a test is positive. Since the interval between exposure—and thus ability to transmit the virus—and a test being able to show that one has been exposed is three to six months, three-fourths of physicians who use frozen semen observe a quarantine period on the use of the semen. Thus, a would-be donor who has a genetic or sexually transmitted disease may represent a threat to numerous women and their offspring, and the payment of a fee for semen introduces into AID a conflict between the financial interests of donors and the health interests not only of their sexual partners but also recipients of their donated semen and the resulting offspring. Many feel that this is a basis for mandatory screening of donors.

An elitist twist to AID was proposed some years ago by Nobel Laureates Hermann J. Muller and others. It was their idea to create a bank of semen taken from the greatest intellects and leaders of the world. Women seeking to have exceptional offspring could apply to such a bank of frozen potentialities for AID in pursuit of superior children. Such a bank exists, and there is reason to think that some children have been produced with its contents. However, the jury is still out on whether the offspring are any more able than would be expected from a normal cross-section of the population, and it is certainly a trend that has not gained widespread acceptance.

A final area to be discussed is that of the possibility created by AID for widows and other single women, including those involved in lesbian relationships, to conceive and bear children without sexual contact with males. The OTA estimates that 5.6 percent of patients requesting artificial insemination did not have a relationship with a male partner. Confronted with a knowledgeable, well-situated single woman who asserts her right to reproduce, and possessed of techniques making that possible without the entanglements of sexual relations, gynecologists may find it difficult to maintain rationally that these techniques are only for the use of married women whose husbands cannot impregnate them. For such treatments (particularly AID) are not truly therapies for male infertility; they are ways of enabling a woman to have a child whose husband cannot perform that essential function. A woman without a husband faces precisely the same difficulty as a woman with an infertile one, and it may appear unjust to deny the unmarried woman the right of conception simply because she is unmarried. Human ingenuity being what it is, it would be possible to have a marriage of convenience with an infertile male lasting just long enough to qualify for AID, or even more simply to induce a male acquaintance to provide a plastic baggie containing the makings of one's future offspring.

Nonetheless, when asked if they would be likely to reject an unmarried recipient without a partner, 61 percent of surveyed physicians indicated they would. This pattern has prompted the opening of sperm banks committed to providing AID to any healthy woman or couple regardless of marital status, and one exists with an explicit commitment to providing services to single and lesbian women. The Sperm Bank of Northern California in Oakland also actively seeks freely given sperm from donors who are willing to be contacted by their offspring.

Recipients for AID are frequently screened too for drug and alcohol abuse, for various serious diseases such as gonorrhea, syphilis, hepatitis, and cytomegalovirus, and for psychological conditions associated with child abuse. Where such conditions are present, a sperm bank or physician may refuse the service until the condition is adequately treated.

REVIEW OF THE SELECTIONS

Artificial insemination has become such a widespread practice in the United States that, apart from the Vatican selection in the introductory chapter, it is difficult to find reasoned opposition to it. It is therefore something of a surprise to discover that enormous opposition attended its introduction into medical practice, with its employment regarded as equivalent to adultery (because of the role of the physician) and the offspring of AID stigmatized as illegitimate. Opposition to artificial insemination has been even stronger in Canada and Great Britain.

The chief roots of such opposition have appeared to feminists to be males' anxiety over determining the paternity of their wives' offspring, and the challenges to the rules of inheritance posed by children deliberately conceived through AID.

Gena Corea's selection details something of the history of the development of AID and its introduction in Europe and North America, and is particularly revealing in chronicling the reactions of medical, religious, and legal writers to AID and its use by women who wish children without the complications of husbands or (male) lovers.

The selection by British sociologist Carol Smart develops the logic of paternity and property concerns through an analysis of two Crown-commissioned British reports (the Russell Commission in 1966 and the Warnock Commission of 1985). Her paper carefully untangles biological, social, and legal concepts of paternity and fatherhood, and of maternity and motherhood, and introduces some of the issues extensively debated in feminist literature.

Works Cited

1. Nelson, Hilde Lindemann and James Lindemann Nelson. "Cutting Motherhood in Two: Some Suspicions Concerning Surrogacy." *Hypatia* 4(3), 1989.

2. Office of Technology Assessment, U.S. Congress. *Infertility: Medical and Social Choices.* Washington, D.C.: U.S. Government Printing Office, 1988.

The Subversive Sperm: "A False Strain of Blood"

GENA COREA

Although artificial insemination with donor sperm (AID) has been technologically possible for at least the past one hundred years, the practice has developed at a snail's pace. The fact that AID could be used in a eugenic program to control the "quality" of human beings produced has not been enough to recommend it. It alarmed men that a husband's sperm need not be used to inseminate his wife, that another man's could be. At a symposium on artificial insemination physicians and lawyers held in Chicago back in 1945, one participant suggested that AID was as startling as the atomic bomb and needed legislation accordingly (Greenhill, 1947). Bills were proposed in the Federal Republic of Germany and in Italy in the late 1950s which would have made human AID a criminal offense (Feversham, 1960).

In a paper he wrote in 1953, Dr. Jerome K. Sherman, American pioneer in sperm freezing, wondered why, after the introduction that year of a simple, effective sperm preservation method, many frozen sperm banks were not established. (Even today, only seventeen such banks exist in the United States.) He offers as one possible explanation that "there was a hesitancy on the part of physicians to try something as new as frozen semen, something which introduced another unphysiologic factor into the insemination procedures" (Sherman, 1973).

But there has been no comparable hesitancy on the part of physicians to try something as new as the conception of babies in laboratory dishes, a far more complicated procedure. With the first tentative success, in vitro fertilization clinics popped up all around the world. While in 1974, twenty years after the birth of the first child through frozen sperm, the American Medical Association declared that use of frozen human sperm "must still be recognized as experimental," within four years of the first test-tube baby's birth, physicians were proclaiming that in vitro fertilization was no longer experimental (Callahan, 1982).

Gena Corea is an American journalist and lectures on women's health and reproductive technology. She is the author of The Hidden Malpractice: How American Medicine Mistreats Women *(1977, reprinted 1985) and* The Mother Machine: Reproductive Technologies from Artificial Insemination to Artificial Wombs *(1985), and a contributor to* Man-Made Women: How New Reproductive Technologies Affect Women *(1987).*

Sperm banks have developed slowly, not because pharmacrats fear a "new" technology, but because they recognize that artificial insemination by donor sperm poses a threat to the patriarchal family and to male dominance.

Before discussing these threats, let us review the development of this technology. Artificial insemination was possible at all only when the role of sperm in reproduction was grasped. Anton van Leeuwenhoek first described spermatozoa in human seminal fluid but, peering through his microscope in 1677, he did not know the sperm's function.

In 1779, the Italian priest and physiologist Lazaro Spallanzani showed experimentally for the first time that in order for embryos to develop, the egg and seminal fluid must come into actual physical contact. In his laboratory, Spallanzani artificially inseminated frogs, fish and dogs.

With this new knowledge on the sperm's role in reproduction, the first attempt to artificially inseminate a woman was made in 1790. The famous Scottish anatomist and surgeon John Hunter successfully inseminated the wife of a linen draper using her husband's sperm (AIH).[1] In the nineteenth century in Britain, Germany, France and the United States, AIH was reportedly practiced to a limited extent. The first recorded case using donor sperm rather than the husband's took place in 1884 in Philadelphia. In the next forty years, there was some discussion of AID and a few cases were reported in medical journals in the United States and Germany.

It was in the 1930s that physicians in Britain first seriously discussed the possibility of artificially inseminating the wives of infertile men. Small groups of gynecologists inseminated women during the Second World War but few people knew this. The practice was only beginning. A mere fifteen artificial inseminations using the husband's sperm and fifteen using donor sperm were reportedly performed in Great Britain in 1945 (Langer, 1969); by 1960, only an estimated twenty physicians were regularly performing it.

In Holland the practice was embraced no more heartily. From 1948, when the practice began, until 1960, there were fewer than ten AIDs (Levie, 1972). In the United States, 5,000 to 7,000 AID children were born every year, according to a 1960 estimate. Almost twenty years later, that estimate had expanded little: 6,000 to 10,000 births per year (Curie-Cohen, 1979).

The ability to freeze sperm expanded the potential use of artificial insemination. In 1949, A. S. Parkes and two fellow British scientists developed a method using glycerol, a syrupy substance, to protect semen from injury during the freezing.[2]

Farmers employed this method in the breeding industry. The use of frozen human sperm, however, was ignored until 1953 and 1954 when Sherman and his co-workers reported their research. They introduced a simple method of preserving human sperm using glycerol with a slow cooling of sperm and storage with solid carbon dioxide as a refrigerant. They also demonstrated for the first time that frozen sperm, when thawed, were able to fertilize an egg and induce its normal development.[3]

Despite this demonstration, few rushed to establish sperm banks. In the decade after the Sherman reports, only two frozen sperm banks or "cryobanks" opened—one in Iowa City and the other in Tokyo. The first human being conceived with frozen semen was born in 1954. By 1965, a mere twenty-four babies born in the United States and Japan had been conceived through frozen-thawed sperm. (Yet just six years after the first test-tube baby's birth, an estimated 200 babies had been born by in vitro fertilization.) In 1970, the first commercial human sperm cryobank in the United States was established and the largest one in the world, Idant, opened the following year in New York City. By 1973, the clinical use of frozen semen had resulted in only 571 births.[4]

By contrast, use of AID developed rapidly among farm animals. In Russia about 1900, scientists began studies on AID, primarily in cattle and sheep. They immediately saw its usefulness in breeding. They could inseminate thousands of females with the sperm of a few prize animals.

But how to get the sperm? Giuseppe Amantea, professor of human physiology at the University of Rome, had an idea. In 1914, he devised an artificial vagina ("AV," they came to call it) to collect dog semen. Russian scientists soon developed AVs suitable for the stallion, bull and ram. The men would sexually stimulate the bull by exposing him to a teaser animal and allowing him false mounts. Right before ejaculation, they would guide the bull's penis into the AV.

Sometimes an animal could not "serve" the AV. In 1948, scientists developed the electroejaculator, "a useful innovation for collecting from reluctant or disabled bulls and rams" (Bearden, 1980, p. 140). An electrode is placed in the rectum of crippled or old bulls in such a way that the reproductive system is stimulated.

If neither the AV nor electric current methods work, drugs can be injected to induce ejaculation. If all fails, a final option remains: "the recovery of spermatozoa from the male reproductive tract after slaughter."[5]

In 1936 in Denmark, cattle breeders formed the first cooperative AI association for the purpose of sharing the sperm of their prize bulls. The next year, Danish veterinarians developed the method of insemination (recto-vaginal) now widely used.

During World War II, the artificial insemination of farm animals accelerated rapidly and by the late 1940s, there were many AI organizations breeding cows all over the United States. The availability of frozen semen led to the widespread use of AI in the mid-1960s. Today, thirty-seven companies sell cattle semen. In the United States in 1980, 60 percent of dairy cows and 2 to 4 percent of beef cattle were inseminated artificially. These animals have never experienced their natural sexuality.[6]

While pharmacrats were enthusiastic about the use of AID to increase their control over the breeding of farm animals, most viewed the prospect of AID in women with alarm. There are two reasons for this. It poses a threat to patriarchal descent and it provides women with a means of rebellion.

AID desecrates sperm, the holy seed from which blossoms forth the power of the patriarchy. In introducing another man's "donor" sperm into a husband's wife, AID jeopardizes patriarchal descent. How can a man pass on his name and goods to his son if that son is not really *his*?

For many centuries before the establishment of patriarchy, man did not realize that he played any part in the creation of a baby (see Chapter 15). When paternity—the connection between sexual intercourse and the birth of a child—was discovered, man had a motive for subjugating woman.* If he could control his woman, allowing no other man to impregnate her, he could pass his name, power and property down through his sons. In this way, he could achieve immortality and a sense of connection with generations to come.

Subjugated, a woman became chattel, the movable property of men. She served as the womb of her husband and held a status comparable to that of cattle. She was required to bear only "legitimate" children, that is, offspring containing the seed of the man who owned her.

A woman can never legitimate her own child because "legitimacy" is a concept invented by men for men. It controls women who might defy male rules for reproduction. Men punish both rule-breaking women and their out-of-wedlock children. In Colonial America, a woman who bore a bastard could be fined, publicly whipped and bound into indentured servitude.[7] Her bastard child could also be bound into servitude for twenty-one years or even for a lifetime. Bastardy, unlike rape or wife-murder, was an unforgivable crime. Theodore Sedgwick called it "the only crime which good society never pardons. . . . Shame, ridicule, infamy, exile attend it" (Jones, 1980, p. 44). To Jean Jacques Rousseau, the father of the Romantic revolution, bastardy was treasonous. Explaining that a faithless wife is worse than a faithless husband, he wrote:

> She destroys the family and breaks the bounds of nature; when she gives her husband children who are not his own she is false both to him and them, her crime is not infidelity but treason. To my mind, it is the source of dissension and of crime of every kind. Can any position be more wretched than that of the unhappy father who, when he clasps his child to his breast, is haunted by the suspicion that this is the child of another, the badge of his own dishonour, a thief who is robbing his own children of their inheritance? (From *Emile* in Figes, 1970, p. 74.)

To avoid punishments (such as public whippings and enforced servitude) devised by men who thought as Rousseau thought, thousands of seventeenth and eighteenth century women killed their own children. They murdered the babies men labeled "illegitimate." They stuffed their infants into sewers, threw them into rivers, hid them in trunks, buried them in the garden, in the cellar. Many were caught. Many were hung (Jones, 1980, pp. 42–57).

This is the key question AID posed to the patriarchy, the one to which courts solemnly devoted their attention: Is an AID child a "legitimate" child? Even when delivered by a man's wife, the child does not spring from the man's own loins. If an AID child is "illegitimate," has the mother committed adultery in conceiving it? Is an AID child entitled to receive a man's property, the patrimony?

Early on, the answer to that last question was no. Early on, men saw only the threat AID posed to them.

---

*No one knows exactly when paternity was discovered. The observation that males were necessary for reproduction, Elizabeth Fisher suggests, may have been loosely made during the early stages of animal keeping, about 11,000 years ago (Fisher, 1979, p. 192).

"What husband or wife, no matter how intense their longing for an heir, will consent to an injection of strange semen?" Dr. Hermann Rohleder wrote in a 1934 book on artificial insemination. "Thank God that most people still have that much tact, decency and moral feeling."

An Italian physician, he reported, had been entreated by a childless married woman to inseminate her with the sperm of a fertile man. "He told his patient the evil contained in her suggestion," Rohleder wrote, "and pointed out to her that the artificial introduction of the semen of a strange man would be just as much of a sin as if she had herself consorted with a strange man" (Rohleder, 1934, p. 167).

And nine years later, in 1943, a physician wrote in the *American Journal of Obstetrics and Gynecology*: "The happy wife, contented through attaining a baby by means of homologous artificial insemination [i.e., with her husband's sperm], may give voice to her joy and win approbation. But the woman, made pregnant by the use of donor semen, who even whispers out of turn, on a single occasion, becomes a medical curiosity. She is envied by the primitive and wanton-minded, pitied by those gifted with easy fertility, shunned by her relatives and perhaps unfortunately by her own child" (Folsome, 1943).

In early cases, courts in England, Canada and the United States ruled that AID children were illegitimate and that the practice of AID was equivalent to adultery. As such, AID provided grounds for divorce and possible criminal prosecution.

Adultery, then, did not require sex. It was any act that might result in illegitimate conception. A Canadian case dealing with a woman who had allegedly agreed to AID without her husband's consent made that clear. In 1921, the Supreme Court of Ontario defined adultery as "the voluntary surrender to another person of the reproductive powers or faculties of the guilty person."[8] The essential element of adultery is not so much "the moral turpitude of the act of sexual intercourse," as it is "the possibility of introducing into the family of the husband a false strain of blood," the court ruled.[9]

An attorney presenting a paper at that AI symposium in Chicago in 1945 agreed with this ruling. Some courts had held that anything short of actual sexual intercourse—no matter how indecent the acts—did not constitute adultery, attorney James F. Wright pointed out. That fact strengthened the view that it is not moral depravity that is at the core of adultery, he said, "but the invasion of the reproductive function. There can be no adultery so long as nothing takes place which can by any possibility affect that function." Securing a man's property and, thereby, his immortality is really what the adultery prohibitions are all about.[10] It is not surprising then, that Wright indignantly asks from whom the AID child should inherit land and wealth. "Would he inherit from the husband of his mother, when the husband had nothing to do with producing this offspring?" (Greenhill, 1947). AID, Wright declared, should be declared by the courts to be adulterous.

The Superior Court for Cook County obliged him. In 1954, it held that regardless of a husband's consent, AID was "contrary to public policy and good morals," and constituted adultery on the mother's part. A child so conceived was born out of wedlock and was therefore illegitimate. The court added: "As such it is the child of the mother, and the father has no right or interest in said child."

As late as 1963, a court held that an AID child was illegitimate because the sperm donor was not married to the child's mother. Regardless of her husband's consent to AID, the court declared, the woman's insemination had constituted adultery.

In Britain, as in the United States, AID alarmed men. In 1948, a commission of inquiry set up by the Archbishop of Canterbury recommended that AID should be made a criminal offense. In the late 1950s, the British government appointed the Feversham Committee to inquire into AI practices and regulations. The committee, completing its report in 1960, recommended that a woman's conception by AID without the husband's consent be made a new ground for divorce. It found that AID was undesirable because it is a threat to the institution of marriage and to the resulting children. Those AID children, it found, should continue to be labeled illegitimate. "Succession through blood descent is an important element of family life and as such is at the basis of our society. On it depend the peerage and other titles of honour, and the Monarchy itself."[11]

If commissions and courts reacted to AID with distress, the response of male religious and medical leaders bordered on the testicular.* After reviewing the literature on artificial insemination, Dr. Bernard Rubin noted that it evoked "an intense emotional response" which had not changed in almost two hundred years. He thought the writers were unconsciously associating AID with incest. I think he need only have taken the writers literally. Listen to Dr. Rubin summarize their fears:

"It has been stated that AID 'endangers the family,' 'it is socially monstrous,' it endangers 'marriage, family and society.' 'It may well lead to radical revolution in which such concepts as father, brother, family descent, and the like, lose every vestige of their meaning.' There were fears of 'an anonymous world'; 'it should never be recommended.' The British Medical Association felt it was an 'offense against society'" (Rubin, 1965).

Such a response to AID is understandable if we grasp how terrifying to men was the prospect of "an anonymous world," that is, one without genetic continuity for men. "Grieving the loss of genetic continuity" is one of the difficult issues surrounding AID cited by infertility counselor Barbara Menning. She quotes one 30-year-old man who suffered that loss: "I did experience tremendous narcissistic hurt thinking that there would never be a child who looked like me or carried my genes. I recall that when I first considered AID, I had hoped that my wife would deliver a girl, whereas before, I had always expressed no preference. Somehow in my mind a son would highlight my loss because he wouldn't be a small version of me" (Menning, 1981).

AID posed a second threat to patriarchy. It not only jeopardized the mechanism of patriarchal descent, it also provided women with a means of rebellion. If AID were readily available, women could have families with children, but without men. This threatens the family, the community and men, sociologist Jalna Hanmer points out, and patriarchal religious leaders recognize that.

---

*I choose the adjective "testicular" rather than "hysterical" (a word relating to "womb") in respect for the gender to which I here refer.

The Rev. Don McCarthy does: "Should not physicians and other health care personnel be prevented by law from using technology to impregnate unmarried women or
from providing in vitro fertilization for unmarried couples? If the state is concerned to
protect life, perhaps civil law ought to be equally concerned to protect marriage. The
[Roman Catholic] Church stands firmly opposed to non-marital procreation" (McCarthy, 1980).

Men can hardly prevent women from performing AID. No physician is needed, nor
is any complex equipment. "The technique of artificial insemination is simple," Dr.
Wildred Finegold wrote in a 1964 medical text. "In fact, one of the hazards of the
procedure is the ease of its performance."

Hazard to whom? Not to women. Then, to men?

Recognizing that "hazard," one man wrote to the AID Research Project: "God,
you're making us less and less useful and necessary. It is frightening."

As attorney Russell Scott observed in 1981: "If reproduction by AI became the
norm, it would follow that the human male would cease to be socially necessary. . . .
The human species could easily be reproduced from stored sperm, or from sperm
taken from a small number of selected living donors. The social implications of the
disappearance of the historic role of the human male are difficult to imagine" (Scott,
1981, pp. 213–214).

Not surprisingly, men have attempted to limit the access of unmarried women to
AID. Physicians quickly claimed that AI was a "medical" procedure over which they,
and only they, should exercise control. The American Medical Association declared in
1974: "Because human artificial insemination is a medical procedure, the medical
profession should exert its influence and efforts to the fullest extent necessary to
ensure that the procedure is performed only by individuals licensed to practice medicine or osteopathy" (AMA, 1973). In 1980, a committee of the American Fertility Society recommended model legislation which provides imprisonment and fines for nonmedical persons performing AI.[12] Georgia passed a law legitimizing the AID child but
only under certain conditions, among them, that a physician had performed the insemination. If a woman refuses to hire a physician, the child she bears is a bastard; if
she goes to a doctor's office and takes her medicine, her baby is legitimate, sanctioned
by the patriarchal state.

Most laws concerning AID now stipulate that the insemination should be performed by a doctor.

In Quebec, physicians write prescriptions for sperm. It is a "medicine." The
Quebec Order of Pharmacists classified it as such in 1980 so that it could be considered a prescription drug cost under the Medicare program (AMN, 1980).

"In practice, if not in law, it's very similar here," comments Francie Hornstein,
originator of an AID program at the Los Angeles Feminist Women's Health Center.
"You need a doctor to formally requisition the sperm. You can't get it on your own.
You register at the sperm bank. Each time you want to get the sperm, the doctor's
office has to call."

Male medicine has certain criteria for women allowed what it calls the "therapy" of
artificial insemination. The main criteria is that they be married. As attorney Barbara
Kritchevsky observes, the very terms used to describe AI reveal the intent to limit its

use to marriage: There can be no such thing as AIH—artificial insemination by husband—for a single woman.[13]

The possibility that unmarried women could choose pregnancy by AI has been mentioned in the legal literature since the 1940s "with great concern and distaste," Kritchevsky reports. She cites two articles published in 1949 that recommend legislative bans on AI for unmarried women.

Ninety percent of physicians queried in a 1979 survey had never used AID for unmarried women; 10 percent had. Physicians performed fewer than 1 percent of all artificial inseminations for the single (Curie-Cohen, 1979).

Many physicians have simply refused to inseminate them. "We do not offer the program [AID] to single women," doctors noted in *The New England Journal of Medicine* (Strickler, 1975).

Some doctors fear the practice is illegal. (It is not.) Others disapprove of bringing a child into a fatherless home or believe that unmarried women and lesbians should not be mothers. For example, Dr. Finegold believes an unmarried woman's interest in AI is "indicative of psychological distress" (Kritchevsky, 1981).

"I would refuse AID for a spinster," a British fertility clinic director wrote in 1972, "or for a couple of mixed colour or even of mixed religious denomination" (Sandler, 1972).

In 1962, the Royal Dutch Medical Association declared: "Artificial insemination of an unmarried woman is in conflict with the social order, and inadmissible on medical ethical grounds."

Similarly, the Feversham Committee expressed unqualified disapproval of AI for women unattached to men: single women, widows and "married women living apart from their husbands."

But in 1980 a woman challenged the right of physicians to refuse her AID on the grounds that she was unmarried. For such an alleged refusal, she sued a clinic in Detroit. She dropped the suit when the clinic, a division of Wayne State University's School of Medicine, announced that marital status would not be a factor in selecting "patients" for the procedure.

The reaction to this announcement overwhelmed the clinic. For several weeks, the obstetrics and gynecology department at Wayne received more than a dozen calls a day from single women, department chair Dr. Tommy N. Evans reported. "A lot of people have the idea that they can just walk in and get inseminated," Evans told *Ob/Gyn News*, "and that's just not the case at all."[14]

True. So some women began to take AI into their own hands, stating that childbearing was as much a woman's reproductive right as was abortion. "AID has a tremendous potential for expanding the options women have in living their lives," says Hornstein. "I think a lot of people get married solely because they want to have children. And maybe now those people—mostly women—won't feel that they have to get married."

The women using AI come from all walks of life. They are physicians, teachers, nurses' aides, social workers, psychotherapists, business executives, stewardesses, clerical and factory workers, principals, editors and secretaries. Some are feminists, others not at all consciously political.

Ever since approximately 1976, increasing numbers of heterosexual career women have been using AID, Annette Baran, a clinical social worker and co-founder of the AID Research Project, reports. These women are able to take care of themselves. They want a child. They are in their thirties. They have no guarantee they will ever meet, love and marry a man who will also want a child. So they go ahead on their own and bear a baby.

"They're a whole different breed," Baran says. "They're all Virgin Marys. There's no sex involved. They're bragging about it all over the place."

They do not feel like unwed mothers, Baran notes, because they did not get pregnant through an "illicit" sexual relationship. "They share it with their Board of Directors or their friends. They talk to everybody about it. They are very proud that they're a kind of pioneer woman."

Lesbian women started using AID at about the same time. It began small. A lesbian in Vermont wanted a child. A photographer who had graduated from Vassar College and obtained a master's degree from Johns Hopkins, she recalled: "I knew that the technique [AID] existed and that married women with infertile husbands were doing it and I figured maybe I could find a way for myself." For a year she kept careful records of her menstrual cycle so she could predict her ovulation, the optimal time for insemination. "I got very good at that," she observed.

Her physician father is proud of what she has done. "He sees that the choice made sense for me and is proud that I struggled to find a way to make it happen," she wrote on a questionnaire I distributed among lesbian AID mothers. "My mother views it as 'science fiction' and is sad that I did not live out her story-book fantasy of being married, etc. But she is so pleased with her granddaughter that those feelings have not surfaced since I first told her early in the pregnancy."

That same year, 1976, a lesbian in Los Angeles bore an AID baby. Rather than use a sperm bank, she and her lover found donors on their own. Then they went to the Los Angeles Feminist Women's Health Center. Staffer Francie Hornstein showed the women how to examine themselves using a speculum, flashlight and mirror and how to insert the sperm.

"She was the first woman I ever knew who actually went ahead and got pregnant by AID on her own," Hornstein recalls.

The Vermont Women's Health Center, the Los Angeles and the Oakland Feminist Women's Health Centers all now offer donor insemination programs. They began their programs, respectively, in 1975, 1979 and 1982. The Oakland center also has its own sperm bank.

"We've had three health center babies," reports Vermont staffer Dana Gallagher.

Attorney Donna Hitchens, who has written on donor insemination for the Lesbian Rights Project in San Francisco, says that AID is now in fairly extensive use among lesbians. "I'm seeing it a lot, especially in lesbians between 30 and 36 years old," she says. "In the Bay Area, we probably have two hundred children." The first such children in any numbers were born in 1979, she estimates.

A few books and articles offer how-to advice on "alternative fertilization" or "self-insemination," terms the authors prefer to "artificial insemination." They describe how to pinpoint ovulation so the woman can inseminate herself at the optimal time for fertilization. They report how women have found sperm donors (often, through friends) and what problems these women have encountered. Some women, they note, know who their sperm donors are, feeling this knowledge is important should their children someday want to learn about or form a relationship with their fathers. (One woman who filled out my questionnaire wrote that her sperm donor is a co-worker who regularly sees the child, acting as the child's friend, not father.) In many other instances, women try to keep the sperm donor anonymous for fear of a child custody suit by him later.

Gordon Prince of the Department of Child and Family Psychiatry at King's College Hospital in London is one of the many who disapproves of a lesbian using AID. A lesbian's motive for wanting children concerns him, he stated. Possibly that motive stems from aggression? Prince wonders if a lesbian's desire for AID might arise from "a basic hostility to men or to the traditional male pattern of society."* The issue needs study, he concluded. Earlier, in a 1978 case conference on lesbian use of AID, Prince had commented: "The hostility and fear to what we are discussing is very deep" (JME, 1978).

Lesbians know that. Many worry about what effect that hostility and fear may have on their children. Mary N., who eventually bore a son, Andy, is one of them: "The one thing that made us [her partner and herself] take so long in deciding to do donor insemination was fear for Andy's suffering. Was it really fair to him to do this? Finally we decided that if you think something is right—if you believe it is a woman's right to have children regardless of whether she's a lesbian or a celibate heterosexual—then it would be better to do the insemination and fight to make it acceptable. But it still scares us. It's scary thinking that your child is going to have pain."

It is still too early yet to know the full range of difficulties and joys these female-headed AID families will experience. All lesbian mothers who filled out my question-naire or talked with me were very happy they had had a baby through AID. But their responses did indicate some of the complexities of their situations: the insecurity felt by the partner of an AID mother because she, who also loves and mothers the child, may have no legal or socially sanctioned relationship to that child or any right to see the child again if the relationship with the mother ends; a fear that, as lesbians, they will be declared unfit mothers and have their children taken away from them, a fear causing them to be secretive about the AID to the outside world while telling their children the truth about their conception; the guilt any mother feels ("Am I doing it right?") exacerbated, for the single lesbian, by the messages she gets that a single parent family is incomplete and undesirable; the uniqueness of the AID family's rela-tionship with grandparents—often supportive, sometimes uneasy.

Since many of the women started their families independent of physician-con-trolled donor insemination services, they, unlike married couples using AID, are not so readily available for study. Many of the lesbian mothers I talked with thought it would be useful to themselves, to other lesbians considering AID, and to AID children

---

*In a brilliant analysis of heterosexuality as an institution, Adrienne Rich writes that part of the lie promulgated by that institution is "the frequently encountered implication that women turn to women out of hatred for men" (Rich, 1980).

to have information about their experiences compiled, perhaps by one of themselves. Aware of societal hostility and of the effect that hostility might have on the way any study of themselves was constructed and its results evaluated, they would be careful about which researchers they allowed into their lives.

Notes

1. Hunter artificially inseminated the linen draper's wife before it was understood that the essential requirement for fertilization was the entry of the sperm into the egg. Martin Barry, an English embryologist, suggested this possibility in 1840. It was seen for the first time in 1854 in frogs (Timson, 1979).

2. In 1776, Spallanzani was perhaps the first to report the effects of cooling on human sperm, noting that sperm cooled by snow became motionless. In the nineteenth century, Mantegazza experimented unsuccessfully with freezing sperm. From 1938 to 1945, a number of scientists observed that some human sperm could survive freezing and storage at temperatures as low as 269 degrees below 0°. Under the Parkes method, developed in 1949, a mixture of semen and glycerol is poured into a container that looks like a drinking straw. Then it is chilled in liquid nitrogen to 383 degrees below zero. Before use, the semen is thawed.

3. About 67 percent of the sperm they froze survived after storage for at least three months.

4. In 1963, Sherman introduced a new method to freeze-store human sperm using the vapor of liquid nitrogen for freezing and its liquid for storage. He reported that the survival rate of thawed sperm with this new nitrogen-vapor method was superior to that with the original "dry-ice" method.

   Not all sperm survive either freezing process, however. Moreover, the conception rate for frozen sperm is estimated to be anywhere from 15 to 33 percent lower than that of fresh sperm. The length of time sperm can be stored also remains controversial. Evidence suggests that, with time, the sperm's motility (ability to move) declines. While pregnancies after ten years' storage have been reported, such reports of pregnancies using sperm in long-term storage are sporadic and do not provide data on success rates. No long-term follow-up of children conceived with frozen sperm has ever been conducted. Sources for the section on frozen sperm include: AMA, 1974; OGN, 6/1/80; Bunge, 1954.

5. Artificial insemination is not widespread outside the cattle industry. However, CBS reported that in 1978, the following animals were created by AI: 136 million turkeys; 300,000 swine; 35,000 horses; and 3,000 goats (McMullen, 1979).

6. Interview with spokesman for the National Association of Animal Breeders, July 1, 1981.

7. A more recent punishment for out-of-wedlock mothers has been the loss of their children through adoption. In recent years, these "birthmothers" have begun to organize and to declare that many of them had not wanted to surrender their children to strangers. Denied all forms of social and economic support, they had had little choice. Carole Anderson of Concerned United Birthparents wrote of the situation in the 1960s: "In order to convince us to surrender, they told us we would be ruining our children's lives by keeping them. Children of single parents, they said, would be ridiculed at school as bastards, or grow up to be homosexual because they lacked a father image, or would live in poverty forever because no decent man would marry us." In the 1960s, Anderson reported, most high schools and colleges expelled pregnant students. Employers rarely hired single mothers. Even if mothers could get jobs, few could find day-care centers. "Denied education, denied jobs, and denied any knowledge of financial assistance, few of us had any option but to surrender our children," Anderson wrote. Some of those social conditions had changed by 1981. The attitude toward unwed mothers became less punitive. Schools encouraged pregnant students to continue their studies. Subsidized day care and job training were available to some single mothers. While in 1970, more than 90 percent of single mothers had surrendered their children, by 1981, fewer than 10 percent did so (Anderson, 1981).

8. The case was Orford v. Orford. It, along with subsequent cases discussed, are reported on in these articles: Kritchevsky, 1981; Katz, *Appendix*, 1979, pp. 5–6. British courts sometimes ruled differently on this issue. See Scott, 1981, p. 206.

9. A 1939 editorial in the *Journal of the American Medical Association* (JAMA) observed: "The fact that conception is effected not by adultery or fornication but by a method not involving sexual intercourse does not in principle seem to alter the concept of legitimacy. This concept seems to demand that the child be the actual offspring of the husband of the mother of the child." If the husband's semen was used, the child would seem to be legitimate; if not, illegitimate, JAMA argued. (It suggested that a couple adopt its AID child to safeguard its inheritency.) (JAMA, 5/6/39)

10. The comments of an unnamed woman who, in a recent year, was artificially inseminated with donor sperm, reveal her failure to understand that the unfaithful act consists—not in sexual pleasure without her husband—but in using his property (i.e., her own body) to produce children that are not his: "I asked my husband repeatedly to assure me that I was not going to commit an unfaithful act. Despite his wholehearted support, I could not really believe him." She adds that she was glad he was present on the first day of insemination. "I am so glad he could witness my terror, that he heard the physician ask me three times to relax before he could even get the speculum in, that he realized this experience was certainly not sexually enjoyable for me" (Menning, 1981).

11. Feversham, 1960. The form recommended by Britain's Medical Defense Union for authorizing the doctor to inseminate a wife with donor sperm required the couple to assure the doctor that the birth of an AID child to them "will not defeat the claims of any person to any titles, estates, interests or funds."

12. As of August 1981, the American Fertility Society had not formally approved the model legislation.

13. AIH also refers to "artificial insemination homologous," use of the husband's sperm. AID is also called "artificial insemination heterologous," use of a donor's sperm. The use of the terms "homologous" and "heterologous" in these contexts is curious. Certainly the terms do not scientifically describe the procedures.

    A husband's sperm is considered homologous to his wife. My medical dictionary partly defines homologous as: "Derived from an animal of the same species but of different genotype, as a homograft." A husband is a being of the same species as his wife?

    Heterologous means: "1. Made up of tissue not normal to the part. 2. Derived from an individual of a different species or one having a different genetic constitution." A man who is not a particular woman's husband is "of a different species" to that woman?

    Una Stannard's work gives some insight into what is going on here. In her book, she points out that not so long ago, when a woman married, she was considered to become a part of her husband in ways so literal we can scarcely grasp it today. The woman was subsumed within her husband's person; she became an actual part of his body, his womb which produced his children (see Stannard, 1977). She was "homologous" to him, "heterologous" to all other men.

14. OGN, 12/1/80. Dr. Tommy Evans, chair of the obstetrics and gynecology department at Wayne State, is quoted in this article as saying that by settling out of court "we at least limited the scope of this thing. We avoided setting a legal precedent that could be applied to other institutions." Dr. Evans noted that although the clinic is obligated to abide by the agreement, no physician can be compelled to perform any medical procedure against his principles. Attorney Kritchevsky doubts that the suit will have much effect on fertility clinic practices.

Bibliography

1. AMA. 1973, June. Human Artificial Insemination: Report of the Judicial Council. Adopted by the American Medical Association House of Delegates, June 1974.

2. Anderson, Carole, with Sue Campbell and Mary Anne Cohen. 1981. Eternal Punishment of Women: Adoption Abuse. Pamphlet available from Concerned United Birthparents, P.O. Box 573, Milford, Mass. 01757.

3. Bearden, H. Joe, and John Fuquay. 1980. *Applied Animal Breeding*. Reston, Va.: Reston Publishing Co., Inc.

4. Bunge, R. G. and J. K. Sherman. 1954. Frozen human semen. *Fertility and Sterility* 5: 193–194.

5. Callahan, Sheila. 1982. In vitro fertilization no longer considered experimental. *Ob/Gyn News* 17(9).

6. Curie-Cohen, Martin, Lesleigh Luttrell, and Sander Shapiro. 1979. Current practice of artificial insemination by donor in the United States. *NEJM* 300(1): 585–590.

7. Feversham, Earl of, Chairman. 1960, July. Report of the Departmental Committee on human artificial insemination. London: Her Majesty's Stationery Office.

8. Figes, Eva. 1970. *Patriarchal Attitudes*. Greenwich, Conn.: Fawcett Publications, Inc.

9. Fisher, Elizabeth. 1979. *Woman's Creation*. New York: McGraw-Hill Book Co.

10. Folsome, Claire E. 1943. The status of artificial insemination. *American Journal of Obstetricians and Gynecologists* 45(6): 915–927.

11. Greenhill, J. P. 1947. Artificial insemination: its medicolegal implications: A symposium. *American Practice*, I(5): 227–241.

12. JAMA. 1939, May 6. Artificial insemination and illegitimacy. *JAMA* 112(18): 1832–1833.

13. JME. 1978. Case Conference, "Lesbian couples: Should help extend to AID?" *Journal of Medical Ethics* 4: 91–95.

14. Jones, Syl. 1980, Aug. Playboy interview: William Shockley. *Playboy*.

15. Katz, Barbara F. 1979, May 4. Legal implications of in vitro fertilization and its regulation. *Appendix*.

16. Kritchevsky, Barbara. 1981. The unmarried woman's right to artificial insemination: A call for an expanded definition of family. *Harvard Women's Law Journal* 4(1).

17. Langer, G., et al. 1969. Artificial insemination: A study of 156 successful cases. *International Journal of Fertility* 14(3): 232–240.

18. Levie, L. H. 1972. Donor insemination in Holland. *World Medical Journal* 19(5).

19. McCarthy, Don. 1980, May. Parenting and technology. *Boston Pilot*.

20. McMullen, Jay, reporter. 1979, Oct. 30. Transcript of *CBS Reports: The Babymakers*.

21. Menning, Barbara Eck. 1981. In defense of in vitro fertilization. In H. Holmes, B. Hoskins, and M. Gross, eds., *The Custom-Made Child?* Clifton, N.J.: Humana Press.

22. OGN. 1980, Dec. 1. Suit impels fertility clinic to alter stand on marital status. *Ob/Gyn News*.

23. OGN. 1980, June 1. "Vasectomy insurance" misleading because future fertility of sperm not guaranteed. *Ob/Gyn News*.

24. Rohleder, Hermann. 1934. *Test Tube Babies*. New York: Panurge Press.

25. Rubin, Bernard. 1965, Aug. Psychological aspects of human artificial insemination. *Archives of General Psychiatry* 13.

26. Sandler, Bernard. 1972. Donor insemination in England. *World Medical Journal* 19(5).

27. Scott, Russell. 1981. *The Body as Property*. New York: Viking Press.

28. Sherman, J. K. 1973. Synopsis of the use of frozen human semen since 1964: State of the art of human semen banking. *Fertility and Sterility* 24(5): 397–412.

29. Strickler, Ronald C., et al. 1975. Artificial insemination with fresh donor semen. *NEJM* 295(17): 848–853.

30. Stannard, Una. 1977. *Mrs. Man*. San Francisco: Germainbooks.

31. Timson, John. 1979, Dec. 13. Lazzaro Spallanzani's seminal discovery. *New Scientist*.

"There is of course the distinction dictated by nature": Law and the Problem of Paternity

CAROL SMART

Reproductive technology is not a new phenomenon. Apart from technologies designed to prevent conception, the technology of artificial insemination using donor semen (AID) has been available in Britain for over fifty years. Yet we are clearly experiencing an escalation in the speed of development of new technologies which necessarily raises vexed questions for feminists who are concerned to prevent the exploitation of the reproductive capacity of women. It is important to recognize that these 'new' technologies are being developed at a moment in history when there is a re-emphasis on fatherhood, growing demands from anti-feminist men's organizations for greater control over children and shifts in policy to decrease the legal status of mothers in the realm of child custody.

It is not my intention in this chapter to locate the development of 'new' technologies of reproduction in their economic and social context, albeit that that is a necessary task. Rather I wish to trace how the problem of paternity has been dealt with by the law in order to draw lessons to help us deal with the contemporary problems of fatherhood. It is perhaps important to define what I mean by the terms paternity and fatherhood. Although these terms are often used synonymously, I shall use paternity to refer to the legal status of men who are deemed to have fathered certain children. Paternity alone does not automatically bring rights of custody or control over children unless the father is married to the mother of the children. By fatherhood I shall mean the actual biological or genetic relationship between a man and his 'offspring'. When referring to men's role in parenting, which may occur independently of a biological link, I shall use the term social fatherhood.

Carol Smart *is Lecturer in Sociology at the University of Warwick, England. Formerly she was Director of the National Council for One-Parent Families, and she has carried out research at the University of Sheffield and the Institute of Psychiatry, London. Her recent publications include* The Ties that Bind *and* Women in Law, *which was co-edited with Julia Brophy. She has also written widely in the field of feminism and criminology.*

These definitions may appear to be unnecessarily complex and confusing but they are unfortunately necessary. This is because, unlike motherhood, fatherhood has posed complicated problems for a legal system that has based the ownership and inheritance of property on descent through the male line—on that is, patrilineal and primogenital ordering. Paternity has been a continuing 'problem' for the patriarchal family in Western Europe (and undoubtedly elsewhere) and this is manifest in the tortuous complexity of the legal system designed to protect the descent of property and privilege. The following passage from the *Report of the Committee on the Law of Succession in Relation to Illegitimate Persons* (known as the Russell Report, 1966) gives some insight into the legal maze.

> There is of course the distinction dictated by nature between the association between a bastard and his mother and that between a bastard and his father; and this distinction has both an evidential and a familial aspect. Nature permits that a man may produce more bastards more secretly. Facts dictate that it must be generally far more difficult to establish the paternity of a bastard than the maternity: blood tests can sometimes deny an alleged paternity but at present cannot to any significant extent establish it: the facts of birth normally establish maternity. (Russell, 1966, p. 5)

This passage reveals the way in which apparent biological truths are used to give substance to a purely legal and social ordering of parenthood. It alleges that the paternity of illegitimate children is problematic and, by inference, that the paternity of legitimate children is not. I shall unravel this convoluted thinking below, but it is important in these introductory remarks to make plain the fact that the relationship between men and children in English law has been mediated by marriage. The biological relationship, although extremely important, has not been the primary factor. I shall therefore trace the way in which law has sought to 'attach' men to children (and in some instances has 'detached' them), in order to challenge the growing biologism of men's claim to children, engendered in part by reproductive technologies but also by the assertion of 'autonomous' motherhood. (By this latter concept I mean motherhood without the support of the 'traditional' nuclear family structure.)

There is a danger that the moral panic arising from a fear of the disruption of the idealized nuclear family will only serve to increase the power of men in the family by the extension of the legal concept of paternity and the enhancement of paternal rights. Moreover the new technologies themselves extend the influence of the state, through law and medicine, to restrict 'autonomous' motherhood. In other words, the price to pay for the reward of children becomes conformity to the nuclear family ideal. A paradox therefore arises in which a quest to control biological reproduction engenders new forms of biological determination.

Although I shall concentrate on paternity and fatherhood, it is also the case that the new technologies present a challenge to ideas about, and the legal definition of, maternity. With the advent of egg donation it is possible for women to carry to term infants that are genetically unrelated to them. At the same time conception in the petri dish, as opposed to the uterus, not only allows subfertile couples to have their 'own' children, it allows men, for the first time in history, to be absolutely certain that they are the genetic fathers of their future children. In view of this it becomes increasingly important to understand the role of law in extending paternity or in protecting maternity.

It may seem ironic, however, to be expressing concern over the 'extension' of the legal status of paternity and the need to protect the position of mothers, at a time when it appears that fathers are extremely badly done by when it comes to legal battles over children. To judge by the mass media and men's groups like Families Need Fathers, it would seem that the law favours women and that there is now a need to 'redress the balance'. However I hope to show here that mothers do not have more 'rights' than fathers; for example, mothers tend to get legal custody of children only because they are the ones doing the caring when marriages break down. On the contrary I shall try to show that the law operates to reinforce the patriarchal family from which men benefit disproportionately. Attempts to extend men's rights over children and to assert legal paternity are not so much a claim for 'equal rights' as a reassertion of patriarchal authority in the family.

'There is of course a distinction dictated by nature'

The issue of paternity is most clearly articulated in the law on illegitimacy. For example, the Russell Report presumed that the difference between legitimate and illegitimate children was self-evident. It assumed that paternity was a problem only in cases of illegitimacy because of the biological facts of conception and birth. It also assumed that it was the difficulty over ascertaining paternity that led fathers and not mothers to 'jettison' illegitimate children. To unravel the ideological content of these statements it is important to distinguish between so-called 'blood' ties and marriage ties. Throughout the history of law in this area these ties have overlapped confusingly, at times being treated as synonymous and at other times being separated rigorously.

The 'blood' tie is of course the biological or genetic link between parents and children. This extends to ties with other 'blood' relatives such as uncles and aunts, grandparents and so on. In our culture the 'blood' tie is apparently given ideological primacy (blood is thicker than water etc.). However it is the paternity of a child, rather than the 'maternity', that provides the link with the kinship network. In English common law the illegitimate child was '*filius nullius*' which meant it was the child of no one. S/he had no legal relationship to her mother, father, grandparents or siblings. In the legal sense the illegitimate child did not exist. Biological links were therefore immaterial as far as the common law was concerned. (This was gradually changed in practice, however, and from 1841 the mothers of illegitimate children were entitled to the sole custody of their children. The position of fathers did not change.) Hence the English legal tradition was prepared to ignore 'blood' ties under certain circumstances.

The marriage tie is a legal construct. It is a means of uniting biologically unrelated (or only distantly related) couples and their kinship networks. It is *marriage* and not the blood tie that confers automatic paternity on men and creates a legal relationship between children and their fathers. Marriage is the traditional means by which law recognizes the relationship between men and children. It is no longer the only means but it remains the most important one. As I shall discuss below, marriage could establish paternity in defiance of the 'true' biological relationship between men and children. Paternity was not dependent upon proof of fatherhood, only proof of marriage. Hence the law on paternity has never followed strictly the biological relationship between men and children. So whilst biology is important it has not been of overriding importance. This is significant where there is a growing presumption that law should follow biology and a belief that the biological relationship between 'fathers' and children is and always has been sacrosanct.

Constructing Paternity

The legal category of illegitimacy is crucial to an understanding of the construction of paternity because it is here that biological fatherhood and legal paternity most clearly come adrift. Whilst the legitimate child had an automatic relationship with its father, the illegitimate child has had to struggle over many centuries to establish a legal relationship with its biological father. This is because the legal relationship, once established, meant that the father was obliged to contribute in some way to the upkeep of the child. At various moments in history the state would help mothers to extract maintenance (through affiliation orders) from their former lovers; at other times the Poor Law Guardians were only interested in keeping the money to recompense the parish for the maintenance of the 'bastard'. At yet other times the state absolved men altogether of any financial responsibility for bastard children. At all times, however, the position of the mother and the child was a weak one and the father's obligations varied only according to the state's concern to protect public spending. Hence he was required to acknowledge his children and pay maintenance when their dependency began to cost the state (for example the parish) too much money. By the same token, men were absolved of this liability when it was felt that the dire financial consequences of having children outside marriage should be used to deter women from getting pregnant. (In fact such policies merely led to a dramatic rise in infanticide and concealed births.)

Even the recent history of affiliation orders is a dismal one. Not only have the courts traditionally been restricted in the amounts they could award to mothers for their illegitimate children, but the criminal nature of the proceedings, which until 1959 were heard in open court alongside criminal offences, was so stigmatizing that women were extremely reluctant to go to court. Marsden (1969) has documented how humiliating women found the proceedings and there is evidence that the magistrates' courts are still regarded as dispensers of inadequate and second-class justice in domestic matters (Smart, 1984).

One of the main problems of using the courts to secure financial provision for illegitimate children has been the difficulty of proving paternity. On one level there has been the problem of establishing a biological link at moments in history when the technology to achieve this was unavailable. Until the 1980s blood tests were only useful as a way of 'disproving' paternity. In other words they could only establish that a man was *not* the father of the child. They could not prove that a man *was* the biological father. On a rather different level, the mother's evidence as to paternity had to be 'corroborated in some material particular by other evidence'. (This wording dates from the earliest Poor Law legislation.) This requirement for corroboration, like the requirement in cases of rape, is based on a belief in the mendacity of women. The Russell Report (1966) for example states that 'There are grounds for supposing that there are cases in which the mother successfully selects the man who is the best prospect'. The report does not clarify what these 'grounds' are, and it would seem that there is little evidence to substantiate this prejudice. In fact there is rather more evidence to substantiate women's reluctance to go to court at all. Marsden, for example, documents how the National Assistance Board (now the Department of Health and Social Security—DHSS) bullied unmarried mothers to try to extract the name of the putative father, and how its officers pressurized mothers into going to court. It is by no means certain that these practices have ended.

Nor was it difficult for alleged fathers to rebut 'accusations' of paternity. It was generally only necessary to allege promiscuity or to bring to court other witnesses who would claim to have had intercourse with the mother for the accusation to fail. The English courts did not have a system of making a number of men pay maintenance where any of them could be the biological father, so there was no deterrent to false allegations. Women therefore took a considerable risk in going to court. Not only would their circumstances become public knowledge but their damaged 'reputations' could be even more irreparably harmed.

Putative fathers therefore had little to fear from the laws of affiliation unless they provided support voluntarily or admitted paternity. In appearance the law sought to enforce the father's obligations to his biological child(ren), but in practice the law was organized to dissuade mothers from going to court, and ultimately offered them a pittance in the form of maintenance for the trouble of going.

Clearly the law had little real interest in attaching men to illegitimate children except to recoup public expenditure, but it showed even less interest in other important legal proceedings. An illegitimate child, for example, could not claim on its father's intestacy until 1969. Moreover, for the purposes of adoption the putative father is still not regarded in law as a parent with rights to consent or dissent unless he has a custody order or is the child's legal guardian. In spite of the rhetoric of the law little has been done yet to attach men to their illegitimate children. Indeed it is possible to argue that it has protected men from the obligations of paternity, while leaving the stigma and the punitive financial consequences of child-rearing to mothers. (As I shall point out below this situation may soon change to the greater detriment of the mothers of illegitimate children.)

The situation regarding legitimate children is rather different.

The 'Presumption of Legitimacy'

Common law gave the men who fathered legitimate children absolute 'father right' which meant that the 'paterfamilias' had absolute control over the lives of his children whilst, in legal terms, mothers had none. All the duties and obligations of parenthood rested with the father, as did all the rights and privileges (see Strachey, 1978). This absolute patriarchal power was gradually modified in the nineteenth century through the introduction of legislation on the guardianship of infants (Brophy and Smart, 1981).

Whilst the law gave considerable power over children to married men, at the same time it made it extremely difficult for men to rid themselves of their formal obligations to these children. These fathers were in exactly the opposite position to the fathers of illegitimate children. This was a result of what is known as the 'presumption of legitimacy'.

The common law presumed that all children born in wedlock were legitimate, but it went further than a mere presumption in practice. Until the introduction of the 1949 Law Reform (Miscellaneous Provisions) Act neither husband nor wife was allowed to give evidence of non-access (i.e., a lack of sexual intercourse) which would bastardize a child born during the marriage. In a case in 1777 the judge, Lord Mansfield, stated:

> But it is a rule, founded in decency, morality, and polity, that [the spouses] shall not be permitted to say after marriage, that they have had no connection, and therefore that the offspring is spurious; more especially the mother, who is the offending party. (*Goodright ex Dim. Stevens* v. *Moss* et al., 1777, 2Cowp 591, p. 594)

The law in fact operated a dual standard as to the conditions under which children might be bastardized. On the one hand it appears that there was a reluctance to bastardize children if this meant that they would no longer be financially supported by the 'father'. For example in cases where wives were found 'guilty' of adultery this would not bastardize their children as it would be presumed that the husband could still be the biological father.

Yet there were cases where this strict application did not apply and these all tended to involve the inheritance of property rather than the issue of maintenance. So, where the husband was a man of property there was a tendency to bastardize children who were likely to have been fathered by another man. In more modest cases, for example those involving pauper children, the courts were less ready to absolve the man's responsibility.

Nonetheless, the point is that it was extremely difficult for a husband to divest himself of paternity until the law was changed by statute in 1949 (Law Reform [Miscellaneous Provisions] Act). If a child was to be bastardized the husband had the burden of proof, which had to be established 'beyond all reasonable doubt'. And the law tended to hold this rigid position even in the face of the growing use of reliable contraceptive methods or in the light of an 'admission' by the mother that the child was not her husband's.

Clearly the law in these cases was operating against the interest of individual men. It seems that it was serving a 'higher' goal, namely that of preserving the patriarchal family. Hoggett (1981) for example, has argued:

> The institution of marriage may well have been devised in early societies in order to establish a relationship between man and child. A man may derive spiritual, emotional and material advantages from having children, but whereas motherhood may easily be proved, fatherhood may not. A formal ceremony between man and woman, after which it is assumed that any children she may have are his, is the simplest method of establishing a link. It also enables him to limit his relationships to the offspring of a suitable selected mate. (Hoggett, 1981, p. 119)

This analysis is very persuasive, not least because throughout history the law has deliberately ignored evidence that husbands are unlikely to be the fathers of their wives' children. If marriage was the only method of attaching men to children, it was clearly meant to be an indelible method, impervious to indications of biological incompatibility.

The change of law in 1949 does not indicate that legislation had become more sensitive to a biological imperative however. Certainly with the growth of technology to ascertain paternity through blood tests and the reduction in the dire consequences of being found to be illegitimate, the law risked losing all credibility if it did not alter its doctrine on the presumption of legitimacy. But at the same time there was a growth in social fathering which also blurred the distinction between legitimate and illegitimate children, once thought to be so clear-cut and so desirable.

Undoubtedly law kept legitimate children firmly attached to their fathers in order to maintain a familial system of support of dependents. However with the increasing divorce rate in the 1970s and the creation of stepfamilies, and with the growth of cohabitation without marriage, other methods of ensuring that men assumed responsibility for dependent children developed. Without having to establish marital or biological ties, the concept of the 'child of the family' made all men responsible for the support of children whom they had treated as members of their family. As with the history of affiliation orders, this measure developed mainly to protect public expenditure and to prevent children, abandoned by their biological fathers, becoming dependent upon state benefits. This development was however wrapped in the rhetoric of the 'welfare of the child' and presented as a means of protecting children.

In large measure this development abolished the legal significance of paternity and legitimacy whilst enshrining men's responsibilities towards children. (The legislation also applies to women although women are less frequently in a position to provide maintenance or an inheritance.) Nonetheless, as I shall argue below, the issue of paternity has reappeared in another form in contemporary family law, namely in relation to children conceived through artificial insemination by donor (AID).

The Unique Position
of AID Children

The child conceived by AID is, legally speaking, illegitimate. As the law currently stands the donor is responsible for contributing towards the financial maintenance of the child and the child could claim provision from the estate of its genetic father. This legal 'right' is, however, unenforceable in practice because of the anonymity of the donor.

The illegitimate status of the AID child is almost always obscured by the practice of the husband and wife, in collusion with the medical profession, of naming the husband as the father on the child's birth certificate. In so doing, however, the couple are committing an offence which has given rise to considerable concern (Law Commission, 1979). It has been argued that the law should be changed to make the AID child legitimate and that a child in this situation does not 'deserve' the status of illegitimacy. For example Mayo (1976) has argued:

> To call AID children illegitimate (as well as being unjust to them and a misnomer) is inconsistent with the policies behind the idea of legitimacy—monogamous marriage, family stability, aversion to illicit sexual relationships, property inheritance. These policies are promoted not infringed by the introduction of an AID child, born after thorough planning and careful thought, into a stable and hitherto childless home. (Mayo, 1976, p. 24)

This form of 'special pleading' for the AID child is a relatively new development. When the technology was first introduced the legal profession and the Established Church took an extremely dim view of the practice. For example the Archbishop of Canterbury's Committee on Artificial Human Insemination (1948) took the view that it should be made a criminal offence. It was held to undermine the very foundation of marriage, and to be a means of foisting spurious children on an unsuspecting world. The Royal Commission on Marriage and Divorce (Morton, 1956) recommended that AID without a husband's consent should be a new, separate ground for divorce.

> In our view, if a wife accepts artificial insemination by a donor without the consent of her husband she is doing him a grave injury, an injury which, in its possible consequences, is as serious as that of adultery. The intention is, and the result may be, to father a child on the husband without his knowledge. (Morton, 1956, p. 31)

The Feversham Committee (1960), a government committee set up to report on AID, reflected the views of these earlier reports. It refused to recommend that the AID child accepted by the husband should be legitimate and continued to regard AID as a threat to the very basis of family life and society. The Committee did, however, acknowledge that the law should not totally disregard the welfare of the AID child. The doctrine of the 'best interests of the child' was gaining credibility in cases of divorce and was therefore, in theory at least, seen as relevant in all cases involving children. This doctrine, however, did not apply to illegitimate children until considerably later than 1960 and the Committee was not prepared to disregard the distinction between legitimate and illegitimate as a method of safeguarding the interests of 'innocent' AID children. Basically the interests of AID children were not regarded as sufficiently weighty to risk undermining the basis of marriage. Their status in law therefore remained unchanged.

By the 1970s this view of AID as a threat to marriage and society waned. The position typified by Mayo above became increasingly dominant. Instead of being a threat to the ideologically acceptable family, AID was seen as a way of enhancing family life for the childless. It was childlessness itself that was becoming the 'problem'. Childlessness was in fact the very antithesis of the nuclear family ideal.

According to this logic, the illegitimate child born outside wedlock or born of an extramarital affair was in quite a different position to the AID child who was 'wanted' by both husband and wife. (It was, and possibly still is, widely assumed that the illegitimate child was not 'wanted' by anyone, least of all its father.) The fact of being wanted, and consequently *acknowledged* by the husband has become the crucial element in the argument for legitimizing AID children. In other words, the fact that the husband wants to assume the legal status of paternity is the overriding factor.

A similar trend has occurred with illegitimacy. For example the 1926 Legitimacy Act allowed children born illegitimate to be legitimized if the child's biological parents married. Hence in choosing to marry, the father could assume the paternity of the child and, in addition, erase the stigma of illegitimacy. Of course, it is an oversimplification to argue that paternity as a legal status merely reflects the wishes or choices of men. As the cases involving the presumption of legitimacy reveal, men certainly could not divest themselves of the responsibilities of paternity at whim. Nonetheless, at different historical moments, certain elements of the law relating to paternity have come extremely close to this position. Basically, however, family law appears to strive to preserve marriage as the basis of family life (Smart, 1984).

The Law Commission's (1979) proposals on AID are a good example of this focus on the patriarchal family. In their Working Paper they argued that AID children should be regarded as legitimate because the mother had had no personal relationship with the donor (so it was not really adulterous), because the husband had agreed to the procedure (this was assumed, as women need to have their husband's permission before AID is provided), and because the genetic father is unknown. The transformation of a marriage into a nuclear family by means of AID was therefore condoned. However, the Law Commission did not envisage that this presumption of legitimacy could be extended to the AID child born to an unmarried woman. In this case, not only is the 'accepting' husband missing, but a single parent would not constitute a 'proper' nuclear family. Undoubtedly the Law Commission, like the Warnock Committee some years later, presumed that AID would not in any case be available to single women.

Since the introduction of the technology of AID, views on its possible effect on family life have been transformed—even though the law has yet to be changed. This transformation has taken thirty years to reach the point at which it might produce legal changes. But its significance has now been overtaken by further and more dramatic advances in reproductive technology. For example, egg donation and in-vitro fertilization now so dominate the debates on infertility, that AID has been subsumed into a renewed panic over the preservation of family life. Ironically the old arguments over the dangers of AID are now being rehearsed in relation to other methods of infertility treatment. The legal issues may not be identical, but the Warnock Committee appears to be as preoccupied with questions of inheritance, primogeniture and the preservation of 'stable' nuclear family life as was its predecessors thirty or more years ago. Before discussing the limitations of Warnock, however, I wish to look at more general developments in family law which have affected the respective statuses of motherhood and fatherhood.

Recent Developments
Concerning Children

Children are an increasingly important group as far as legislation on marriage and the family is concerned. Although legislators and lawyers expressed concern over children in earlier times, since the end of the Second World War there has been a marked trend towards giving greater priority to children's welfare as a principle to guide judicial decisions and law reform. This is particularly noticeable in the field of divorce. Although judges in the last century voiced the rhetoric of children's welfare, it is not until the second half of the twentieth century that the welfare of children began to take precedence over the legal 'rights' of parents.

It is of course important to recognize that the meaning of the 'welfare' of children is subject to interpretation, and, as Brophy (1985) has shown, this judicial interpretation is very ideological. Notwithstanding this, it is clear that during the latter half of the twentieth century judges increasingly regarded mothers as the most appropriate custodians of children on divorce. The common law doctrine of absolute father right was abandoned and judges increasingly voiced the benefits of mother love (as long as the mother was not 'promiscuous' or a lesbian). Hence, while children have become more of a focus, the relative statuses of motherhood and fatherhood have changed and developed. These developments are best outlined in the fields of illegitimacy and divorce.

Illegitimacy

Until the last quarter of the twentieth century the position of the unmarried mother was so undesirable that her parental obligations were seen as little more than part of her stigma and rejection. Having sole custody rights (in practice from 1841, although this was not put into legislation until the 1975 Children Act) was more a form of legal punishment than a concession. This has changed however. The growth of cohabitation leading to a situation in which illegitimate children are born into an unmarried but nonetheless two-parent household, and the rise in the illegitimate birth-rate have contributed to a number of social changes. The mother of an illegitimate child is no longer in a completely different position from other lone mothers (with the partial exception of widows). Although there may still be some stigma attached to being an unmarried mother, the state does not penalize her financially any more than it does divorced or separated mothers. So the disadvantages have diminished yet she is in a *stronger* position *vis-à-vis* her children than the divorced or separated mother because she is entitled to their sole custody.

The unmarried mother can exercise all parental rights herself, as long as the courts have made no order to the contrary. The married mother on the other hand, holds these parental 'rights' in common with her husband. She is entitled to sole custody only if a court has awarded her such an order. This difference can be extremely important when there is conflict over children, or when men attempt to exercise power over women through their children.

Shortly after the passage of the 1975 Children Act, the fathers of illegitimate children began to recognize that they could not exercise the same rights over children as married men. At the same time unmarried mothers began to recognize the advantages of their status which allowed them to have children without the disadvantages of marriage and beyond the control of men. Hence the traditional position of the 'putative' father wishing to deny paternity at all costs and, in the terms of the Russell Committee, jettisoning the child, began to give way to a situation in which fathers wanted not only the legal status of paternity but all the 'rights' of married fathers.

This transition, which is by no means complete or universal, is epitomized by the concerns of the Law Commission in its Working Paper on illegitimacy (1979). Their document, which is meant to consider the position of the illegitimate child, is in effect, a treatise on the wrongs of unmarried fathers and how they can best be modified. They state:

> From a strictly legal point of view, the father of an illegitimate child is today probably at a greater disadvantage than the child himself [*sic*]; and while many fathers may take little or no interest in their children born out of wedlock, other fathers who have lived with the mother for perhaps many years are clearly affected by the discrimination. (Law Commission, 1979, p. 14)

The Commission lists all the discriminations 'suffered' by the unmarried father and concludes that the best method of eradicating these wrongs and eliminating the problem of illegitimacy, was to give all biological fathers automatic parental rights on a par with the mother of an illegitimate child. Under this proposal the unmarried mother would have to go to court if she wanted sole custody or did not wish the father to exercise his rights. These rights include not only actual custody, but the right to decide whether the child should have medical treatment, which school the child should go to, where the child should live and what the child's name should be.

The Law Commission has since abandoned this proposal because of the strength of adverse reaction they received. Nonetheless, the Working Paper is an important document inasmuch as it points to, and legitimizes, a growing disquiet over the supposed power of mothers. For example, in the Working Paper the Law Commission acknowledged that there might be unmeritorious fathers (for example, rapists), who should not be able to exercise untrammelled authority over their biological offspring. They went on to state:

> But we think that the decision to exclude a father from all parental rights and duties is so important that it should not be the mother's alone; the final decision should lie with the courts, which are bound to regard the welfare of the child as paramount. (Ibid., p. 29)

This passage reveals the underlying concern that women should not be entitled to exercise parental rights exclusively without the prior permission of the courts. It reveals a concern that mothers will exclude fathers maliciously and without consideration for the interests of their children whilst, at the same time, it minimizes the possibility that fathers might harass and unduly interfere with the lives of mothers attempting to bring up their children. Although the Law Commission acknowledged the possibility of unmeritorious fathers, it was clear that their crimes would have to be very serious to outweigh the 'justice' of giving unmarried fathers equal rights.

The Working Paper was particularly vexed at the situation in which an unmarried mother could refuse to have the name of the child's biological father on the birth certificate. This was a practice they wished to see ended, and in their later recommendations (1982) they did not rescind the proposal that all fathers should have the right to be named. (This of course excludes donors for AID whom the Commission view in a different light.) They state,

> It seems to us that if a man is obliged to accept the financial obligations of paternity it is reasonable that he should be entitled, if he wishes, to have the fact of his fatherhood recorded (on the birth certificate). (Law Commission, 1982, p. 115)

In other words the Law Commission recognized, and sought to legitimize, the economic power of men. There is little in this sentiment about the welfare of children, it simply reflects the power of money.

The Law Commission's first proposals on illegitimacy (1979) sought to abolish the status by enhancing paternity and attaching biological fathers automatically to all children. However the aim to improve the position of the unmarried father ran counter to their ideas on AID children. The last thing the Commission wished was inadvertently to give donors full parental rights. Hence with AID, the biological link immediately became unimportant, being overridden by the desirability of social fatherhood in a two-parent family household. It would seem that the biological father is expendable in some, but not all circumstances.

Divorce

There is a presumption that the courts favour mothers when it comes to decisions on the custody of children on divorce. This presumption is not altered by the weight of evidence which suggests that whilst judges subscribe to the ideology of motherhood, the courts in fact, in the vast majority of cases, only give legal recognition to custody arrangements previously decided by the parents themselves. It is also the case that the courts are more influenced by current arrangements which they are unlikely to wish to disrupt for fear of unsettling the children involved. This is known as the status quo effect (see Eekelaar and Clive, 1977; Brophy, 1985).

In spite of serious doubts that the courts do operate a system of maternal preference, it has become such a firm belief that there is now a growing reaction against it. This has taken the form of a demand that all custody decisions on divorce should award parental rights jointly to both parents. Actual care and control of the child would still tend to go to the mother under this arrangement, but the father would be able to make decisions about schooling etc. If the parents could not agree they would have to return to court to get a judicial decision.

This development (see the Booth Committee Report, 1985) is, like the developments on illegitimacy, linked to a disquiet about the power of mothers if they have sole custody. It is feared that the bitterness of a mother may deny a child the right to know and see its father. This disquiet is closely related to the development of a school of thought in psychology which now argues that a child must *know* and *interact* with its biological father to grow up to be a stable and well-adjusted (heterosexual) adult (Isaacs, 1948; Green, 1976; Wallerstein and Kelly, 1980).

To a large extent this idea is already enshrined in legislation. The 1975 Children Act gave adopted children the right to trace their genetic parents on the grounds that it is important that every person should be allowed to know his or her parentage. This legislation gives priority to the biological tie and is based on theories of psychological adjustment and development.

Not all theories of child development accept the thesis that a child must know its biological father to be a well-adjusted adult. Indeed some argue that even in cases of divorce where children know their fathers well, it may be harmful to the child's development for the courts to order access to the non-custodial parent. Goldstein, Freud and Solnit (1980) have argued the case that the custodial parent ought to be entitled to decide whether or not the other parent retains contact with the children in cases where there is conflict. This idea is the total antithesis to current developments in custody and access. Divorce courts in the United Kingdom and the United States are increasingly asserting that access to the non-custodial parent is a right of the child, a right that is necessary to ensure proper development. This means that unwilling children are forced to meet their fathers, or that children may be severely disturbed by access visits.

Thus, while the court appears to be protecting the interests of children in enforcing access and joint custody in cases of conflict, it is in fact reasserting paternal authority. The issue of a child's surname after the divorce of its parents is one small example of this process.

A Child's Name

There have been conflicting judgements on whether a child should adopt the surname of a 'reconstituted' family (i.e., the name of the mother's new husband or cohabitee) or whether it should retain its father's surname. A divorced mother does not have the right to change a child's name without the consent or agreement of her former husband, although in practice many probably do. The reasons for changing the name may be to save embarrassment at the child's school or to enable the child to feel a part of a new family. Nonetheless, some judges have taken severe exception to this and have argued that a child must retain this link with its biological father (Evans, 1978; Parry, 1978; Fortin, 1980). For example in one case cited by Evans the judge stated

> But to deprive the child of her father's surname, in my judgement, is not in the best interests of the child because, I think, it is injurious to the link between the father and the child to suggest to the child that there is some reason why it is desirable that she should be called by some name other than her father's name. (Evans, 1978, p. 113)

Although the courts no longer operate a straightforward paternal preference in this matter, the courts will insist on a child retaining its father's name if the judge decides that this is in the child's interests. As the quotation above reveals, some judges may perceive the welfare of children in very narrow ways.

W(h)ither Paternity?

The law appears to be moving in two conflicting directions at the same time. In the cases of divorce and illegitimacy there is a growing emphasis on the importance of biological fatherhood and paternity. In the case of AID, however, the opposite is occurring, and the legal concept of the 'child of the family' seems to ignore the importance of legal paternity altogether. Underlying both of these developments, however, is the legal antipathy shown towards women mothering children alone and the goal of properly attaching men to children to prevent women exercising too much independence. It would seem that the law is agnostic on the issue of whether women do all the caring for children, but it takes a strong view if women try to detach children from men, and by implication, from the nuclear family.

If these apparent contradictory trends are examined more closely it is possible to see that they in fact lend support to a particular family structure, namely one in which there is 'a heterosexual couple living together in a stable relationship, whether married or not' (Warnock, 1985, p. 10). In other words, the primary aim of law is to link biological fathers to children where it is the biological father who is most likely to reproduce the ideal nuclear family structure. Where the biological father is not available, or is unsuitable (for example, the Law Commission's unmeritorious father), the social father will suffice. Where there is a biological father and a social (step)father (as in the case of divorce and remarriage) the law preserves the rights of the biological father in the 'best interests of the children'. In other cases where there is both a biological and a social father (as with AID) the tendency is to ignore the biological father and to invest all the rights of paternity in the social father who will be the head of a two-parent family.

The advent of the new reproductive technologies has, in itself, neither strengthened nor weakened the law's ability to attach men to children. Rather I hope I have shown that the methods have altered, and the emphasis on biological links has undergone transformations, whilst remaining highly salient. However the development of the new technology does have implications for 'maternity'. For the first time the law must contemplate the idea that a woman may bring to term offspring derived from the ovum of another woman. In this case the 'fact of birth' is no proof of genetic connection.

Whilst AID, adultery and other practices that cast doubt on the paternity of children have posed considerable problems for the legal system, it is unlikely that egg or embryo transplants will pose similar problems unless the procedure interferes with patrilineal inheritance rights. Basically the law has not been interested in maternity as a vehicle of 'rights' for women in the way that paternity has always implied 'rights' for men. To a large extent the law has seen women solely in terms of whether they produce legitimate children and then whether they care for children adequately. The fact of mothering children has never involved a question of rights except, as I have outlined above, in relation to the punitive consequences of illegitimacy. Once mothers began to demand certain rights from the law, the parameters of debate changed; the law became interested only in the welfare of children and asserted that parental rights were an inadequate concept when dealing with minors.

So it is for the first time that the law must look at this issue in terms of deciding which woman in a surrogacy arrangement should be the legal 'mother'. *The Warnock Report on Human Fertilisation and Embryology* (1985) has recommended that a woman who gives birth following egg or embryo donation should be regarded in law as the mother of the child. In this respect their recommendations follow closely the long-standing recommendations on AID, namely that the mother's husband should be regarded in law as the father of the child. However the different legal statuses of paternity and maternity become apparent when the Committee turns its attention to inheritance and succession. The Committee states 'The use by a widow of her dead husband's semen for AIH is a practice which we feel should be actively discouraged' (Warnock, 1985, p. 55). It goes on to recommend that

> legislation be introduced to provide that any child born by AIH who was not *in utero* at the date of the death of its father shall be disregarded for the purposes of succession to and inheritance from the latter. (Ibid., p. 55)

The Committee makes the same recommendation in respect of children born following IVF, using a frozen embryo where the husband is dead before the embryo is *in utero*.

There are no recommendations restricting the inheritance rights of children born of these same methods where the husband is alive but where the biological mother is dead. Should a widower elect to implant the egg or embryo of his dead wife into an infertile second wife, the child born as a consequence will not be disinherited or ignored for purposes of succession.

In effect the Warnock Report attempts to create a new form of illegitimacy, but one in which the child has fewer rights than illegitimate children born today without the help of new technology. At least these children can claim from the estate of their biological fathers.

The case of posthumous embryo, egg or sperm donation may be relatively rare although it has clearly worried the Warnock Committee because it attaches such importance to the legal consequences affecting inheritance through the male line. But whilst making recommendations on this subject, the Committee did not even consider the legal position of the child born, with the assistance of reproductive technology, to the mother without a male partner, or to the lesbian. This was because the Report recommends that only *stable heterosexual couples* will be able to benefit from this form of infertility treatment.

In this respect, the Warnock Report is no more progressive than was the Russell Report of 1966. Its aim is to preserve the narrow ideal of patriarchal family life. What is more it is far more limited than existing legislation on adoption which allows single women and men to adopt children. Presumably the Committee's logic would argue that it is more in the interests of children to be adopted into 'unconventional' households than to remain in care, but that 'as a general rule it is better for children to be *born* into a two-parent family' (Warnock, 1985, p. 11, emphasis added).

Concluding Remarks

Discussions on reproductive technologies in feminist literature have mainly focused on the issue of male/medical control over the technology and the exploitation of women's reproductive capacity. There has been little on how it affects the issue of fatherhood and paternity and the meaning of these concepts in terms of control over women and children. There is a growing awareness of the centrality of children to an understanding of the position of women. In recent years this has been linked to the problem of custody of children on divorce (Brophy, 1985; Sevenhuijsen and de Vries, 1984) as well as to the issue of illegitimacy (Rights of Women Family Law Subgroup, 1985). It is vital that the women's movement does not ignore these crucial issues. The fact that the Warnock Report proposes that 'single' women should be excluded from new forms of medical help for infertility is extremely important; and it should not be overlooked that there are proposals to recognize new forms of paternity whilst continuing to deny certain rights to children who inconveniently upset the rules of inheritance. What is more, whilst women still want children we should not ignore the abysmal status of maternity in law. It may be that a demand for total and automatic rights over children is misplaced whether the demand comes from men or women. It is important, however, that as law is created in this area that the position of mothers is not relegated to third place behind fathers' rights and the welfare of children.

In spite of the fact that reproductive technologies contain the possibility of rendering biological or 'blood' ties immaterial, it remains the case that the legal parameters outlined for its development still give priority to paternity. It is more than an irony that maternity is legally insignificant whilst motherhood is so important for the actual physical and emotional care of children. The importance of paternity seems to be in an *inverse relationship* to the amount of physical and emotional care provided by fathers. As long as this remains unchanged women will be powerless in the face of the reassertion, by men, of their claim to children. Reproductive technologies increase the opportunities for relatively privileged men and women to have children, but as long as the technology is contained within legal parameters that prioritize the patriarchal family, it does nothing to challenge existing notions of fatherhood and motherhood. In fact, in ideological terms, it adds to the celebration of the biological, nuclear family that affects us all. In this respect the development of the legal concept of paternity outlined here, and the recommendations of the Warnock Committee should give rise to concern. This is not so much for the vision of a brave new world peopled only by men and 'mother-machines', but for the way in which these developments will bind women more securely to the confines of the patriarchal, nuclear family—not through marriage as in the past, but for the sake of children.

Bibliography

1. Booth, The Hon. Mrs. Justice. 1985. *Report of the Matrimonial Causes Procedure Committee*. London: Her Majesty's Stationery Office.

2. Brophy, J. 1985. "Child Care and the Growth of Power: The Status of Mothers in Custody Disputes." In Brophy and Smart (eds.), *Women in Law*.

3. Brophy, J., and C. Smart. 1981. "From Disregard to Disrepute: The Position of Women in Family Law." *Feminist Review*, 9.

4. Brophy, J., and C. Smart, eds. 1985. *Women in Law*. London: Routledge and Kegan Paul.

5. Eekelaar, J., and E. Clive. 1977. *Custody After Divorce*. Oxford: Center for Socio-legal Studies.

6. Evans, W. 1978. "Changing a Child's Name After Re-marriage." *Family Law*, 8.

7. Feversham, the Earl of. 1960. *Report of the Departmental Committee on Human Artificial Insemination*, Cmnd. 1105. London: Her Majesty's Stationery Office.

8. Fortin, J. 1980. "The Nature of the Right to Select a Child's Surname." *Family Law*, 10, 2.

9. Goldstein, J., A. Freud, and A. J. Solnit. 1980. *Beyond the Best Interests of the Child*. London: Burnett Books.

10. Green, M. 1976. *Goodbye Father*. London: Routledge and Kegan Paul.

11. Hoggett, B. 1981. *Parents and Children*. London: Sweet and Maxwell.

12. Isaacs, S. 1948. *Childhood and After*. London: Routledge and Kegan Paul.

13. Law Commission. 1979. *Family Law: Illegitimacy*. London: Her Majesty's Stationery Office, Working Paper 74.

14. Marsden, D. 1969. *Mothers Alone*. London: Allen Lane.

15. Mayo, M. M. 1976. "Legitimacy for the AID Child." *Family Law*, 6.

16. Morton, Lord. 1956. *Report of the Royal Commission on Marriage and Divorce*, Cmnd. 9678. London: Her Majesty's Stationery Office.

17. Parry, M. L. 1978. "Changing a Child's Name after Re-Marriage—A Reply." *Family Law*, 8.

18. Rights of Women Family Law Subgroup. 1985. "Campaigning Around Family Law: Politics and Practice." In Brophy and Smart (eds.), *Women in Law*.

19. Russell, Lord Justice. 1966. *Report of the Committee on the Law of Succession in Relation to Illegitimate Persons*, Cmnd. 3051. London: Her Majesty's Stationery Office.

20. Sevenhuijsen, J., and P. de Vries. 1984. "The Women's Movement and Motherhood." In A. Meulenbelt, et al. (eds.), *A Creative Tension*. London: Pluto.

21. Smart, C. 1974. *The Ties That Bind: Law, Marriage, and the Reproduction of Patriarchal Relations*. London: Routledge and Kegan Paul.

22. Wallerstein, J., and J. Kelley. 1980. *Surviving the Breakup: How Children and Parents Cope with Divorce*. London: Grant McIntyre.

23. Warnock, M. 1985. *A Question of Life: The Warnock Report on Human Fertilisation and Embryology*, Cmnd. 9314. London: Her Majesty's Stationery Office.

CHAPTER 2

Fertility Drugs, GIFT, and IVF

CASES FOR
PRELIMINARY DISCUSSION

Case 2.1

Janet Cosmos, a divorced college professor in her mid-thirties, had had no children during her five-year marriage. The diagnosis of infertility due to fallopian tube scarring caused by an STD (sexually transmitted disease) given her by her husband had been the final straw that ended a marriage that had been troubled since the first year by his extramarital escapades, and that destroyed her regard for that institution. Now in the fourth year of a stable, monogamous relationship with her lover, George Starr, she turns to medicine for assistance in having a child of her own.

She consults with a gynecologist about surgical repair of her scarred fallopian tubes, indicating that it is her intention, when they are repaired, to have George father her child out of wedlock. She indicates that, in her view, marriage is a sham and that it is precisely the fact that neither has made a formal, legal commitment that makes her trust George's commitment; but that, if he should ever betray her, she wants him to have no legitimated claim on their child.

Case 2.2

Maria Gonzales, a 31-year-old married woman, has a long-standing fertility problem: oligomenorrhea, or infrequent and scanty menstruation. Her religion, Catholicism, forbids her to employ artificial means (such as GIFT or IVF) of conceiving, but does permit medical treatment of her fertility problem.

Physicians at a fertility clinic treat her with a fertility drug, clomiphene citrate; she becomes pregnant via natural insemination by her husband and is overjoyed. However, ultrasonography discloses in the fourth month that she is carrying seven fetuses, whose very number makes it impossible for the pregnancies to go to term. She is advised that it is virtually certain the babies will be born very prematurely, and that the odds of all surviving are negligible. Moreover, there is considerable likelihood that those who do survive early delivery, if any, may have reduced body weights, chronic breathing problems, reduced IQ, and other problems associated with the pressures of so many occupants of the uterus plus seven separate placental structures.

The doctors indicate that it may be possible to selectively reduce the number of fetuses to two which, although they are likely to be born somewhat early, would have a far greater chance at survival and normalcy than if the multiple pregnancy is allowed to continue. Mrs. Gonzales consults her priest, who advises her that to consent would be a heinous sin, since it would involve killing five in order to save two, and using an evil means to a good end is inherently immoral.

Case 2.3

Sally Morgan is 46 years old and has been divorced for 10 years. She has one child, a 25-year-old daughter. Recently she married Frank Charlton, a 49-year-old childless widower. They would like to start a family of their own, but she is now infertile.

Mrs. Charlton consults a university IVF program, where she is told that she is not a suitable candidate for the procedure because of problems with her production of ova. However, her husband's sperm could be used to fertilize an egg cell from an anonymous donor. The embryo could then be implanted in Mrs. Charlton and carried to term.

Since Mrs. Charlton would like her child to be genetically related, her daughter offers to donate the egg to be utilized in the IVF process. Each of the daughter's cells contains 50 percent of her mother's genetic material; therefore the baby would have one-half of that amount, or 25 percent. In this manner, the child would be genetically related to Mrs. Charlton. Mrs. Charlton would be in the unusual position of being both (gestational) mother and (biological) grandmother to the child; her daughter would be both its (biological) mother and half-sister.

—Modified from a case presented by David Fassler, "When Baby's Mother Is Also Grandma—and Sister," *Hastings Center Report* 15, no. 5 (October 1985): 29.

Case 2.4

Mr. and Mrs. Diaz had wanted a child for all of their 15 years of marriage, but had been unable to conceive despite extensive analysis and treatment. They contacted a new Australian clinic that had just started in vitro fertilizations, and the clinic determined that Mrs. Diaz was a good candidate for the procedure.

Mrs. Diaz went through a period of hormone stimulation to mature several ova simultaneously, and was then subjected to a surgical procedure to remove the ova by aspiration. They were then mixed with Mr. Diaz's semen in a petri dish, where each of the ova was fertilized. All appeared normal, so one was selected for implantation, and the rest were cryopreserved, frozen for possible future use in case the implantation attempt was not successful.

The first attempt at implantation failed, and the Diaz couple was terribly disappointed. However, several frozen embryos were still viable and available, and they resolved to try again after a brief vacation. The couple was tragically killed in an airplane accident while on vacation just before being scheduled to attempt a second implantation.

The problem arose as to the legal status of the frozen preimplantation embryos, a problem that had not even been anticipated in the contract between the parents and the clinic. Were they heirs to the considerable estate? Were they the property of the fertility clinic? Could they be implanted in host women who wanted them? If they were so implanted, would they stand to inherit a portion of the estate, with their gestational and rearing parents free to administer their wealth? Perhaps fortunately, the embryos passed beyond the point of viability before these legal issues could be resolved.

REVIEW OF THE ISSUES

Male infertility yielded sooner to technical assistance than female infertility. Problems of female infertility have proven more resistant to medical advances, perhaps in part because of the dominance of male physicians in fertility research but also because of the greater complexity of the female reproductive system. Female sterility may be due to a number of factors, from lack of quantities of natural hormone sufficient for maturing egg follicles, to endometriosis and other STDs resulting in chronic pelvic inflammatory disease, to blockage of the fallopian tubes as the result of injury, surgical sterilization, or disease, to uterine abnormality. As in the case of male infertility, some of these problems yield to surgical or hormonal therapy.

The two most common, surgically correctable causes of female infertility are endometriosis and blocked or scarred fallopian tubes. Endometriosis appears to involve the presence of small pieces of the endometrium, the normal uterine lining, in abnormal locations such as the fallopian tubes, the ovaries, or the peritoneal cavity. While its etiology is not fully understood, it appears sometimes to be caused by endometrial material that is sloughed off the uterine wall during menstruation and then is forced back up through the fallopian tubes. Areas of chronic inflammation develop around the sites where endometrial material lodges, interfering with normal hormonal regulation of the reproductive cycle. Both medical and surgical techniques exist for dissolving or removing these areas.

Fallopian tubal blockage may occur for a number of reasons, but is frequently due to inflammation or scarring from an STD or other disease of the pelvic area. Treatment of the disease medically may open the tubes, but sometimes surgical removal of scar tissue must be attempted. Typical costs of surgical procedures for repairing causes of female infertility run from $1,200 for laser laparoscopy for endometriosis to $3,500 for tubal surgery.

Other major causes of female infertility are amenorrhea, oligomenorrhea, and luteal phase defect (LPD). Amenorrhea, or the absence of menstruation, and oligomenorrhea, or infrequent, scanty menstruation, have a number of causes, including extreme physical activity, as in dancers and athletes, and anorexia, malnutrition caused by obsessive preoccupation with weight loss. LPD involves failure of the endometrial lining of the uterus to develop properly after ovulation. All of these disorders also involve ovulation dysfunction. Drugs that induce ovulation (the so-called fertility drugs, such as gonadotropins and clomiphene citrate), as well as drugs that promote normal endometrial growth (such as progesterone), are employed to treat these disorders. Fundamentally, these are synthetic hormones designed to supplement what has been diagnosed as a subthreshold level of the hormones necessary to ripen and release ova, and their administration is sometimes unpredictable. The costs of the drugs themselves can run from $30 to $588 per month.

It was not uncommon during the 1970s and 1980s to read of a woman giving birth to four or more premature infants, as a result of having received fertility drugs. Frequently one or more of these children failed to survive the experience of prematurity, and those that did survive succeeded in doing so only with enormous expenditure of costly neonatal technology, with the result not always a normal child.

The phenomenon of a multiple pregnancy, whether due to natural or artificial causes, together with the substantially increased risk of premature delivery, has prompted some obstetricians to employ the technology of fetal monitoring to identify those fetuses in a multiple pregnancy at greatest risk for abnormality, and to "selectively reduce the pregnancy"—that is, selectively abort one or more of the fetuses so as to increase the chance for the remaining ones to come to full term. Such abortions are viewed as a form of triage, designed to increase the chances of some by denying the chances of others; however, they possess an active, interventionist character that strikes many as morally different from simply yielding to the hopelessness of a case (how that difference is assessed as a moral one, is, of course, frequently the point of contention).

Selection is thought to be nonarbitrary when it is based on evidence of identifiable defects in some of the offspring, and thought even to be a kind of therapy in defense of the lives and health of those fetuses not aborted, to whom the very multiplicity of siblings poses a grave risk. At the same time, such measures are inherently desperate, based precisely on the kinds of decision making that hospital allocation committees found so difficult before the federal government's provision of virtual universal access to dialysis.

Part of the difficulty here is the inability to make such selection very early in the gestational period, and even to control how many ova are released and fertilized. Other new techniques offered increased control of that process, as well as the possibility of therapy for the many women whose infertility was due to physical blockage of the fallopian tubes that could not be surgically reversed.

GIFT is the technique of extracting female gametes, called oocytes or ova, using laparoscopy and aspiration, from follicles stimulated to "ripen" through the use of one of several fertility drugs, and inserting one or two of them together with sperm into a catheter from which they are transferred into the end of a fallopian tube. The procedure is then repeated in the other fallopian tube, if possible. The procedure is thus thought to approximate most closely the conditions of natural fertilization, is less expensive and technically challenging than IVF, and may be used to overcome certain problems of fertility in either the male or female partner. Surveys found the technique to be successful on average in 29 percent of attempted cases, ranging from 10 percent to 56 percent effectiveness based on the type of infertility, at an average cost of $3,500 (OTA, 1987, pp. 297, 141).

GIFT is relatively safe and appears to offer slightly more favorable odds than IVF. In addition, some couples prefer it because the fertilization is "natural"—that is, it occurs at the place where fertilization naturally occurs, in the fallopian tubes. The procedure does carry the risk of multiple pregnancy, although, given the naturally low incidence of fertilization coupled with whatever other factors in an infertile couple might make for reduction in that percentage, the frequency of multiple pregnancy is quite low. It also involves a general anesthetic for the surgical procedure, posing to the woman the risks of general anesthesia. Finally, it does not permit either sex selection or other diagnosis of genetic or chromosomal abnormalities in preimplantation embryos, nor identification of defects in the fertilizing ability of sperm or eggs—all of which are possible with IVF.

IVF utilizes the same medical and surgical techniques for harvesting eggs as employed by GIFT. The eggs are then placed in a sterile fluid culture medium in a glass container, into which sperm are introduced. Fertilization takes place in the glass container (hence *in vitro*, or "in glass" fertilization). The fertilized ovum, or preimplantation embryo, is then examined and tested during several days of cell division to detect abnormalities. If found to be abnormal, the preimplantation embryo is discarded. But if normal, the embryo is introduced through the vagina into the uterus. If the embryo successfully implants in the uterine wall, pregnancy has occurred and technology has circumvented the blockage in the fallopian tubes that prevented sperm from reaching the egg.

The procedure requires careful monitoring of the ovulatory cycle for months prior to the release of ova from follicles, biochemical manipulation of the ovaries to stimulate multiple release, an invasive surgical procedure to remove released ova, and an expensive laboratory cell culture technique not normally available to the typical obstetrician. The average cost of IVF through two complete cycles was $9,376 in 1986; however, since a couple is likely to come to IVF only after medical drug treatment for diagnosed oligomenorrhea has failed and complete infertility evaluation and surgical repair has failed, the approximately 11 percent of infertile couples who proceed to IVF will have spent at least 4.5 years and $22,217 in order to achieve pregnancy in 25 percent of the cases.

There is the additional risk to the woman of ectopic pregnancy (where the embryo is accidentally flushed back up into the fallopian tube and implants there, and rupture of the tube occurs as the embryo grows, causing massive internal bleeding and possibly death) in introducing the embryo into the uterus (Corea, 1986). A tubal pregnancy occurs in 2 to 17 percent of IVF procedures, probably depending on how high the catheter is placed in the uterus (OTA, 1988, p. 131).

A failure of the fertilized ovum to implant in the uterus would necessitate a repeat of the entire cycle, and thus reexposure of the woman to the risks of infection and ectopic pregnancy inherent in the full procedure, as well as further preoccupation with tracking the ovulatory cycle and loss of time for harvesting ova. Thus, in the early years of this technique's development, women undergoing IVF might be subjected to four or more repetitions of the cycle of harvesting, fertilization, and implantation before achieving pregnancy.

It was thus a welcome merging of the techniques of cryopreservation and IVF that was permitted by the discovery that early-stage embryos could successfully be frozen to arrest their development, then later thawed and implanted without damage. For this permitted harvesting of several ova in one procedure through prior administration of fertility drugs, fertilization of them all, and then cryopreservation of those normal ones not to be used in the initial implantation effort. Medicine's defense of the procedure was thus based on minimizing the risk of harm to the woman. Rather than expose the woman to repeated months of monitoring, multiple hormonal manipulations, and multiple surgical procedures, one of each would normally suffice. Because unfertilized ova tend not to cryopreserve well, fertilization followed by cryopreservation of a reserve supply serves to minimize the need for repeated applications of the procedure as well. Finally, medicine has generally taken the position, at such early stages of development, that there is only the one existing patient whose interests bear on the medical decisions to be made.

Such principled justifications, however, struck substantial portions of the public struggling to integrate the new technology into its institutions as little more than rationalizations. Serious questions were raised about the necessity for preservation of many preimplantation embryos, and medicine was criticized as erring on the side of excessive preoccupation with the interests of the woman. The issue was most forcefully brought home by the tragedy of the Diaz couple who sought IVF in an Australian clinic.

Medicine's response has been to walk more carefully the thin line between necessity and excess, reflecting increased skill with the procedures: The number of ova permitted to be fertilized is now typically no more than would be implanted at one time in the woman—usually two. Thus, if both are normal she can look forward to twins; if one is abnormal, it is discarded and a single child hopefully will result.

The questions posed by the new IVF technology did not end with the possibility of the Diaz's tragic case, nor even with the troubling issue of what was to be done with unused preimplantation embryos not needed in order to achieve a woman's pregnancy. With the IVF technology, it would be possible for one woman to act as surrogate gestational mother for another's biological child, then return the newborn to its biological parents. Such embryo transfer simply employs as the receptacle for the selected embryo a different uterus than that normally intended with IVF.

Such an application of the technique could serve as a kind of therapeutic option for a couple wishing to have "their own" child but unable to do so because of, say, a surgical removal of the wife's uterus (where the ovaries were left intact). The woman's ovaries would be stimulated to produce several ova, just as in IVF; these would be harvested and fertilized with the husband's sperm in vitro, just as in IVF; but they would be implanted in the uterus of another woman, perhaps a sister or daughter or other individual contracted for the purpose, and carried to term in and by the host. The host would then go through labor and delivery and surrender the child to its "rightful" parents, receiving their thankful gratitude and any coverage of expenses or other remuneration for her trouble they had contracted, or cared, to provide. ET thus appeared to be a technology implicit in IVF, only requiring manipulation of the reproductive cycles of two women instead of just one. However, substantial social, psycho-logical, and ethical differences have emerged as we have gained experience with gestational surrogacy. These and even more complex issues associated with so-called surrogate motherhood will form the focus of the next chapter.

REVIEW OF THE SELECTIONS

Arthur Caplan's thoughtful piece challenges us to answer a host of philosophical and ethical questions involved in the various forms of assisted reproduction and their integration into or exclusion from medical and social practice. What is the moral status of ova, sperm, and embryos, and how does that affect what we may do to them? Shall we regard infertility as a disease for which medical treatment is appropriate? Are services to correct infertility appropriate in a country with liberal abortion policies, inasmuch as such services aim at creating wanted children while unwanted fetuses are destroyed, where an alternative would be to match unwanted prospective children with infertile couples desiring children? Shall infertility technologies be made avail-able to those who want but cannot afford them, or limited to those who have private insurance coverage or personal income sufficient to pay for them? Is it legitimate to donate or receive ova for IVF and implantation in a woman not biologically related to the prospective offspring? How shall the possible uses of IVF be regulated, if at all? Caplan's useful presentation of these and related questions helps set the stage for the arguments in succeeding selections.

LeRoy Walters addresses a number of Caplan's questions in the course of reviewing and analyzing some 15 statements by medical, religious, or governmental bodies on IVF and ET. His essay is included because of its useful function of drawing together in review the variety of positions taken on these issues, underscoring the enormous diversity of reasoned opinions—sometimes entertained at different points in time by the same organization—that have been offered as the basis for personal decisions, professional practices, and social policies.

As an example of the many debates occurring between scholars on the questions Caplan raises, papers by Hans Tiefel and Richard Zaner are included. Tiefel takes a conservative approach, arguing that the potential for harm to embryos of the research necessary to develop the IVF technology is sufficient to raise a decisive moral objec-tion both to such research and to clinical uses of IVF and ET. Tiefel's essay usefully contrasts the interests of adult humans in having children with the interests of "pro-tectable humanity" in not having the risk of harm imposed except where some direct therapeutic benefit is intended. He weighs these contrasting interests and finds the scales to be tipped against IVF and ET, echoing a principle articulated by Leon Kass that "one cannot ethically choose for the would-be-child the unknown hazards that he must face and simultaneously choose to give him life in which to face them."

Richard Zaner examines these conservative claims and defends IVF and ET against them. In an essay exemplifying the detailed examination of argumentation with which critical thinking is synonymous, Zaner probes Tiefel's arguments concerning risk, the impossibility of meeting the requirement of informed consent in fetal research, and the moral status of the fetus. He offers a diagnosis of the compelling character of Tiefel's arguments, and concludes with a discussion of the question of whether IVF and ET constitute therapeutic procedures for a treatable medical condition.

Works Cited

1. Corea, Gena. *The Mother Machine: Reproductive Technologies from Artificial Insemination to Artificial Wombs*. New York: Harper & Row, 1986.
2. Office of Technology Assessment, U.S. Congress. *Infertility: Medical and Social Choices*. Washington, D.C.: U.S. Government Printing Office, 1988.

The Ethics of In Vitro Fertilization

ARTHUR L. CAPLAN, Ph.D.

Assisted Reproduction— A Cornucopia of Moral Muddles

There has been an explosion in recent years in the demand for and resources devoted to the treatment of infertility in the United States. Many parents have benefited from the availability of new techniques such as artificial insemination, microsurgery, fertility drugs, and the various forms of what is generically known as "in vitro fertilization." At the same time, increases in the demand for and allocation of resources to the medical treatment of infertility raise profoundly disturbing and complex moral issues.

The scientific status of the current generation of infertility interventions remains unclear. Some commentators assert that it is obvious that artificial reproduction is still in its infancy. Others, usually more directly involved in providing the technology to patients, avow that the level of success is so high that many forms of artificial reproduction can be viewed only as therapies. The issue of whether medicine is capable of treating infertility is important not only for scientific reasons but also because basic moral issues concerning informed consent, liability for untoward results, and public policies concerning reimbursement pivot around the answer. Where should artificial reproduction be placed on the experiment/therapy continuum?

Little consensus exists either within the medical profession or among the general public as to the moral status of the entities that are the objects of a great deal of medical manipulation in any attempt to treat infertility: ova, sperm, and embryos. The ethics of manipulating, storing, or destroying reproductive materials raise basic questions about the moral status of possible and potential human beings.

It is not even clear whether infertility is or ought to be viewed as a disease requiring or meriting medical intervention. Many of the causes of infertility and many of the

Director, Center for Biomedical Ethics, University of Minnesota, Minneapolis.

possible remedies are as much a function of social, cultural, and economic factors as they are physiologic or biologic abnormalities. Attitudes about conception, child rearing, and the nature of the family are greatly influenced by social and ethical beliefs concerning individual rights, the duties of marriage, and the desirability of passing on a particular set of genetic information into the next generation.

The treatment of infertility also raises basic questions concerning equity and justice. These fall roughly into two broad categories: questions of social justice and questions of individual justice.

Questions of Social Justice

At the social level, increasing amounts of scarce medical resources are being invested in the provision of services for those suffering from impaired fertility. It is estimated conservatively that the United States is now spending more than 200 million dollars annually on medical interventions intended to correct infertility. In the years from 1981 to 1983, more than 2 million visits were made to physicians in private practice by those seeking assistance regarding procreation.

Not only are many persons seeking help, but also an increasing proportion of medical resources are being devoted to this problem. The number of programs offering in vitro fertilization doubled in 1984 alone from 60 to 120. Private clinics whose sole interest is the provision of services to treat infertility have opened in many areas of the country.[9]

Increases in both the supply and demand for medical services to treat infertility can be expected to continue. The number of persons seeking medical assistance is still far below the number of persons in the general population estimated to have serious impairments of fertility.

The expenditure of scarce funds for health resources is not the only social issue raised by technologic progress with respect to reproduction. It is not uncommon for fertility services to be located in the same building, if not on the same floor, as services devoted to the termination of pregnancies. If this situation were not ironic enough in itself, it is surely odd to contemplate increases in the resources devoted to the alleviation of infertility at a time when millions of children in the United States and around the world lack parents as well as the basic necessities of life.

In the United States itself, there are still thousands of children who cannot be placed with either foster families or adoptive parents. This situation raises obvious issues of social justice and individual rights, particularly when many of the children requiring adoption have special physical, cognitive, and emotional needs.

Issues regarding the priority that should be given to the development of fertility-enhancing services are made all the more pressing at a time when both federal and state governments have been moving rapidly to institute cost-containment measures such as prospective payment and reimbursement by diagnosis related groups (DRGs). These efforts are likely to curtail sharply access to proven therapeutic services for the elderly, the disabled, and the poor, who depend on public expenditures for their care.

Questions of Individual Justice

At an individual or familial level, access to infertility services frequently is limited to those who can pay for them, either out of pocket or, in some cases, through private insurance. Access to services also is constrained by patient awareness of the existence of medical options, geography, and the ability to bear the often onerous financial, psychosocial, and time commitments associated with many of the available forms of assisted reproduction.

The proper role of the law and of the state in influencing or controlling individual decisions concerning reproduction is also a matter of much disagreement and dispute. Traditionally, American courts have been loathe to countenance any interference with matters pertaining to the family and individual decisions concerning procreation. As one philosopher has observed, parental decisions concerning children have been seen as "a right against all the rest of society to be indulged within wide limits, . . . immune from the scrutiny of and direction of others."[15]

However, in recent years, federal and state law has begun to acknowledge a powerful state interest in the welfare of children, particularly newborns. Child abuse statutes in many states have recently been revised and strengthened. The federal government has expressed its wish that children born with handicaps or congenital defects receive access to the same opportunities for medical assistance and treatment as would be available to other children. The traditional assumption in American law and morality that privacy provides an inviolate shield against intervention by other parties or the state has weakened somewhat in the face of increasing concern about protecting the interests of especially vulnerable human beings such as newborns and children and assuring that no one is subject to invidious discrimination on the basis of handicap, race, sex, or ethnic origin.[12]

The Growing Demand
for Medical Assistance
in Procreation

Infertility is a major problem in the United States. Almost one in six couples who have tried to conceive a child for 1 year fail to do so. Although the overall incidence of infertility appears to be relatively stable, the demand for infertility services is increasing rapidly.

The increase in demand for medical assistance in conceiving children is due to a variety of factors. Many couples have chosen to delay conception, thereby exposing themselves to the increased risks of infertility associated with aging. There appears to be some increase in the number of women encountering iatrogenic fertility problems as a result of difficulties associated with various forms of birth control, such as intrauterine devices (IUDs). More women have entered the work force and, as a result, have been exposed to reproductive hazards and pollutants that may adversely affect fertility. Increases in the incidence of sexually transmitted diseases, especially pelvic inflammatory disease, have also produced a higher incidence of infertility among some subgroups within the general population.

The causes of increased demand for fertility services are not confined to physiologic factors. Couples who might have considered adoption in earlier decades are now turning in increasing numbers to the medical profession for assistance with respect to conception. Moreover, there has been a dramatic increase in the availability of infertility services in the United States. Advances in diagnostic techniques such as laparoscopy and hormonal and genetic analysis also allow health care professionals to identify with increasing reliability those suffering from impairments in fertility.[8]

Attitudes toward human variability, the desirability of marriage and family, and the importance of biologic kinship between parent and child also play a powerful role in influencing the demand for medical assistance with respect to infertility. There is some evidence that parental expectations concerning pregnancy and reproduction have changed drastically during the past decade.

Lawsuits against and malpractice rates among those engaged in obstetrics have increased dramatically in recent years. Our society has come, whether wisely or not, to expect physicians to facilitate the conception of optimally healthy children at the conclusion of every pregnancy.

The power of medical intervention to influence procreation and reproduction challenges social norms concerning human differences and variability that are, at best, poorly understood by social scientists and moral philosophers. A growing emphasis on perfection in procreation and child rearing contributes to a situation in which those who are disabled, dysfunctional, or merely different from the norm may encounter increasing difficulties in securing social acceptance and material security. The availability of technologic methods for detecting and eliminating disease and disorder early in pregnancy as well as technologic methods for facilitating procreation in those for whom this would not have been an option in earlier times means that personal autonomy and individual choice are enhanced. However, it may also mean that such gains are purchased at the cost of lowering public tolerance for differences and diversity among individual human beings and about decisions concerning child-bearing, child rearing, childlessness, and disability.[12]

In Vitro Fertilization: A Case Study

Perhaps the most controversial and provocative of all the new forms of medically assisted reproduction available today is in vitro fertilization. Although it has been common practice for decades in the United States as well as in other nations to utilize sperm donated by either spouses or strangers for the purpose of facilitating procreation, it is only in the past 10 years that efforts have been made to utilize donated ova by various means in order to facilitate reproduction.

It is not merely the novelty of in vitro fertilization that makes it worthy of special comment and ethical reflection. The fact that in vitro fertilization is a technology that severs the traditional link between gestation and maternal identity raises serious and novel issues for both the law and morality. The prevailing ideology of equality, at least with respect to opportunity, in the United States makes it easy to overlook the fact that one of our society's most basic and fundamental beliefs about reproduction and the family is that the mothers of children are undeniably that, the mothers. Although it is true that artificial insemination by donor (AID) raises questions about paternal identity, the fact is that paternal identity, whether men like to admit it or not, has always been subject to a certain degree of uncertainty—with or without artificial insemination by donor.

Prior to the appearance of in vitro fertilization, there has never been any doubt, much less any empiric reason for doubting, that the woman who bore a child bore a direct familial relationship to that child. It is difficult to know exactly what the social reverberations of a technology capable of severing the tie between genetic relationship and gestation will be. However, the fact that this new technology can change a previously basic and undeniable reality of the human condition makes this particular technology worthy of serious and special moral consideration.

Standard In Vitro Fertilization

In vitro fertilization actually refers to a family of procedures that all involve the fertilization of an ovum outside of the human body. In the most commonly utilized technique, which might be termed "standard in vitro fertilization," one or more eggs are removed from the ovaries using a syringe known as a laparoscope. Egg cells are exceedingly small, so that the process of retrieval requires considerable skill and experience.

In many but not in all centers in which standard in vitro fertilization is practiced, the ovaries are stimulated artificially by hormones administered to the donor to produce more than one egg in the menstrual cycle. The eggs that are removed are subjected to microscopic inspection to determine which appears to be structurally most sound. One or more of the eggs is then fertilized in vitro using the husband's or a donor's sperm. The egg or eggs are then observed until they have grown to the eight-cell stage in an artificial medium. A decision is then made as to which of the developing embryos will be reimplanted into the prospective mother's womb.[3,18]

Reimplantation or, as it is often termed, "embryo transfer," also requires careful monitoring of the prospective mother in order to ascertain the optimal time for reimplanting the egg back into the uterus. Timing is critical to the success of reimplantation.

In some centers, some of the embryos that are produced are frozen for later use should the initial attempt at reimplantation fail. Techniques for freezing fertilized eggs at very low temperatures are well developed. The decision to freeze a fertilized egg allows for further efforts at reimplantation, but it also raises questions about the disposition of unused embryos.

The first successful use of standard in vitro fertilization took place in Britain in 1978. Since that time, nearly 1000 infants have been born utilizing this technique in the United States, Australia, the Netherlands, and a number of other countries. The procedure generally costs between $3000 and $5000 per attempt. Several attempts are often required in order to achieve pregnancy. One recent report stated that out of 24,037 oocytes collected, 7722 resulted in fertilized embryos that were reimplanted in the mother's uterus. From this group, 590 children were born, among which were 56 twins, 7 triplets, and 1 set of quadruplets. These multiple births were a result of the simultaneous reimplantation of more than one embryo in order to increase the likelihood of a successful implantation and birth.[10]

These data indicate that the pregnancy rate achieved is about 25 per cent, although the number of pregnancies resulting in a liveborn child is less than 10 per cent. These figures are low, but it should be noted that they do not differ all that much from the rates of pregnancy and birth associated with sexual intercourse between fertile parents.[14]

Nonstandard In Vitro Fertilization

The techniques utilized in standard in vitro fertilization allow for a startling number of permutations and combinations with respect to the donors of sperm and eggs, the choice of a recipient to receive the embryos that result, and the choice of individuals to parent the children who are born as a result of these techniques. Donors of sperm or eggs may or may not be persons who are married. Women who cannot produce viable eggs or who for some reason are unwilling or unable to undergo the procedures necessary to perform laparoscopy may ask another woman to supply eggs for in vitro fertilization.

It is also possible to utilize women other than the biologic donor to serve as the "gestational mother" for a fertilized egg. These women may carry an embryo to term and then either keep the resulting child or turn it over to another party—either the biologic donor or yet another person or persons. Because it is possible to freeze embryos, it is also possible to utilize in vitro fertilization techniques to produce a child after the death of the biologic donors or without the knowledge and consent of the biologic donors.

Nonstandard in vitro fertilization techniques allow for a division of the roles of mother and parent that was, quite simply, impossible before the appearance of these techniques. It is now possible to produce a child who has one set of biologic parents who may be either alive or dead and who provide eggs and sperm, another person or persons who are involved in pregnancy and gestation, and still a third person or persons who serve as the actual or social parent(s) of the child![20]

The fact that it is now possible to separate the biologic, gestational, and social aspects of mothering and parenting introduces a range of further novel possibilities concerning fertilization, reproduction, and birth. For example, frozen embryos not utilized for in vitro fertilization are available for research directly related to in vitro fertilization techniques or other medical purposes involving therapies not related to procreation (for example, the development of embryos in order to produce and harvest useful organic materials). Nonstandard in vitro fertilization techniques raise the possibility of remuneration of women for their services as either egg donors or gestational mothers, or, as the role is often termed, surrogates. The availability of standard and nonstandard in vitro fertilization techniques may facilitate the application of genetic engineering either for therapeutic purposes, aesthetic reasons, or even eugenic goals.

Major Policy Issues Raised by In Vitro Fertilization

The development of in vitro fertilization techniques of various types poses a direct and pressing challenge to public policy. At present, in vitro fertilization is still a relatively new medical modality, and as such, there are many aspects of the techniques utilized, including hormonal induction of ovulation, the freezing and storage of embryos, and the development of optimal media for embryo growth, in which further research is necessary. Little is known about the long-term psychosocial impacts of in vitro fertilization on children born by these methods or on the families who raise children produced by either standard or nonstandard in vitro fertilization techniques.[18]

Little formal supervision and regulation has been exercised to date by local, state, and federal authorities in the United States over the provision of in vitro fertilization as a therapy. At present, the only form of control over those who provide in vitro fertilization exists in the form of peer regulation through professional societies and individual collegial review. Few courts have ruled on matters pertaining to in vitro fertilization, and there are few legislative statutes that govern either research or therapy in this area.[2]

In 1975, a federal law required the creation of an Ethics Advisory Board (EAB) with the Department of Health, Education and Welfare (now Health and Human Services). In June 1979, the EAB issued a report on the scientific, ethical, legal, and social aspects of in vitro fertilization that concluded that the conduct of research pertaining to in vitro fertilization was ethically acceptable and worthy of monetary support by the federal government.[7] However, those who have served as the secretary of the Department of Health and Human Services have chosen not to respond to the report or to extend the life of the EAB. The EAB was disbanded at the end of 1979. Because its approval is necessary for any research protocols to receive federal funding, to date, no American research or clinical trials on in vitro fertilization have received any federal dollars. A key recommendation of the EAB was that a model statute be drafted to clarify the rights of in vitro fertilization donors, offspring, parents, and medical professionals. No subsequent efforts have been made to draft such a statute.

It is interesting to note that 23 states have enacted laws prohibiting "fetal research or embryo research." Some states also prohibit the performance of autopsies or research procedures on abortuses, miscarried fetuses, or stillborn fetuses. No state has enacted legislation or regulation governing the conduct of medical facilities identifying themselves as in vitro fertilization clinics or fertility clinics. Minimal standards for in vitro fertilization programs have been developed by the American Fertility Society,[1] but these standards have not yet received explicit legal or legislative recognition.

Other nations have established commissions or committees at the national level to examine in vitro fertilization. In England, the Department of Health and Social Security established a commission under the leadership of Dame Mary Warnock to conduct an inquiry into human fertilization and embryology. This commission issued a detailed report in July 1984.[18] This report addressed such topics as artificial insemination, in vitro fertilization, surrogacy, the freezing and storage of reproductive materials, and the use of embryos for research.

The Warnock commission issued a list of more than 60 recommendations concerning artificial techniques for assisting human reproduction. Among these were a call for the creation of a new licensing authority to regulate both research and therapy pertaining to artificial insemination by donor and both standard and nonstandard forms of in vitro fertilization, a 14-day limit on the use of frozen embryos for either research or therapeutic purposes, the need to obtain consent from the donor for any interventions pertaining to frozen embryos, and, perhaps most controversially, the criminalization of surrogacy. Similar studies reaching somewhat different conclusions have been issued recently by committees in the Netherlands, Canada, and Australia.[17]

Perhaps the most glaring public policy question arising in the United States today is whether there is any need for legal, legislative, or regulatory action at the federal, state, or local level with respect to in vitro fertilization and its associated technologies. These regulatory interventions might take the form of bans or moratoriums on various forms of in vitro fertilization research or therapy, modifications of existing state laws to clarify the legal status of in vitro fertilization, or statutes intended to recognize and spur the development of research and therapy regarding in vitro fertilization.

The heated and critical reaction that greeted the appearance of the Warnock commission's report in the United Kingdom should give pause to those in the United States who believe that the time has come to initiate any form of regulation or legislation with respect to in vitro fertilization. The Warnock report has been strongly criticized by various members of Parliament in the United Kingdom who believe that its recommendations are too permissive, by prominent scientists and scientific societies who worry that it is too restrictive in its recommendations concerning research, and by a number of legal authorities concerning its stance on such matters as surrogacy and the commercialization of in vitro fertilization.[14, 19]

Although there is certainly a need for both federal and state bodies to encourage and solicit further study of the many moral and legal issues raised by in vitro fertilization, there would not yet appear to exist the empiric or valuational foundation for establishing regulatory policies that could command consent and compliance from health care professionals, researchers, or those who wish to avail themselves of in vitro fertilization for various reasons. Such forums as the Congressional Office of Technology Assessment, the newly formed Committee on Life and the Law in New York state, or a reconstituted President's Commission for the Study of Ethical Problems in Medicine and Biomedical and Behavioral Research, whose mandate expired at the end of 1983, would appear to be ideal forums for attempting to attain the consensus requisite for the implementation of rules and regulations governing the application of medical knowledge and skills to as sensitive and as fundamental an arena of human experience as human reproduction. These bodies could attempt to grapple with some of the basic ethical issues that still have not received sufficient public deliberation and reflection.

Major Ethical Issues Raised by In Vitro Fertilization

There is a tendency in the existing literature on in vitro fertilization to move directly to arguments about the moral implications of the nonstandard forms of the technique.[13, 16] In many ways, this is understandable, because as noted earlier, the permutations and combinations of nonstandard in vitro fertilization techniques do allow for the separation of biologic, gestational, and parental functions, especially with respect to women, that pose enormous challenges to the legal system.

However, although issues pertaining to the moral acceptability of surrogacy, the desirability or undesirability of commercial relationships in nonstandard and standard forms of in vitro fertilization, and the policies that should be followed with regard to matters such as inheritance where in vitro fertilization embryos and children are concerned raise obvious moral and legal conundrums, it is not clear that these issues are actually the pivotal ones raised by advances in in vitro fertilization techniques. I suspect that moral matters regarding in vitro fertilization in terms of both research and therapy will actually hinge on the answers that are given to the following questions:

1. Is infertility a disease?
2. What counts as fair and equitable access to in vitro fertilization?
3. What is the moral status of a human embryo?

Is Infertility a Disease?

One common definition of disease often found in medical literature is that disease represents any deviation from the existing norms that prevail for human functioning.[4] Certainly, infertility, although not uncommon, is uncommon enough to qualify as abnormal or deviant relative to the average capacities and abilities of the human population.

Nonetheless, defining disease as abnormality has its own significant problems, not the least of which is that such a definition makes any physical or mental state at the tail ends of normal distributions diseases by definition. Thus, the state of being very tall, very smart, very dark-skinned, or very strong all qualify as diseases according to the abnormality criterion.

One way of avoiding including too much in the disease category is to restrict the definition of disease to those states that represent biologic dysfunction. According to this view, infertility would qualify as a disease because the relevant organ systems are not functioning as they presumably were designed to do.

However, again, a strictly biologic definition of disease flounders on empiric grounds. Not all dysfunctional bodily states constitute sources of symptoms or even problems for those who possess them. One can be afflicted with any number of dysfunctional states and attributes over the course of a normal life span without either knowing or caring very much about them one way or another. It seems odd to argue that a person who does not want children and who also has a low sperm count should be labeled as diseased.

Perhaps the most satisfying way to handle the problem of defining disease is to attempt a definition that captures both physiologic and patient perspectives. Disease would appear to refer to those dysfunctional states that a person recognizes or, if left untreated, will eventually come to recognize as dysfunctional either due to impairments in abilities or capacities or as a result of noxious symptoms.[5]

Using a definition that recognizes both the biologic and psychosocial aspects of disease, it would appear defensible to argue that infertility is a disease that falls reasonably within medicine's purview. Although not all persons afflicted with fertility problems find this state distressing or limiting, many certainly do. Furthermore, although it is true that fertility and the ability to have children is a desire that is strongly mediated by social and cultural values, it is also true that this desire comes as close as can be to constituting a universal desire that can be found among every human society.

Indeed, it is the pervasiveness of the importance assigned to the ability to have offspring that provides one of the empiric warrants not only for labeling infertility as a disease but also for assigning its care and treatment a relatively high priority with respect to other disease states. If it is reasonable to include the capacity to bear children among those abilities and skills that constitute basic human goods, such as cognition, locomotion, and perception, infertility not only is a disease but also is one that should receive special attention and concern from physicians and those concerned with health policy.

What Counts As Fair and Equitable Access to In Vitro Fertilization?

If it is true that infertility is a disease that adversely affects a basic and important human capacity, it would seem important to assure access to efficacious and safe diagnostic, therapeutic, and palliative health care services that may contribute to the enhancement of this capacity. Indeed, infertility would appear to constitute so severe an impairment of a basic human capacity that, other things being equal, access to such services should not be contingent upon the individual patient's or family's ability to pay.

However, the major issue requiring resolution with respect to justice and equity in the allocation of resources for the diagnosis and treatment of infertility is not how much to spend or who should foot the bill, but rather whether the diagnostic and therapeutic techniques now in existence are safe and efficacious. Until the requisite empiric information for analyzing this issue has been obtained, it would be unethical to divert resources from other medical interventions already known to be safe and efficacious.

Moreover, although high priority should be accorded to the treatment of infertility, it should not be assumed that in vitro fertilization and other techniques are the only techniques that can be utilized to cope with the dysfunctional consequences of infertility or that the demonstration of a need for services thereby entails that any and all health care practitioners who wish to engage in treatment are thereby entitled to do so. Equity and fairness demand that those afflicted with the disease of infertility be aware of all options available to them, including adoption and foster parenting, and that public policy facilitate the utilization of these options. Equity and fairness also require that the resources devoted to in vitro fertilization and other techniques be used in the most efficient manner possible. This may require that diagnostic and therapeutic services be regionalized and that funding be restricted to those centers that can demonstrate a high level of safety and efficacy with regard to in vitro fertilization techniques.[11]

What Is the Moral Status of a Human Embryo?

One of the most perplexing issues raised by the evolution of in vitro fertilization is the need to examine the moral standing that should be accorded to an embryo. Arguments about research on embryos and about the storage and disposition of embryos will ultimately pivot upon the moral status that should be accorded to these entities.

In general, the scientific and medical communities have tried to shy away from the suggestion that science has anything much to say about the questions of when life begins or what counts as a human being. Recent Congressional hearings on the question of the definition of life produced a barrage of disclaimers, dodges, and apologies from those scientists called upon to testify.

The unwillingness of many members of the scientific and medical communities to address squarely the issue of when life begins and what counts as a human being is perhaps not surprising. After all, the definition of human life raises theologic and psychologic issues that are difficult and disturbing to contemplate.

However, it is important to note that members of the scientific and medical communities have not been reticent about an analogous issue—when does human life end. The existence of brain death statutes in most states is evidence of the fact that the biomedical community has been willing to offer its expert opinion as to both the definition of death and the criteria that should be followed to assess whether a particular person meets this definition.[6]

The issues of when life begins and what entities count as human beings demand similar degrees of courage and attention from the biomedical community. Although biomedical scientists may not be able to formulate definitions of life and personhood among themselves that can command societal assent, they surely have a role to play in participating in the formulation of definitions and criteria that society will have to establish in order to cope with the existence of in vitro fertilization.

Two lessons should be learned from other attempts to define life and personhood in such arenas as the debates about abortion and animal experimentation. First, no single property is likely to serve as a distinct boundary for establishing the existence of personhood or even life. The criteria used in a definition are more likely to constitute a family or cluster of concepts.

Second, the definition of life and the criteria used to assess its presence do not end moral matters. Knowing when life begins and when personhood or humanity can be attributed to a particular entity provides only the starting point for arguments about what to do with embryos. It is still necessary to consider the rights, duties, and obligations of donors, prospective parents, and health care professionals in deciding what is to be done with and to embryos. However, it will not do for the biomedical community to continue to adopt an ostrich-like posture and proclaim that it has nothing whatsoever to contribute in the way of empiric information that might facilitate the formulation of an answer to the question of what moral status should be accorded to human embryos.

Conclusion

The evolution of medicine's capacity to assist those afflicted with impairments of fertility is an exciting and commendable prospect. However, enthusiasm for the techniques and for the benefit they can bring to those afflicted with a disease that impairs a fundamental and universally valued human capacity should not blind us to the fact that these techniques are still new, relatively poorly understood, and surrounded with uncertainty as to their efficacy and safety.

In vitro fertilization is not only a scientific and financial challenge to society but also a moral challenge. The possibility of separating the functions of biologic, gestational, and social parenting raises dilemmas of policy, law, and regulation that have never before faced humankind. However, insufficient attention has been given to some of the basic moral issues that underlie much of the current fascination with and fear of in vitro fertilization. Given the implications of this technique for basic social institutions such as the family, kinship, and parenting, it is imperative that our regulatory, legal, and legislative responses to it be wise. We as a society must look much more carefully before we take a leap in any particular regulatory or legal direction.

References

1. American Fertility Society: Minimal standards for programs of in vitro fertilization. Fertil. Steril., *41*:12–13, 1984.

2. Annas, G., and Elias, S.: In vitro fertilization and embryo transfer: Medicolegal aspects of a new technique to create a family. Family Law Quarterly, *17*:199–223, 1983.

3. Blank, R.: Making babies: The state of the art. The Futurist, *19*:1–17, 1985.

4. Caplan, A., and Engelhardt, II, T. (eds.): Concepts of Health and Disease. Reading, Massachusetts, Addison-Wesley, 1981.

5. Caplan, A.: Is aging a disease? *In* Spicker, S., and Ingman, S. (eds.): Vitalizing Long-Term Care. New York, Springer-Verlag, 1984, pp. 14–28.

6. Culver, C., and Gert, B.: Philosophy in Medicine. New York, Oxford University Press, 1982.

7. Department of Health, Education and Welfare: Protection of Human Subjects: HEW Support of Human In Vitro Fertilization and Embryo Transfer. Washington, D.C., Government Printing Office, 1979.

8. Grobstein, C., Flower, M., and Mendeloff, J.: External human fertilization: An evaluation of policy. Science, *222*:127–133, 1983.

9. Henahan, J.: Fertilization: Embryo transfer procedures raise many questions. J.A.M.A., *252*:877–882, 1984.

10. Hodgen, G.: The Need for Infertility Treatment. Testimony in Hearings on Human Embryo Transfer, Subcommittee on Investigations and Oversight, Committee on Science and Technology, U.S. House of Representatives, August 8, 1984.

11. Institute of Medicine: Assessing Medical Technologies. Washington, D.C., National Academy Press, 1985.

12. Murray, T., and Caplan, A. (eds.): Which Babies Shall Live? Clifton, New Jersey, Humana, 1985.

13. Robertson, J. A.: Procreative liberty and the control of conception, pregnancy and childbirth. Virginia Law Review, *69*:20–80, 1983.

14. Sattaur, O.: New conception threatened by old morality. New Scientist, *103*:12–17, 1984.

15. Schoeman, F.: Rights of children, rights of parents and the moral basis of the family. Ethics, *91*:6–19, 1980.

16. Wadlington, W.: Artificial conception: The challenge for family law. Virginia Law Review, *69*:126–174, 1983.

17. Waller, L., et al.: Report on the Disposition of Embryos Produced by In Vitro Fertilization. Victoria, Australia, Committee to Consider the Social, Ethical and Legal Issues Arising from In Vitro Fertilization, August 1984.

18. Warnock, M.: Report of the Committee of Inquiry into Human Fertilization and Embryology. London, HMSO, 1984.

19. Warnock Proposals in trouble. Nature, *313*:417, 1985.

20. Working Party, Council for Science and Society: Human Procreation: Ethical Aspects of the New Techniques. Oxford, Oxford University Press, 1984.

Test-Tube Babies:
Ethical Considerations

LeROY WALTERS, Ph.D.

This essay is based on 15 statements by medical, religious, or publicly appointed bodies on in vitro fertilization (IVF) and embryo transfer (ET). The 15 statements span the period from 1979 through 1985; they represent the points of view of groups from Australia, Western Europe (including the United Kingdom), Canada, and the United States. The aim of the essay is to analyze the ethical and public policy issues raised by the 15 statements.

The 15 public statements, arrayed in chronological order, are the following:

1. The report of the U.S. Department of Health, Education, and Welfare (HEW) Ethics Advisory Board (May 1979).[16]

2. The report of a working party to the Australian National Health and Research Council (August 1982).[3]

3. The submission of the Catholic Bishops of Victoria, Australia, to the Waller Committee (August 1982).[5]

4. The interim report of the Waller Committee in Victoria, Australia (September 1982).[17]

5. The statement of the British Medical Research Council (November 1982).[9]

6. The report of the British Royal College of Obstetricians and Gynaecologists (March 1983).[12]

7. The submission to the Warnock Committee of a joint committee established by the Catholic Bishops of the United Kingdom (March 1983).[6]

8. The submission of the British Royal Society to the Warnock Committee (March 1983).[13]

9. The interim report of a working group to the British Medical Association (May 1983).[4]

Director, Center for Bioethics, Kennedy Institute of Ethics; Associate Professor, Department of Philosophy; Adjunct Professor, Department of Obstetrics and Gynecology, Georgetown University, Washington, D.C.

The research for the essay was supported in part by a grant from the Joseph P. Kennedy Jr. Foundation.

10. The report on donor gametes by the Waller Committee (August 1983).[18]

11. The recommendations of an advisory subgroup to the European Medical Research Councils (November 1983).[7]

12. The statement of the American Fertility Society (January 1984).[1]

13. The Warnock Committee report in the United Kingdom (July 1984).[8]

14. The final report of the Waller Committee in Victoria, Australia (August 1984).[19]

15. The report of the Ontario Law Reform Commission (1985).[10]

Even this rather long list of statements is not exhaustive for the years from 1979 to the present. For example, it does not include the report of the Demack Committee from Queensland, Australia, nor does it include all of the testimony formally submitted to the Warnock Committee in the United Kingdom and the Waller Committee in Victoria, Australia. At the same time, however, the list is representative of the spectrum of views expressed during this period and does not exclude any of the most-cited statements on IVF and ET.

The analysis that follows is divided into two parts. First, 18 issues that were prominently featured in the early statements are examined. These issues can be called first-generation issues. Second, eight new clinical issues that have been raised in some of the more recent statements on IVF and ET are considered. These issues are termed second-generation issues.

First-Generation Issues

From 1979 through the early 1980s, eighteen issues predominated in public-policy statements on IVF and ET. These eighteen issues are presented in the first column of Table 1. The combination of the fifteen statements and eighteen issues produces a 270-cell matrix, as displayed in Table 1. The four options within each cell of the matrix are Yes, No, Not Resolved (NR), and Not Discussed (—).[20]

The constellation of yes and no answers on the matrix is not random; rather, it represents a series of moral *Gestalten*, or patterns, on the ethics of IVF and ET. Four major positions can be identified.[20]

The Natural-Reproduction Only Position This first viewpoint, represented by column three in the matrix, holds that any separation of the lovemaking and procreative aspects of sexual intercourse is ethically unacceptable. Thus, IVF and ET are disapproved, even if the gametes are provided by husband and wife, because fertilization occurs in the laboratory as a result of technical procedures rather than in the Fallopian tube following coitus. For the same general reasons, artificial modes of contraception would also be considered ethically unacceptable by this first position.

The Clinical IVF Without Donation Position According to a second viewpoint, clinical IVF is ethically acceptable if it employs only the gametes of a married couple and if IVF is employed as a matter of necessity. This position is represented by column seven of the matrix. The donation of sperm or egg cells is rejected by this view, either because it represents the intrusion of a third party into the marital relationship or because it confuses the genetic lineage of offspring. This position may or may not be associated with the view that early human embryos are protectable entities and that all developing embryos should be transferred.

The Clinical IVF Only Position   This third position differs from the second only in its acceptance of gamete donation in cases of necessity. Such cases would include situations in which one or both members of a married couple are incapable of producing gametes that are reproductively competent, at least in the context of sexual intercourse. Also included in the notion of "necessity" might be cases in which one or both members of a married couple were at risk for transmitting a known, serious genetic defect. This third position is represented in the matrix by column 10. All clinical interventions involving IVF are considered ethically acceptable; only research with early human embryos is considered to be unacceptable. Like position two, this position may or may not be correlated with the view that all developing embryos should be transferred.

The Clinical IVF and Laboratory Research Position   Unlike the previous three positions, this fourth position accepts the moral legitimacy of laboratory research with early human embryos and the nontransfer of such embryos. According to this viewpoint, we have no moral obligations to protect early human embryos from harm, or the obligation to protect early human embryos from harm is outweighed by other, more important obligations. On the matrix this position is represented by columns 13, 14, and 15, among others.

One can distinguish between conservative and liberal proponents of position four. For example, some groups explicitly permitted a wide variety of experimental manipulations (see columns six and eight), while other groups either rejected such manipulations or came to no resolution about them (see columns 11 and 13). Moreover, although the matrix does not reflect this parameter, the groups differed in their views on the permissible time period during which early human embryos may be cultured for research purposes.

The matrix reveals a rather clear trend toward the acceptance of position four, the Clinical IVF and laboratory Research Position. In fact, three of the four publicly appointed bodies—those in the United Kingdom, Victoria (Australia), and Ontario (Canada)—have adopted this fourth position (see columns 13, 14, and 15).

Second-Generation Issues

Several clinical issues that are not represented on the matrix have been discussed by at least some of the institutional bodies listed there—particularly the last three groups. If added to the matrix, these issues would follow E under "Therapy" in the first column. On two of these second-generation issues there is substantial consensus; on the remaining six, ethical controversy continues.

Table 1. Contrasting Viewpoints on the Ethics of In Vitro Fertilization and/or Embryo Transfer

	(1) HEW	(2) (Austr.) NH & MC	(3) Catholic Bishops (Austr.)	(4) Waller I (Austr.)	(5) (British) MRC	(6) (British) RCOG
Therapy						
(A) Acceptability in Principle	Yes	Yes	No	Yes	Yes	Yes
(B) Freezing of Embryos	—	Yes	No	Yes	No	Yes
(C) Donation of Oocytes	No	Yes	No	NR	—	Yes
(D) Donation of Embryos (In Vitro Fertilization)	No	—	—	No	—	Yes
(E) Donation of Embryos (In Vivo Fertilization)	—	—	—	—	—	—
Laboratory Research						
(F) Acceptability in Principle	Yes	Yes	No	NR	Yes	Yes
(G) Donation of Embryos for Research	Yes	Yes	—	—	Yes	Yes
(H) Freezing of Embryos	—	—	—	—	Yes	Yes
(I) Interspecies Fertilization	No	—	No	—	Yes	—
(J) Division of Embryos (Cloning)	—	—	—	—	—	Yes
(K) Nuclear Transfer (Actual Cloning)	No	Yes	—	—	—	—
(L) Gene Repair	—	—	—	—	—	Yes
(M) Harvesting of Embryonic Cells for Transplant Purposes	—	—	No	—	—	Yes
(N) Production of Pathenogenones	—	—	—	—	—	—
(O) Teratogenic Studies	—	—	—	—	—	—
(P) Interspecies Fusion of Embryos	No	—	No	—	—	—
General Issues						
(Q) Disposal of Embryos	—	Yes	No	Yes	Yes	No
Related Issue						
(R) Surrogate Motherhood	No	NR	No	No	—	No

— = Not Discussed.

NR = Not Resolved.

[1]If research beneficial to embryo itself.

[2]Irish MRC had strong reservations.

[3]Norwegian MRC limited to embryos following IVF.

[4]Norwegian MRC limited to infertility studies.

[5]Norwegian MRC disapproved.

[6]Majority view.

[7]For fertility testing; developmental limit: 2 cells.

[8]Majority view; acceptable only if spare embryos used.

(7) Catholic Committee (UK)	(8) Royal Society (UK)	(9) Br. Med. Assn.	(10) Waller II (Austr.)	(11) European MRCs	(12) American Fertility Society	(13) Warnock (UK)	(14) Waller III (Austr.)	(15) Ont. Law Ref. Comm.
Yes	Yes	Yes	Yes	Yes	Yes	Yes	Yes	Yes
Yes	No	Yes	Yes	—	Yes	Yes	Yes	Yes
No	—	Yes	Yes	—	Yes	Yes	Yes	Yes
No	—	Yes	Yes	—	Yes	Yes	Yes	Yes
—	—	—	—	—	—	No	NR	Yes
Yes[1]	Yes	Yes	NR	Yes[2]	Yes	Yes[6]	Yes[8]	Yes
—	Yes	Yes	—	Yes[3]	Yes	Yes	Yes	Yes
—	Yes	Yes	—	Yes	Yes	Yes	Yes	—
No	—	—	—	Yes[4]	—	Yes[7]	—	—
No	Yes	Yes	—	—	—	NR	Yes	—
No	—	Yes	—	—	—	NR	—	—
—	Yes	Yes	—	—	—	NR	NR	—
No	—	—	—	—	—	—	—	—
No	—	—	—	—	—	NR	—	—
—	Yes	—	—	—[5]	—	NR	—	—
—	—	—	—	—	—	—	—	—
No	—	Yes	NR	—	Yes	Yes	Yes	Yes
No	—	No	NR	—	—	No	No	Yes

Noncontroversial Issues

The Screening of Gamete Donors   The question of donor screening first rose in the context of artificial insemination by donor (AID). The traditional rationale for such screening has been to reduce the chances of transmitting genetic disease or infection. With the emergence of AIDS as a human disease and one case report of the transmission of infection with the AIDS-related virus through AID,[14] this traditional rationale takes on new urgency. Recent statements have unanimously advocated the screening of donors and the long-term confidential maintenance of records that would allow for the recontacting of the gamete donor for serious medical reasons.

The Freezing of Oocytes   Because of their concern about possible multiple pregnancies, some centers that offer IVF and ET limit the number of embryos transferred during a given ovulatory cycle. If the number of cleaving embryos exceeds this limit, a "surplus-embryo" problem arises. The freezing of such excess embryos may provide one approach to this problem, but the long-term cryopreservation of embryos raises ethical problems in its own right. An alternative approach that would avoid the surplus-embryo problem would be to freeze oocytes not needed for fertilization in a given cycle. In principle, this approach would have the dual advantage of allowing for the retrieval of the maximum available number of oocytes per cycle, while at the same time permitting the fertilization and transfer of only some of the fertilized oocytes in a given cycle. In practice, the safety of oocyte cryopreservation remains to be demonstrated. Two recent statements have supported oocyte freezing.[8, 19]

Controversial Issues

On six new clinical issues there remains a substantial amount of ethical controversy. In most cases one can identify a liberty-oriented viewpoint that emphasizes privacy rights and resists regulation by third parties. The contrasting viewpoint is usually welfare-oriented and advocates external regulation for either paternalistic or nonpaternalistic reasons.

The Screening of Prospective Social Parents   This issue concerns the potential role of health professionals in attempting to assess the fitness of particular individuals or couples to participate in IVF programs. Possible grounds for the exclusion of particular individuals from participation could include the following: a history of child abuse; poverty; the single status of a female candidate; the nontraditional character of an applicant couple (for example, a lesbian couple); or the unmarried status of a heterosexual couple.

    A liberty-oriented approach to this issue would argue as follows. Whoever wishes to bear or beget a child with the aid of medical assistance should be free to seek, and should be able to find, such assistance—provided that he or she can pay for the assistance. In contrast, a welfare-oriented view would advocate at least some screening of prospective social parents to prevent harmful consequences—to the parent or parents themselves (a paternalistic reason), to potential offspring, or to society more generally. An example of the welfare-oriented view would be a program that limits IVF to heterosexual married couples or even to stably married heterosexual couples.

The Ontario Law Reform Commission report contains the most detailed discussion of this issue. A majority of the commission recommended that "stable single women and stable men and women in stable marital or nonmarital unions should be eligible to participate in an artificial conception program."[10] The Ontario commissioners argue that the capacity of a parent or two parents to provide "a proper home environment for the child" should be the principal criterion for participation and that judgments about such capacities should not be left to the discretion of individual physicians but rather should be based on published government regulations.[10]

The Sale and Purchase of Human Gametes   A liberty-oriented approach to this issue would argue that individuals and commercial sperm (and, in the future, oocyte) banks should be free to buy and sell gametes, so long as certain minimal safety standards are met. In contrast, a welfare-oriented view would argue that a voluntary, nonprofit system for donating and distributing gametes may prevent foreseeable harms, and, in any event, better symbolizes social solidarity.

Of the fifteen statements under discussion, the British Warnock Committee report has devoted the most detailed attention to the sale and purchase of gametes. In the tradition of Richard Titmuss[15] the Warnock Committee recommends the establishment of a voluntary, nonprofit system for collecting and distributing gametes in the United Kingdom.[8] Thus, the Warnock Committee implicitly adopts the model of organ procurement and distribution in its attempt to resolve this issue.

Elective Use of the New Reproductive Technologies   On this issue, a liberty-oriented approach would argue that whoever wishes to employ the new reproductive technologies should be free to do so, without regard to infertility status or genetic indications. According to this view, resort to the Repository for Germinal Choice by a fertile couple seeking to produce a "better" baby is ethically acceptable. Similarly, contractual arrangements by couples who are capable of conventional reproduction to have a surrogate carrier substitute for the wife during gestation are, on this view, ethically legitimate.

The welfare-oriented view would restrict the use of clinical IVF and ET to cases in which substantial medical indications exist, for example, infertility or genetic problems. This restriction could be adopted for one or more of the following reasons: (1) to conserve a scarce medical resource for those most in need of it; (2) to prevent the exploitation of poor women; or (3) to reduce the chances that human reproduction will be degraded to the level of the cattle-breeding industry.

This issue has been addressed only indirectly by most of the fifteen statements being analyzed. Many simply assume that the new reproductive technologies will be resorted to only in cases of necessity. Others, by denying the ethical legitimacy of commercial transactions in human reproduction, would render some elective arrangements, for example, surrogate carrier arrangements, infeasible. Most of the fifteen statements oppose the use of the new technologies for social reasons or mere convenience. They thus adopt the welfare- rather than the liberty-oriented view.

Anonymity v. Identification in Cases Involving Third Parties   The liberty-welfare contrast may not apply neatly to this issue. What one may be confronting is contrasting viewpoints on what policies are in the best interests of (that is, promote the welfare of) prospective social parents, third parties, and offspring. Further, the liberties of various moral agents may point one toward different resolutions of this problem. Nonetheless, this issue can be construed in liberty or welfare terms.

According to the liberty-oriented view, prospective social parents should be free either to know or not to know any third parties involved in medically assisted reproduction. Similarly, the offspring of such third-party arrangements should be at liberty to decide whether or not they wish to become acquainted with any third parties. The welfare-oriented view would argue that third-party arrangements will be less complicated and more likely to succeed if the gamete donor or surrogate carrier remains anonymous.

This issue is reminiscent of current debates about adoption policy. The recent statements that have taken an explicit position on anonymity versus identification in the clinical IVF context have advocated anonymity.

Quality Control in Programs Offering the New Reproductive Technologies   The liberty-oriented approach to this issue would argue that clinics involved with the new reproductive technologies should be free to operate and advertise for clients, subject only to such general moral obligations as truth-telling and promise-keeping and general standards of good medical practice. The welfare-oriented approach to this question can take at least two forms. According to one welfare-oriented viewpoint, clinics offering IVF should be *certified* by a pertinent professional organization, for example, the American Fertility Society. A second welfare-oriented viewpoint is that such clinics should be *licensed* by public bodies, for example, departments of health. The goal of both welfare-oriented viewpoints is to promote high standards of practice and to protect potential parents and their offspring from avoidable harm.

The Warnock Committee goes furthest in the direction of licensing, that is, proposing the establishment of a statutory licensing authority to oversee both clinical IVF and laboratory research on human embryos.[8] The Waller Committee assumes that all hospitals that conduct IVF programs have been especially authorized by the Victoria Minister of Health to conduct such programs.[19] The Australian committee proposes that, in addition, a Standing Review and Advisory Body on Fertility, Reproduction, and Related Matters be established in the state of Victoria.[19] In contrast, the Ontario Law Reform Commission recommends that both spheres of government regulation and spheres of professional self-regulation should be created to oversee the new reproductive technologies.[10]

Insurance Coverage for the New Reproductive Technologies   According to the liberty-oriented approach to this issue, people who wish access to the new reproductive technologies are free to find and pay health professionals who will then try to assist

Table 2. Recent Issues in Clinical IVF

	(13) Warnock (UK)	(14) Waller III (Austr.)	(15) Ont. Law Ref. Comm.
(E_1) Screening of Gamete Donors	Yes	—	Yes
(E_2) Freezing of Oocytes	Yes	Yes	—
(E_3) Screening of Prospective Social Parents	—	—	Yes
(E_4) Sale and Purchase of Gametes	No[1]	—	No[2]
(E_5) Elective Use	No[3]	—	—
(E_6) Anonymity of Third Parties	Yes	Yes	Yes
(E_7) Quality Control	Yes	Yes	Yes
(E_8) Insurance Coverage	Yes	—	—

[1]Advocates movement toward a system in which donors are paid only for their expenses
[2]Advocates payment only for "reasonably incurred expenses"
[3]In the discussion of gender selection

them. Similarly, they are free to shop for insurance plans that will cover such services. In contrast, the welfare-oriented approach argues that society has a moral obligation to assist couples who are involuntarily infertile because such infertility seriously disrupts their life-plans and diminishes their happiness.

In this case the welfare-oriented approach presupposes a relatively robust public health insurance system (or at least a publicly guaranteed health insurance system) and then makes the judgement that services to combat involuntary infertility should receive a relatively high priority within that system. The Warnock Committee and Ontario Law Reform Commission reports devote the most sustained attention to the problem of involuntary infertility;[8] the Warnock Committee advocates better organization and, perhaps, more generous funding of infertility treatment programs.[8]

A matrix depicting the positions of three major recent statements on the eight new issues in clinical IVF appears as Table 2.

Analysis

Careful study of Table 2 reveals a general pattern in the responses of the three recent statements. All three statements tend to adopt the welfare-oriented approach to the six controversial clinical issues (numbers E_3 to E_8). That is, the statements accent the need to protect prospective social parents, offspring, third parties, and society as a whole from potential harm. No public statement of a liberty-oriented approach has been published as of this writing. However, U.S. practice in at least some programs and the writings of two leading U.S. scholars[2, 11] reflect strong sympathy for at least some aspects of the liberty-oriented approach.

Conclusion

Between 1979 and 1985 at least 15 public and private committees and commissions issued public statements of the ethics of IVF and ET. Insofar as such bodies received public input, reasoned carefully, and justified their conclusions, their statements provide a useful resource for future deliberations about an important bioethical topic. The reports of these bodies over a period of approximately 7 years also help us to see how ethical thinking about the new reproductive technologies has evolved—at least in the Western industrialized world.

References

1. American Fertility Society: Ethical statement on in vitro fertilization. Fertil Steril 41:12, 1984

2. Andrews LB: New Conceptions: A Consumer's Guide to the Newest Infertility Treatments, Including In Vitro Fertilization, Artificial Insemination, and Surrogate Motherhood. Revised edition. New York, Ballantine Books, 1985

3. Australia, National Health and Medical Research Council, Working Party on Ethics in Medical Research: Ethics in Medical Research. Canberra, Australia, Australian Government Publishing Service, 1983

4. British Medical Association, Working Group on In-Vitro Fertilisation: Interim report on human in vitro fertilisation and embryo replacement and transfer. Br Med J 286:1594, 1983

5. Catholic Bishops of Victoria [Australia]: Submission to the Committee to Examine In Vitro Fertilization. Unpublished document, August 6, 1982

6. Catholic Bishops' Joint Committee on Bio-Ethical Issues [Great Britain]: In Vitro Fertilisation: Morality and Public Policy. Unpublished document, March 2, 1983

7. European Medical Research Councils, Advisory Subgroup: Human in-vitro fertilisation and embryo transfer. Lancet 2:1187, 1983

8. Great Britain, Department of Health and Social Security: Report of the Committee of Inquiry into Human Fertilisation and Embryology (Chairman: Mary Warnock). London, Her Majesty's Stationery Office, July 1984

9. Medical Research Council [Great Britain]: Research related to human fertilisation and embryology. Br Med J 285:1480, 1982

10. Ontario Law Reform Commission: Report on Human Artificial Reproduction and Related Matters. 2 vols. Toronto, Ministry of the Attorney General, 1985

11. Robertson J: Procreative liberty and the control of conception, pregnancy and childbirth. Va Law Rev 69:405, 1975

12. Royal College of Obstetricians and Gynaecologists [Great Britain]: Report of the RCOG Ethics Committee on In Vitro Fertilisation and Embryo Transfer. London, Chameleon Press, March 1983

13. Royal Society [Great Britain]: Human Fertilization and Embryology, London, Royal Society, March 1983

14. Stewart GJ, Cunningham AL, Driscoll GL, et al: Transmission of human T-cell lymphotropic virus type III (HTLV-III) by artificial insemination by donor. Lancet 2:581, 1985

15. Titmuss RM: The Gift Relationship: From Human Blood to Social Policy. New York, Random House, 1972

16. U.S. Department of Health, Education, and Welfare, Ethics Advisory Board: HEW Support of Research Involving Human In Vitro Fertilization and Embryo Transfer. 2 vols. Washington, DC, HEW, May 4, 1979

17. Victoria, Australia, Committee to Consider the Social, Ethical and Legal Issues Arising from In Vitro Fertilization (Chairman: Louis Waller): Interim Report. Unpublished document, September 1982

18. Victoria, Australia, Committee to Consider the Social, Ethical and Legal Issues Arising from In Vitro Fertilization (Chairman: Louis Waller): Report on Donor Gametes in IVF. Unpublished document, August 1983

19. Victoria, Australia, Committee to Consider the Social, Ethical and Legal Issues Arising from In Vitro Fertilization (Chairman: Louis Waller): Report on the Disposition of Embryos Produced by In Vitro Fertilization. Melbourne, FD Atkinson Government Printer, August 1984

20. Walter L: Ethical issues in human in vitro fertilization and embryo transfer. *In* Milunsky A, Annas GJ (eds.): Genetics and the Law III. New York, Plenum Press, 1985, pp. 215–225

The Joseph and Rose Kennedy Institute of Ethics
Center for Bioethics
Georgetown University
Washington, D.C. 20057

Human In Vitro Fertilization

A Conservative View

HANS O. TIEFEL, Ph.D.

Ethical objections to both the means and ends of clinical in vitro fertilization and embryo transfer, as well as of nonclinical applications, are analyzed and evaluated. Morally important but inconclusive arguments consider these procedures to be unnatural or harmful to women. The decisive objection to clinical uses lies in the possible and even likely risk of greater than normal harm to offspring. A discussion of the need and right to have children, and of the relationship of this procedure to abortion and to freezing embryos, concludes the analysis of clinical uses. The ethics of research applications of in vitro fertilization hinges on the status of the embryo. After prefatory conceptual clarification, this article argues for the inclusion of human embryos within protectable humanity, which makes nontherapeutic research unjustifiable. Public decision making and federal research funding are discussed.

(*JAMA* 1982;247:3235–3242)

The extracorporeal engendering of human life that led to the birth of Louise Brown in 1978 struck the world as an awesome medical achievement. Even 3½ years later, the 15th—but this nation's first—child so conceived was fittingly welcomed as the "miracle in Norfolk" (*Washington Post*, Dec 31, 1981, p A-14).

This striking accomplishment offers hope to many of the circa half-million American women whose obstructed or missing Fallopian tubes had seemingly ruled out any chance of having children of their own. Relatively few of the more than 6,000 couples who have applied at the Eastern Virginia Medical School, however, can be helped there or at the other three American clinics.

Two authorities on issues of in vitro fertilization and embryo transfer, LeRoy Walters, PhD, director of the Kennedy Institute's Center for Bioethics, and John D. Biggers, DSc, PhD, the Harvard specialist in human reproductive biology, therefore called for federal support for test-tube conceptions a week after the birth of Elizabeth Carr

From the Department of Religion, the College of William and Mary in Virginia, Williamsburg.

Reprint requests to the Department of Religion, the College of William and Mary in Virginia, Williamsburg, VA 23185 (Dr. Tiefel).

(*Washington Post*, Jan 4, 1982, p A-3). The national government should stop turning its back on childless couples who want babies, according to Dr Walters, particularly since the US Department of Health, Education, and Welfare Ethics Advisory Board had concluded in June 1979 that such funding is "acceptable from an ethical standpoint."[1] The nationwide hearings on whether to lift a 1974 moratorium on such funding, held by the Ethics Advisory Board in 1978 and 1979, elicited similar recommendations. Particularly, medical professionals hope "to break the log jam of prejudice and law, at both state and federal levels, that at present denies infertile couples the blessing of a child by this remarkable method."[2]

This article opposes such recommendations on moral grounds by arguing that this new technology may be a mixed blessing, that federal funding may be blocked not by prejudice but by moral doubts, and that a more cautious or conservative position is justified by valid objections to both means and ends of test-tube babies. I begin with an analysis of objections to the means, specifically the charge that in vitro fertilization and embryo transfer are unnatural and therefore morally wrong.

Unnatural Procreation

The condemnation of this technology as unnatural has at least five meanings, only the last two having moral weight.

1. This procedure may be deemed unnatural simply because it is strange, untried, and even startling. But the same holds true of most scientific breakthroughs and therefore has psychological rather than ethical significance.

2. *Unnatural* may also refer to artificiality: such begetting is not according to nature. Yet our lives are full of ersatz and are the richer for it. When we are personally afflicted with nature's shortcomings, we hope that technological genius will do nature one better. Moreover, resignation to our own impotence may be even more unnatural. In vitro fertilization may therefore be defended as a saving detour. It is no more questionable in its artificiality than any novel alternative that takes us where we want to be.

3. A more profound meaning of *unnatural* lies in its objection to the boundless and therefore illegitimate expansion of science. Insatiable scientific scrutiny will rob us not only of mystery but of respect for the beginning of human life. The Reverend Jerry Falwell expresses this widespread apprehension that scientists are "delving into an area that is far too sacred for human beings to be involved in" (*Washington Post*, Dec 29, 1981, pp A-1, A-16).

It is indeed true that science knows only problems and challenges, not mysteries. The empirical eye beholds no value. But it is also true that the more we know scientifically, the more we become aware of what we do not know—a conclusion not wholly devoid of humility. And those who regard the beginnings of human life with humanistic or religious eyes will see more mystery the deeper they look. Scientific familiarity with early forms of human life need not breed contempt. Our blindness to humanizing and revering visions of life may arise rather from our naive premise that the scientific way of looking is the only way to see.

4. *Unnatural* may also imply serious violations of the dignity of persons and of marital and parental relationships. Obtaining semen for fertilization by masturbating may offend as an unnatural act. Some theologians deplore an unnatural separation of procreation from sexual union. In discussing the papal condemnation of in vitro fertilization, a Catholic writer insists that "the natural forces and laws which govern the begetting of human beings need to be respected," and "what God has united—the procreative and unitive aspects of sexual intercourse—let no man put asunder . . . by technological procreation."[3]

This principle condemns both artificial means of birth control and in vitro fertilization. Yet this norm of nature—invoked in the name of God rather than of its more likely source in medieval philosophy—stands in need of serious revision on both counts. The truth of the inseparability of sexuality and procreation may be intuitively known. But to those who are invincibly ignorant on this point, it appears both more rational and more loving to separate with harmless prevention what otherwise might lead to unintended results. Similarly, both reflection and charity might recommend the separation of procreation from sex with a Petri dish to fulfill the natural desire for offspring.

The perverseness of that version of natural law that condemns in vitro fertilization appears clearly and ironically in the fact that the couples who are here accused would be overjoyed if they could but link their sexual union with procreation. A more reasonable vision of both the working of God and of nature recognizes greater human freedom, in which persons become co-workers with God, jointly improving on an impaired nature.[4]

Similar objections to extracorporeal conception appear in Protestant objections to the assault on "the nature of human parentage by putting the bodily transmission of life completely asunder from bodily lovemaking."[5] It is unnatural for the hand of technology to grasp what for all time has emerged from a loving human embrace.

Granted that it would be unnatural if one could do it in the old-fashioned way but preferred the clinical method. As it stands, the charge is simply unconvincing that this medical help violates the nature of lovemaking or parenting. An adoption analogy applies instead: the extra trouble gladly borne expresses parental caring and reassures all doubters.

5. The last meaning of the charge that this new technology is unnatural refers not to means but to ends, namely, to the fear that this innovation may prove harmful. Such harm would be widely conceived: mental or physical, emotional or social, possible or actual, detracting from health or worth of any or all parties. That, in my judgment, is the crucial issue, especially as it pertains to the offspring. But that problem is more familiar under the rubric of risk or harm.

Risk to the
Would-be Mother

LeRoy Walters succinctly describes the kinds of risks to the woman in in vitro fertilization and embryo transfer:

> (1) pretreatment of the woman with hormones to induce superovulation, a therapy which occasionally produces ovarian cysts; (2) removal of oocytes by means of laparoscopy, a surgical procedure which requires general anesthesia; (3) potential damage to the uterus during embryo transfer . . . (4) the risks which accompany careful monitoring of the pregnancy, for example, the risks of amniocentesis . . . (5) the risk of ectopic pregnancy.[6]

The second of these seems to be the most important. But to assess that risk, one needs statistics of normal impregnation. Biggers concludes that, normally, one can expect between 69% and 78% embryonic loss, which is consistent with data showing that it takes an average of four months of regular inseminations to achieve pregnancy by artificial insemination or four months of sexual activity to achieve normal pregnancy.[7] Thus even under normal conditions, the required number of embryo transfers will, on average, be four times as great as the number of births one can expect.[8]

The success rates for laparoscopies and embryo transfer have been much lower. In their early work, Edwards and Steptoe claimed two births out of 68 laparoscopies. Biggers concluded in February 1981 that when an ovum is discovered, the probability of obtaining a live birth by the Steptoe-Edwards method was about 0.044.[9] That appears to have been the method that yielded 30 failures to impregnate 30 patients in 1980 for Drs Howard and Georgeanna Jones in Norfolk.

With fertility-inducing drugs, however, the odds apparently improve. More than one ovum can be obtained, which allows more than one embryonic implant. In 1981 the Norfolk clinic reported six pregnancies in some 50 tries. Australian results have similarly improved.[10-12] Steptoe claimed that as of Oct 31, 1981, out of 436 laparoscopies, 337 implantations, and 74 pregnancies, eight babies had been born and 48 women were still pregnant (*Washington Post*, Dec 23, 1981, p A-24).

Despite such improvements and the prospects of better odds in the future, the success rate still resembles lottery statistics more than promising therapy. Infertile couples, perhaps misled by their own desperation and unqualified news stories, present themselves as patients when their role is more that of subjects in clinical trials.

Even if the meager success rate is explained to couples and they consent to the odds, there are moral limits to surgical risk, time, resources, and stress on human relationships. The fact that prospective parents say that they will do anything to have a baby of their own is not necessarily a moral justification. "Doing anything" may not only be inimical to oneself but neglects ties and duties to others. To use an odd example, one research team supports the claim that a pregnancy actually resulted from their transplant by stating that "the patient abstained from intercourse during the entire treatment cycle as a result of her own firm and deliberate decision."[13] There is no word whether the husband shared in that decision, which seemed to benefit only the researchers. Similarly, one wonders if the delivery of these babies by cesarean section is always necessary and should be one of the risks of this procedure.

Low success rates, repeated risks, disruption of lives, unneeded impositions, and financial and emotional costs to would-be parents as well as to those supporting them are serious moral problems. But all such liabilities are voluntarily assumed by those who hope to benefit from this technology. That is not true for the would-be child.

Risk to the Would-be Child

Is there risk to a child conceived in vitro and transferred in embryo form into the uterus? It seems that nobody knows for sure. A recent review of the probability of producing a congenitally abnormal baby is offered by Biggers.[9] His conclusion, that the danger of increased congenital defects is not high, seems to be based on the spontaneous elimination of most abnormalities before birth rather than on assurance of no increase in abnormal embryos. But there is no guarantee that this would happen,[14,15] assuming that such loss is reassuring and of little moral relevance.

When the count of children so conceived was 21, only one was reported to have been born with a serious defect, which will be repaired by cardiac surgery, according to the *Washington Post* (Jan 4, 1982, p A-3). But Walters' conclusion that the procedures do not pose "unreasonable risk"[16] is both sanguine and premature.

Not only are there insufficient data about the effects on humans, but the relevance of in vitro studies on animals is in doubt. Thus, some researchers (Mastroianni, Brackett, Gould) call for more animal studies, while others (Soupart, Biggers) dismiss that as irrelevant. The Ethics Advisory Board found a golden mean by giving its imprimatur to both animal and human studies.

In any case, knowledge about risk requires long-range human studies, decades in which to follow up children so conceived into reproductive age and through a normal life span. Not only time but sufficient numbers are required. Schlesselman, in a careful statistical study, concludes that 99.3% to 99.5% of chromosomal abnormalities are eliminated in vivo through spontaneous abortion or fetal death. Such low survival rates of abnormal fetuses imply that even a doubling of abnormalities of in vitro implantations would result in only two or three additional abnormalities per 1,000 live births. Thus, "a large number of births would be required to provide a definitive assessment of risk."[8] The morally crucial answer to the question of risk to the would-be child thus requires a great number of births and much time. The answers seem a long way off, and we must make moral judgments without the benefit of knowing all the facts.

Several responses to this factual uncertainty of risk are troubling. Ethicists have stated repeatedly that risk to the child conceived in vitro would be acceptable if it is no greater than risk to children conceived in vivo. But it is not helpful to say that when no one knows the actual risk. Here ethicists avoid the dilemma.

Others recommend that if couples with recessive defects decide to have children, then the assumed lower risk of in vitro fertilization must be acceptable.[9] Or, since "it is not general practice in this country to interfere with reproductive options facing couples who may be at increased risk for having abnormal offspring,"[17,18] it is held to be right to inform and to accede to a couple's decision here as well.

This acceding role of medical conscience is the opposite extreme of paternalism. Implementing the couple's choice unavoidably makes the physician a part of that decision. But surely the physician should be neither father nor slave, but a responsible participant. If medical judgment anticipates harm, he is obligated to keep patients "from harm and injustice" by virtue of the Hippocratic oath.

Medical proponents of extracorporeal fertilization also offer ethical relativism as a way of overcoming the problem of risk. Individual wishes become king. The fact that a couple wants this procedure is held to make it morally right. For example, one researcher claims that "childless couples' rights to utilize whatever methods and techniques are available to produce wanted offspring far exceeds and surpasses the rights and privileges of the critics who would condemn and suppress scientific work directed toward helping them to accomplish this aim."[14]

Disregarding the lese majesty against science, this is ethical relativism, where individual choice or preference settles moral issues. Medicine should avoid such quicksand, for shifting individual preferences offer no solid support for the objective values undergirding medicine and research. If one lets go of objective and universal values to defer to dubious patient choice, one also relinquishes the heart of medicine, whose life is the objective value of healing and of doing no harm.

A Proposal for the Ethics of Risk

How, then, is one to assess the moral issue of unknown risk to the would-be child? The subject, the would-be child, must first be clearly defined lest we confuse our responsibilities to existing and to future children. For offspring who are actually on the way, we must allow great risk when that is the only option for their continued existence. To the would-be child that is not yet conceived, we have no such obligation. Our responsibilities to living offspring, before and after birth, should not be undercut by the risks they face. But offspring who are concepts rather than conceptions may not claim that immunity. We literally do not owe them a living.

Though no one knows for sure, there is some justification for deeming in vitro fertilization to be harmful to offspring thus conceived. The great embryonic and fetal loss, compared with natural pregnancies, is good reason for saying that this mode of begetting is more dangerous. Moreover, the dimensions of risk may not even be known. To a layman there are repeated surprises in the way in which risk studies appear about therapies that were long thought to be safe. Even medical professionals seem surprised by the latent effect of thalidomide or diethylstilbestrol. To create an artificial environment, to handle, stimulate, and disturb human life at its very beginning when its building blocks are being laid, is to risk damage to the finished construct, even for those few structures that survive spontaneous collapse and demolition.

As best we can, we owe every child a fair chance at physical and mental health. This principle, which is so often misused to justify the destruction of seriously ill fetuses or newborns, is fittingly applied to the would-be child. We must weigh the chances for the well-being of the child while we yet have a choice about initiating this life. Would-be parents have moral obligations to a would-be child. The resolve to have a child of one's own must be tied to a love that seeks the best for that child. To be sure, no parents can guarantee health to future offspring. Nor can they secure safety from nuclear war, a harmful environment, or other dangers over which they have little or no control. But every parent owes every child-to-be reasonable care not to take chances with its health, as every obstetrician explains to every mother-to-be. And the uncertain risks inherent in in vitro fertilization are definitely avoidable by abstinence from this particular technology.

It makes good moral sense never to beget offspring when would-be parents cannot reasonably ensure a future child a fair chance at health. When there are untried risks and even indications of greater than normal risk, "one cannot ethically choose for a child the unknown hazards that he must face, and simultaneously choose to give him life in which to face them."[19] For would-be mothers to undertake risks and burdens for themselves and for consenting partners is one thing. For them knowingly to place future children at risk is quite another. No one has the moral right to endanger a child while there is yet the option of whether the child shall come into existence. That is the crucial and decisive ethical argument against the clinical use of in vitro fertilization. That also makes this procedure unnatural in the sense of being possibly harmful to human beings.

It is misleading and flippant to object that we should ask the children so conceived what they thought of the risks as objections to their being conceived. For if they turn out to be healthy, they are lucky winners in this technological gamble. If handicapped, they would only have the choice between their burdened life or no existence at all. Whether they say yes or no, the moral choice for actually existing children should generally be for life. That is why the choice exists only for would-be children. The dilemma of risk before conception cannot be resolved after the fact.

Ramsey[20] made the crucial moral point about risk to the future child a decade ago. That seems to have made little impact. A survey of the literature yields no medical researcher who thinks that this is one procedure that should not be used. None of the medical experts rejects this risky technology that is being tested even as it is used on women and their babies.[21]

One subtle but significant threat to children so conceived has not yet been mentioned because it is one of the certain rather than likely problems. The suspicion—and guilt on the part of parents—will be unavoidable that whatever health problems develop are the result of this unique genesis. And uncertainty about the future is apt to create anxiety. The possibility of unknown problems yet to come will overshadow the lives of these children, of their parents, and surely also of their medical "creators" and monitors.

The Need and the Right to Have Children

The claim that possible and even likely increased risk to offspring is sufficient reason for opposing this technology seems harsh toward people who desperately want to become parents. That desperation has also been criticized, however, by a surprising coalition of feminists, humanists, and religious moralists who object to social expectations that bind women too closely to their reproductive capacities or make meaningful lives dependent on parenthood. The anxiety of infertile couples is said to result from dehumanizing socialization in which having a child is the ultimate need and in which infertility is seen as personal failure and a sign of worthlessness.

The obvious recommendations of these critics is to reform self-concepts and social expectations rather than to indulge traditional mores. Humanists insist that anyone is endowed with dignity simply because he or she is a person. And in the perspective of biblical faith, one one has value and standing as a child of God regardless of procreative achievement. But I do admit that such liberating insights may be overpowered by ingrained social expectations; human natures are not changed overnight. In any case, having children is surely a great if not a necessary good. Its facilitation may claim sympathy and at least prima facie support.

A second criticism of having to have children is that there are too many children needing parents already. Therefore, "we do not need to improve the supply of children so much as we need to improve their distribution."[22] Our obligations to existing children obviate the need for going to great pains to create others. The solution is to adopt children. It is true that there is a shortage of the "right" children for adoption, since widespread abortion decreases the supply. But we are not about to run out of minority and Third World orphans.

The need to adopt rather than to resort to risky procreation is an extension of the earlier claim that we owe much to existing offspring but we do not owe a living to would-be or wished-for children. That may sound unrealistic, however, since would-be parents in the in vitro programs insist on children genetically their own. Yet this insistence on biologic offspring also comes under heavy attack.

One of the would-be parents who testified at the hearings of the Ethics Advisory Board expressed his opposition to adoption in these words: "I am an individual, I am proud of some of my personal qualities, and maybe we have genetic qualities that we would like to see reproduced. It is a basic human urge to be your own parent."[23] Yet pride is never a good reason for becoming a parent, not only because one never knows how children will turn out but because the motive is self-serving. To be sure, parents often delight in likenesses they see reflected in their children. But that reflection should not be bought at the price of even unknown risk to the well-being of the child. Moreover, it "is not worth opening the hornet's nest of reproductive technology for the privilege of having one's child derive from one's own egg or sperm."[21]

Couples aspiring to be in vitro parents may respond that their quest for a child biologically their own is not an issue of motives or privilege but of rights. *Right* here means entitlement or a service that should be provided. Yet there is neither a moral nor a legal right to have children in a positive or enabling sense. One has the right to try to beget them, but children or chances to have them are not owed to anyone. Calls for federal funding of in vitro fertilization based on rights are as persuasive as demands for printing presses to fulfill the right of free speech.[24] There is no right to have children in this affirmative sense. This holds true not only of the law but of Western religious traditions, in which having children may be a command but is never a right. Children are gifts of God to which believers have no claims, either before or after birth.

In Vitro Fertilization and Abortion

The intentional destruction of embryonic and fetal life evokes criticism. It is true that in vitro programs reject flawed embryos, closely monitor pregnancies, and include amniocentesis and possible abortion. Yet it makes no sense to researchers to implant abnormal embryos, which would either be spontaneously aborted or result in damage to the child. Also, the close control of pregnancies or abortion is usually not compulsory but is left to the discretion of the pregnant woman. No one wants defective offspring. That would be traumatic not only to the child and its parents but to the researchers and their insurers.

A discussion of the morality of abortion is not appropriate here. But in vitro fertilization places abortion in a new light. The would-be parents have gone to such lengths to conceive. Does that persistence and intent create special obligations to the life thus conceived? Or does the willingness to consider and resort to abortion imply that the commitment to a child was not that total after all? One may want a child of one's own for better but not for worse. That may be incompatible with the loyalty that should bind parents to children.

What of the medical mediator? Ordinarily, physicians face abortion requests when they had nothing to do with initiating the life that is now to be ended. But in external fertilization, the physician is the third person without whom it would not have been possible. Does the fact that the clinician has had a hand in the process from the start create special responsibilities to the being thus brought into life? Clinical in vitro fertilization thus uniquely confronts medicine with the tensions between life-giving and death-dealing medical interventions.

The physician's obligation to succeed without a mishap or to avoid research mistakes may well create a conflict of interest with the flawed fetus. Any abnormality in the end result reflects on the procedure and on the researcher/physician. That would be true even if this new technology had nothing to do with the aberration. There is, then, an inherent impetus to jettison any problem pregnancy. The greatest hazard to the unborn may not lie in the vicissitudes of pregnancies as such or in close monitoring but in the physician's desire for a perfect child.[25] There is much disagreement about moral obligations to diseased unborn[26] and even to seriously ill newborns, but in the context of extracorporeal conception, the physician may have a direct stake not in the treatment of the sick but in their termination.

A third problem extends beyond the physician/patient or researcher/subject relationship. Pregnancies, abortions, and births are not only private but public events. Legal and political implications, funding of research, and the use of medical resources make those events public. In regard to public policy, it seems incongruous that our society destroys unborn human life by the millions while also going to great pains to find new ways of creating it. Even strong advocates of abortion must find that morally puzzling, unless, of course, human lives have value only when their bearers wish so and say so.

If one deems consistency toward the value of human embryos to be a virtue, one may also be troubled by the use of intrauterine devices. Since the fertilized human egg is acknowledged as precious in the clinical in vitro setting, should it be discarded without a second thought in birth control?

Freezing Human Embryos

Superovulation yields more ova, more implants, and reduces the need for repeated laparoscopies. But what should be done with "surplus" embryos? Both Australian and British centers have temporarily resolved the problem by "putting it on ice." Freezing was the alternative to discarding the embryos, which could be sustained in no other way.

Freezing also makes sense in another way. The hormones used to induce superovulation may have a detrimental effect on implantation and on early embryonic development. Freezing oocytes or embryos would allow implantation in the subsequent cycle when the woman no longer suffers aftereffects from hormones or from surgery and anesthesia.[27]

A third proposed benefit, recommended by Steptoe and Edwards, lies in banks of frozen embryos for donation to other women, permitting "prenatal adoption" by infertile couples (*New York Times*, Feb 11, 1982, p A-26).

How is one to evaluate this morally? Freezing embryos is particularly unnerving to persons who think that even the earliest forms of human life are special. Here human life is put on hold, as it were. Even if one wants to avoid the judgment that this is unnatural, prolonged freezing may rob a thawed and growing life of its genetic progenitors, of its roots and support. Such a Buck Rogers of the 21st century would lack memories of lost ties, but genuine bonds might well be lost. It is also not too far-fetched to think that once the progenitors are forgotten or gone, these suspended beings may lose their natural protectors to become interesting research material, as may already be happening with embryos incidentally recovered during hysterectomies.

Freezing even for long periods seems to damage only the quantity but not the quality of animal embryos,[28,29] but whether this is true for humans is again unknown. Therefore, the same worries about risk of in vitro fertilization apply here. It would be preferable to freeze ova rather than embryos, since the former are not yet genetically unique lives. And—assuming that the earlier moral arguments against extracorporeal conception will not dissuade anyone—it would be the lesser evil to freeze surplus embryos. The only other practical option, once they have been conjured into existence, is to discard them, a practice that has been described as "a matter solely between a doctor and his plumber."[30] Even if freezing were to entail additional risks, including those of experimentation, it would at least give embryos a chance to live.

As to prenatal adoption, the legal unclarities of who belongs to whom and who owes what to whom would be legion. But again, an acknowledgement of the intrinsic value of the human embryo might also see this mode of life as better than none.

Nonclinical In Vitro Fertilization

This discussion has focused on clinical applications, in which embryo transfer follows in vitro fertilization. Nonclinical uses do not aim at creating offspring but at increasing our understanding of earliest human development. For example, Soupart applied for federal funds to establish genetic risk involved in obtaining preimplantation embryos, using tissue culture methods. His research would focus on the first six days of human embryonic development and would entail the death of embryos.[31]

Nonclinical uses raise the problem of the status of human embryos. That is not problematic in clinical settings, except for the discard and freezing issues, because due care is assured by everyone's expectation that what begins here will soon be one of us in the full sense. But if the embryo is to have no future, can it be treated as human tissue? Is there something about it that would prevent nontherapeutic experimentation? This question was already controversial in fetal experimentation[32] and is predictably difficult here.

The problem, however, is often obscured or avoided by the way in which one refers to the embryo. Prefatory linguistic analysis is therefore essential.

Leading and Misleading Language

Embryo is used as a vague term. It refers both to the "fertilized egg" and to the "developing individual from one week after conception." Persistent use of the first definition tends to reduce this entity to its earlier components. It relegates the growing being to what it was before becoming a genetically unique life form. The same is true of "product of conception" or "product of in vitro fertilization." When researchers speak that way, they may simply be talking shop. When lay persons use such phrases, they refer the embryo to its past and therefore are prone to exclude this being from any future and from inclusion in protectable humanity.

Another way of begging or avoiding the issue of the human status of the embryo is to refer to it as cells, tissues, cellular entities, or human materials. These terms describe us all but would never be allowed to define our status. If that were all the embryo is or should be, there would be no problem. Of course one may experiment with tissue and materials.

Zygote, blastocyst, or conceptus may be more precise, but as all scientific terms, they cannot express human value. To speak scientifically is to use empirical language that cannot accommodate what is special about human beings. To read the technical literature about in vitro fertilization and embryo transfer is to read about mice, monkeys, mammals, and men. Indeed, men are animals biologically, and this is the proper way for scientists to speak. But this shop language resists values and claims about the uniqueness of man. Perhaps if one speaks this language long enough, it becomes definitive and intolerant of tongues that ascribe unique and precious value to humans.

A third example of the tendency of language to lead or mislead is to refer to human embryos as potential life.[25] If it were not life already with all the potential one could ask for, the problem would again disappear. The recent discussions of when life begins are similarly confused. If anything, in vitro fertilization shows that life begins at conception—as if that had ever been in doubt. Some object that life has no beginnings, only ends. But that misleads, for the question is not life per se but the genesis of individual human life. Also, the problem is not when life begins but when it shall have human status, when it shall be important and count as one of us.

A question-begging way of posing the issue of status is to ask whether the embryo qualifies as a person,[33] since *person* usually means a being that can think. Embryos, fetuses, and probably even newborns cannot think. Therefore, they tend to be excluded from protectable humanity and are ranked with lower animals. The question is why *person* rather than perhaps *human being* should be the key term.

Linguistic false leads also emerge from another direction. Opponents condemn "manufacturing test-tube babies." This obscures the facts that procreation has always been in human hands, that the baby merely spent a minute part of its development outside the mother's body and that it is dehumanizing to manufacture babies. The expression "manipulation of life" has similar emotive quality, for, by definition, all manipulation of humans is bad. This, too, shows that we need to watch our language and that all sides are tempted to gain easy victories with verbal sleight of hand.

The Status of the Embryo

The ethics of nonclinical in vitro fertilization hangs on the decision about status. The Ethics Advisory Board agreed "that the human embryo is entitled to profound respect: but this respect does not necessarily encompass the full legal and moral rights attributed to persons."[1] That amounts to a polite bow in the direction of the embryo before dispatching it for tissue cultures. The key question is whether one may use the embryo in nontherapeutic experiments, whether one may use it up. The board said that, at least for 14 days, one may do so. How much profound respect the embryo enjoys as it is being fixed in slides remains in doubt. In any case, the respect due falls short of never using such human life as a means only.

This peculiar use of "respect" also explains the board's strange conclusion that research on human in vitro fertilization was "ethically acceptable" in the sense of still being legitimately controverted. That controversy hinges on embryonic status. Neither the board nor I can prove our beliefs about embryonic status, but I shall nevertheless offer reasons for a more inclusive vision of humanity.

The problem with embryonic status lies partly in our inconsistency. On the one hand, we know that we, at least our bodily selves, began as embryos. If we are special, embryos are special. Even Mr Edwards is reported to have said at the birth of Louise Brown, "The last time I saw the baby it was just eight cells in a test tube. It was beautiful then, and it's still beautiful now" (*Newsweek*, Aug 7, 1978, p 69). That may have been poetic license, but it shows that the value of human beings is linked to our embryonic origin. We also assent to a practical wisdom in the law that allows offspring to bring suit for malpractice against researchers for harm to themselves as embryos.

On the other hand, we acknowledge the value of increased knowledge about earliest human development, such as chromosome constitution of gametes and human infertility. The simplest and most useful way to find out is to experiment, to look through the window that has been opened on early development by in vitro fertilization.[34] Only in this case, our seeing fatally affects the embryo. Such looking may not be done with human beings. We are therefore inclined to exclude the embryo from human status.

This ambiguity growing out of opposing motives was offered to the Ethics Advisory Board by a philosopher who proposed that the status of this being may be judged only in retrospect. If it should be damaged as an embryo and be malformed later, it is fitting to say that the initial harm was an "injury to someone." But if the embryo does not live to term, we may not say that.[35] That ascribes status ("someone") according to what we want to do with the embryo.

Such flexibility is convenient. But historical instances of ascribing human status selectively have not turned out to be our better moments. It is also true that one of the rules of ethics is consistency. If any embryos count as human beings, all do.

It may be a sign of ferment or of poverty in contemporary philosophy, but there is less and less consensus about who counts and why. Handicapped newborns are pushed into the limbo of deferred personhood until we can decide whether they should live.[36] Fetuses are said to have value only when their potentiality is wanted by their progenitors.[37] And a chimpanzee is held to be of more value than a human zygote.[38]

The general trend to restrict humanity to rational and volitional beings may solve a host of medical problems. It cuts the Gordian knot of whether to treat or to protect human beings at the borders of life with a definitional sword that strikes off all who cannot reason. But our medical, humanistic, and religious traditions have been less fierce. We have held and should continue to hold that every human life counts, regardless of capacity. In this more compassionate vision it is fitting to include even the earliest versions of ourselves within the human community.

A Proposal for Embryonic Status

We should be consistent with those perceptions that bind us to our earliest bodily identity. The embryo is indeed someone. The biologic definition of the start of individual human life should coincide with the scope of our ascriptions of human status. The burden of proof should lie with those who would divide them. Nor should we avoid the costly dilemmas that follow from drawing the circle of humanity so widely as to include all human life.

Granted, the embryo looks nothing like us. But appearances undergo great changes in a life span. Granted, the unborn have and should have fewer rights than the born, as children have fewer rights than adults. The minimal rights we should share with even the earliest versions of ourselves are the rights not to be used merely as a means to the ends of others and not to be killed. Even in its initial stages, human beings deserve the kind of respect that excludes dissection and other scientifically promising but fatal designs.

It is true that we reason and decide and embryos do not (or, then we did not). But the potential is there, unless we cut if off. Medicine—in contrast to Hegelian philosophers—has a stake in not tying the status of human beings wholly to mind. We are also our bodies, and our special value inheres in both body and mind. Medicine is dedicated to both physical and mental welfare.

Furthermore, medicine is treating us at ever earlier stages of life. With fetal medicine and surgery it becomes harder to regard the unborn as lacking human status. Those physicians whose expertise constantly expands toward the start of life may regard even unborn lives as precious patients. The intrinsic value of early human lives interferes with the work of researchers, however, who are dedicated to general knowledge rather than to specific patients. Ironically, advancing medical care is impossible without research. Still, therapeutic gain will always lie in the future for researchers who study subjects, not patients. But for physicians—who are devoted to patients here and now, able or disabled, old or young, vocal or mute—it cannot be right to use up lives, even those lives that have just begun.

Comment

Both clinical and nonclinical in vitro fertilization are morally unjustifiable, the former because it entails possible and even likely risk to offspring, the latter because it treats the earliest forms of human life as having less than human standing, disavowing even minimal forms of respect owed to earliest bodily selves.

The cost of these conclusions is to seek alternative solutions for female sterility,[39] to slow down research with human embryos, and to limit experiments with embryos to therapeutic projects.

Pandora's Box

Several ethically troubling variations of in vitro possibilities have not been mentioned. What it means to be a mother becomes more problematic with ovum donation and surrogate or womb mothers. Particularly able or attractive women may donate their ova to enrich the human race, the female equivalent of Nobel Prize semen donors. Genetic alteration of human embryos may no longer be far off now that the embryo is accessible. And animal husbandry may offer clues of what else can be found in this box that has now been opened, which even a distinguished ethics committee was unwilling to keep closed, and which should not be propped open with federal funds.

Decision Making for Federal Research Funds

Recent medical advances have given rise to research projects that Congress is not sure it wants to fund. Advisory commissions have been appointed to explore the ethical soundness of such ventures. The current President's Commission for the Study of Ethical Problems in Medicine and Biomedical and Behavioral Research is the third federal advisory group. It may not last longer than its predecessors, if only because no one can remember its title. But ethicists naturally wish it a long life, for it makes moral problems explicit and decisions publicly accountable. My criticisms of the Ethics Advisory Board should not be taken to imply a rejection of such institutions. Nor should disagreement with its findings detract from an appreciation of its conscientious effort and its dilemma of facing irreconcilable claims.

My objection to each of these commissions is to their composition. Their memberships have always had a majority of medical professionals, usually well-known researchers. But a life commitment to the advancement of medical science will never look kindly on the objection that there may be some research that, while scientifically sound, should never be done—as nontherapeutic research with human embryos.

Such composition of ethics boards creates an inbuilt conflict of interest. It is analogous to loading environmental protection commissions with captains of industry. Nor does any board need so many medical members, for it will solicit expert testimony from outside sources in any case. If such boards are going to be sound and permanent aids to public decision making, they must not compromise their integrity before they start. Imbalance toward professional interests will cast suspicion even on correct moral decisions.

This study was supported by a grant from the Racoon Ridge Foundation.

References

1. Protection of human subjects; HEW support of human in vitro fertilization and embryo transfer. Report of the Ethics Advisory Board. *Federal Register* 1979; 44(June 18):35033–35058.

2. Thompson IE (reviewer), Grobstein C: *From Chance to Purpose: An Appraisal of External Human Fertilization*, book review. *N Engl J Med* 1982;306:51.

3. Moraczewski AS: In vitro fertilization and Christian marriage. *Linacre Q* 1979;46:302–318.

4. Moore JW: Human in vitro fertilization: Can we support it? *The Christian Century*, April 22, 1981, pp 442–446.

5. Ramsey P: *Fabricated Man: The Ethics of Genetic Control*. New Haven, Conn, Yale University Press, 1970, p 136.

6. Walters L: *Ethical Issues in Human In Vitro Fertilization and Research Involving Early Human Embryos*, report to the HEW Ethics Advisory Board. Washington, DC, US Dept of Health, Education, and Welfare, Sept 8, 1978, p 18.

7. Biggers JD: *In Vitro Fertilization, Embryo Culture and Embryo Transfer in the Human*, review for the HEW Ethics Advisory Board. Washington, DC, US Dept of Health, Education, and Welfare, Sept 15, 1978, p 11.

8. Schlesselman JJ: How does one assess the risk of abnormalities from human in vitro fertilization? *Am J Obstet Gynecol* 1979;135:135–148.

9. Biggers JD: In vitro fertilization and embryo transfer in human beings. *N Engl J Med* 1981;304:336–342.

10. And now—test-tube twins on the way, news. *New Scientist* 1980;88:758.

11. Wood C, Trounson AO, Leeton JF, et al: A clinical assessment of nine pregnancies obtained by in vitro fertilization and embryo transfer. *Fertil Steril* 1981;35:502–508.

12. Trounson AO, Leeton JF, Wood C, et al: Pregnancies in humans by fertilization in vitro and embryo transfer in the controlled ovulatory cycle. *Science* 1981;212:681–682.

13. Lapota A, Johnson IWH, Hoult IJ, et al: Pregnancy following intrauterine implantation of an embryo obtained by in vitro fertilization of a preovulatory egg. *Fertil Steril* 1980;33:117–120.

14. Schumacher GFB, Brackett BG, Fletcher J, et al: In vitro fertilization of human ova and blastocyst transfer. An invitational symposium. *J Reprod Med* 1973;11:192–200.

15. *Assessing Biomedical Technologies: An Inquiry Into the Nature of the Process*, National Research Council, Assembly of Behavioral and Social Sciences, Committee on the Life Sciences and Social Policy. Washington, DC, National Academy of Sciences, 1975, pp 13–31.

16. Walters L: Ethicist approves test-tube baby research. *Science* 1982;215:382–383.

17. Transcript of meeting 3 of the US Dept of Health, Education, and Welfare Ethics Advisory Board (testimony of J. D. Schulman), Bethesda, Md, Sept 15, 1978, p 115.

18. Evans MI, Mukherjee AB, Schulman JD: Human in vitro fertilization. *Obstet Gynecol Surv* 1980;35:71–81.

19. Kass LR: Babies by means of in vitro fertilization: Unethical experiments on the unborn? *N Engl J Med* 1971;285:1174–1179.

20. Ramsey P: Shall we reproduce? *JAMA* 1972;220:1346–1350, 1480–1485.

21. Hubbard R: Test tube babies: Solution or problem? *Technol Rev*, March/April 1980, pp 10–12.

22. Transcript of meeting 4 of the US Dept of Health, Education, and Welfare Ethics Advisory Board (testimony of T. Powledge), Boston, Oct 13, 1978, p 63.

23. Transcript of the US Dept of Health, Education, and Welfare, Ethics Advisory Board Public Hearing, San Francisco, Nov 14, 1978, p 89.

24. Nelson JR: In vitro ethics. *The Christian Century*, Jan 27, 1982, pp 78–79.

25. Flannery DM, Weisman CD, Lipsett CR, et al: Test tube babies: Legal issues raised by in vitro fertilization. *Georgetown Law J* 1979;67:1295–1345.

26. Tiefel HO: The unborn: Human values and responsibilities. *JAMA* 1978;239:2263–2267.

27. Frozen test-tube embryos raise hot debate. *New Scientist* 1981;90:747.

28. Lindquist G, Liedholm P: Deep freezing of in vitro fertilized human eggs. *Arch Androl* 1980;5:95–96.

29. Transcript of meeting 3 of US Dept of Health, Education, and Welfare Ethics Advisory Board (testimony of J. D. Biggers), Bethesda, Md, Sept 16, 1978, pp 272–273.

30. Kass LR: Making babies—the new biology and the 'old' morality. *Public Interest* 1972;26:18–56.

31. Transcript of meeting 3 of the US Dept of Health, Education, and Welfare Ethics Advisory Board (testimony of P. Soupart), Bethesda, Md, Sept 15, 1978, pp 143, 148.

32. Tiefel HO: The cost of fetal research: Ethical considerations. *N Engl J Med* 1976;294:85–90.

33. Grobstein C: *From Chance to Purpose: An Appraisal of External Human Fertilization*. Reading, Mass, Addison-Wesley Publishing Co Inc, 1981, p. 37.

34. Grobstein C: External human fertilization. *Sci Am* 1979;340:57–67.

35. Transcript of meeting 4 of the US Dept of Health, Education, and Welfare Ethics Advisory Board (testimony of S. Gorvitz), Boston, Oct 14, 1978, p 266.

36. Marks FR: The defective newborn: An analytic framework for a policy dialog, in Jonsen AR, Garland MJ (eds): *Ethics of Newborn Intensive Care*. Berkeley, Calif, Institute of Government Studies, 1976, pp 97–125.

37. Fletcher J: *Humanhood: Essays in Biomedical Ethics*. Buffalo, Prometheus Books, 1979, p 96.

38. Belliotti RA: Morality and in vitro fertilization. *Bioethics Q* 1980;2:6–19.

39. Hodgen GD: In vitro fertilization and alternatives. *JAMA* 1981;246:590–597.

A Criticism of Moral Conservatism's View of In Vitro Fertilization and Embryo Transfer

RICHARD M. ZANER

In a recent article, Hans O. Tiefel argues for "a more cautious or conservative position" on in vitro fertilization/embryo transfer (IVF/ET) for human beings.[1] His argument is not merely against recommendations for federal support for such programs but is to provide a "decisive" moral objection to this technology itself—whether used therapeutically or for purely research purposes.[2] His major point concerns the supposed "unknown risks" to the offspring. A subsidiary but also key point is that the requirements of informed consent cannot be fulfilled with regard to the offspring.

A good deal of research into animal and human reproductivity has been conducted, with much evidence collected over the past decade from clinical applications of IVF/ET.[2-6] Nonetheless, Tiefel contends, "nobody knows for sure" about possible damages that may result to the infant-product of this technology. Because of this, we are obliged to make moral judgments in the absence of certain knowledge, and this means that an "ethics of risk" is needed. This ethics is guided by two main principles. (1) Every child is owed "a fair chance at physical and mental health," which requires that no parent should "take chances" with the health of any child-to-be. (2) Without clear and certain knowledge, and in the absence of informed consent from such an infant, no risk taking can be tolerated. His conclusion is that only total "abstinence" from IVF/ET is justified ethically.

Tiefel's main argument is derived from Leon Kass's earlier argument. Kass urged that in these prospective experiments on the unconceived and the unborn, "it is not enough to know of any grave defects; one needs to know that there will be no such defects—or at least no more than there are without the procedure." He concluded, "The general presumption of ignorance is caution. When the subject-at-risk cannot give consent, the presumption should be abstention."[7] Tiefel cites and agrees with

Stahlman Professor of Medical Ethics, School of Medicine, Department of Medicine, Vanderbilt University, Nashville, Tennessee 37232.

Kass's principle: "One cannot ethically choose for the would-be-child the unknown hazards that he must face and simultaneously choose to give him life in which to face them."[7]

Parents otherwise unable to bear children have nonetheless earnestly desired to utilize IVF/ET. Like Kass before him, Tiefel regards these desires as unobjectionable in themselves. However, one cannot justify the use of this technology simply by appealing to these desires. To accede to them, Tiefel believes, is to endorse a most unfortunate "ethical relativism." This would devastate medicine: "If one lets go of objective and universal values to defer to dubious patient choice, one also relinquishes the heart of medicine, whose life is the objective value of healing and doing no harm."[1]

Thus, IVF/ET cannot be ethically justified by reference either to the future child or to the parents' desires. The claims of such moral conservatism require careful scrutiny, for they are expressive not only of a prominent view among some ethicists working within medicine but also of a widely held view in our society today.

The Question of Risk to Offspring

Even though the likelihood of possible but unknown risks is the major concern, it is quite difficult to tell just which risks concern Tiefel. At one point he asserts that one must have a "wide conception" of risk: "Mental or physical, emotional or social, possible or actual, detracting from the health or worth of any or all parties."[1]

This "wide conception," however, is not helpful, and not only because it is so sweepingly general and vague. The idea would also commit Tiefel to being opposed to many if not most "natural" pregnancies. After all, it is hardly unreasonable to point out that parents could not possibly know, in advance of initiating a pregnancy, what emotional, social, mental, or other actual or possible "risks" might occur and which would compromise the health or worth of the planned offspring. Or, since a parent knows full well that any offspring, whether "naturally" or "technologically" conceived, will by the mere fact of being human have to face any number of "unknown risks" in life, it follows that Tiefel would apparently have to regard any parent as unethical.

As the wide conception leads to such absurdities and vague generalities, what alternatives does Tiefel give for understanding just what risks must concern us? Although he is surprisingly silent on this issue, one can suppose that there are two sorts: those which might occur because of the technical procedures themselves; and those arising from the purposes and actions of the technicians, researchers, and/or physicians.

1. Which risks should be of concern in the first case? Tiefel at one point cites evidence[8] that there seems to be no pattern of increased congenital defects due to the procedures. Yet, he contends that "there is no guarantee" that such a pattern will not emerge. Nor is there a guarantee that many or most abnormalities present before birth will be expelled spontaneously. Given this "factual uncertainty," hence no guarantee of certainty, IVF/ET must be abandoned. However, the logic of Tiefel's argument at this point, it must be emphasized, would require him to be completely op-

posed to *any* medical procedure which could not offer such a guarantee. This implication is surely unacceptable since it would require the abandonment of most if not all medical procedures—there simply is little, if any, such certainty in medicine.

While Tiefel is content to leave the crucial issue of risk definition so unclear, Kass was not. Also concerned about possible unknown damages from technological manipulations of the preimplanted embryo, Kass was considerably more specific. He mentioned "gross [physical] deformities," "species differences in sensitivity to the physical manipulations," "possible teratogenic agents in a culture medium," "mental retardation," and "sterility."[7]

As reported by Edwards, however, experiments with animals had clearly demonstrated that no embryopathic effect could be ascribed to the researcher's manipulations, the culture medium, and so on. So far as humans are concerned, Edwards reported, "the two most serious risks were [i.e., by 1971] known to be hyperstimulation of the ovary and multiple births. No anomalies other than a low birth weight in multi-pregnancies have occurred in children as a result of these treatments."[3] Moreover, it has been shown not only that the preimplanted embryo is highly resistant to malformations but also that "the fetuses of nonhuman primates are less resistant than human fetuses" in response to various cultures and manipulations.[3] In general, then, there seems no evidence that IVF/ET has resulted in any increase in number or type of abnormality.[5, 6]

Kass's specific concerns were thus addressed directly. The evidence available does not now seem to support the concerns which he expressed—even though it was surely legitimate to worry about these at the time Kass wrote. So far as the question of "certainty" is concerned in such research and clinical applications, Jones's judgment seems the most balanced and warranted: while "abnormalities will undoubtedly be associated with this process, it now seems unlikely that the risk will be substantially greater than the risk following normal fertilization."[6]

2. This brings up the possibility of understanding risk in the second sense: concerns about the purposes and actions of the researcher/physicians using these technical procedures, and those of infertile couples. As this opens up some genuinely murky and sensitive regions, it is essential to be most cautious.

Tiefel remarks with plain dismay that "a survey of the literature yields no medical researcher who thinks that this is one procedure that should not be used. None of the medical experts rejects this risky procedure."[1] This should hardly be surprising, however, since Kass's specific concerns have indeed been responded to directly. What is surprising is Tiefel's continued dismay, and it is this which must be examined.

At one point he makes it quite clear just what concerns him: if we do not protect embryos and fetuses, he believes that they will then "tend" to be ranked with the lower animals. With that, we have opened a veritable "Pandora's box" of evils—and just that, he contends, is inherent to IVF/ET. This "tendency," it seems perfectly clear, is not at all connected with possible risks from the technical procedures; if it were, he could be charged with simply ignoring or underestimating the scientific evidence at hand, or perhaps with asking what cannot be delivered ("guarantees of certainty"). This tendency, on the contrary, is one which he believes is to be found with the *users* of IVF/ET: parents and clinicians who select it to resolve infertility. The issue, then, seems principally a matter of distrust and fear of what these persons might do with this technology.

He suggests, for instance, that the physician's obligation to succeed without mishap, or to avoid research mistakes, may well create a conflict of interest with a flawed fetus. Presumably, this would tend to motivate the physician toward abortion: there is "an inherent impetus to jettison any problem pregnancy."[1] However, as he gives no reasons for the claim of "conflict of interest" or for this supposedly "inherent impetus," we are left with the only credible conclusion: he simply does not believe such physicians can be trusted with the power of such technology.

This conclusion receives direct support from Tiefel's subsequent argument: "the greatest hazard to the unborn may not lie in the vicissitudes of pregnancies as such or in close monitoring but in the physician's desire for a perfect child."[1] Given this "desire," the point seems to be, the physician will "tend" (or be "impelled") to "jettison" anything less than "perfection." In somewhat different terms, the real fear here is the Pandora's box supposedly inherent in such technologies. Once the camel's nose is under the tent, there is no way to keep it from carrying off the whole thing. In short, what concerns him is the "slippery slope": once the first step is allowed, there is no way to prevent sliding down to the horrors at the bottom. The only effective way to stop what this argument contends is "inevitable" is to ensure that not even the first step be permitted. The argument, it needs to be stressed, focuses not on the procedures but on those who use it. I return to this shortly.

About the parents, Tiefel is equally explicit. He asserts, without detectable reason, that to accede to a couple's desire to have their own biologic child is a "quicksand" of "shifting individual preferences," an "ethical relativism" to be avoided at all costs. Such "dubious patient choices" should not be permitted. Indeed, he goes so far as to condemn one parent's desire to have his own biologic child: "Pride is never a good reason for becoming a parent, not only because one never knows how children will turn out but because the motive is self-serving."[1] As was already mentioned, the fact that "one never knows" about a child's future would imply that not even "natural pregnancies" should be permitted. Beyond that, to regard pride in every form as merely "self-serving" seems hardly warranted. To condemn this parent, much less to condemn him and others like him to a condition of childlessness, is little short of plain arrogance.

It is equally unwarranted, finally, to assert without argument that acceding to a couple's desire to resolve their infertility by IVF/ET is equivalent to endorsing "ethical relativism." After all, to act on behalf of what a patient honestly believes is his or her own good could more readily be understood as benevolence. It need hardly be pointed out that the very part of the moral norms of medical practice which Tiefel himself stresses—that is, acting on behalf of the patient's best interests—is precisely what is involved here. To be sure, a patient might not know what these best interests actually are in a given situation. But then one is obliged to give sound reasons for such a claim. In any case, the kind of infertility for which IVF/ET is an appropriate response is neither commonly debilitating nor mentally incapacitating. Hence, it can hardly be claimed that such persons do not and cannot know their own best interests, nor is there any reason to suppose that Tiefel is in any better position to know this than are the parents.

Regarding individual preferences as a shifting quicksand, patient choices as dubious, and physicians as being unwittingly driven by an inherent impetus to achieve perfection, it is quite evident that what concerns Tiefel is not unknown risks stemming from the procedures of IVF/ET but, rather, his considerable distrust of the persons involved.

3. A final possible sense of risk deserves brief comment. Walters suggests that some ethicists object to IVF/ET on the grounds that no laboratory or clinical experiments are capable of providing the amount or kind of evidence needed to assuage moral concern. They have concluded that "the risks of clinical IVF research are not only unknown but unknowable."[2] If this were Tiefel's, or even Kass's, concern, there would obviously be no possible response. There is no answer to a demand for certainty, since medicine is a science or discipline incorporating an element of "necessary fallibility."[9]

Tiefel does not argue for unknowable risks, however. Rather, he contends that "the morally crucial answer to the question of risk to the would-be child thus requires a great number of births and much time."[1] Therefore, *only* further factual investigations are appropriate for satisfying his concern. Now, not only does this stance (contra the abstention Tiefel argues for) require such research, but, in fact, the evidence to date gives far greater weight to IVF/ET than to Tiefel's claims.

The Question
of "Consent" and
"Moral Status"

The appeal to unknown risks seems mainly a straw man. To ask for certainty is to ask for what cannot be given and would forbid any clinical trial, any experimentation and scientific research—since the very point of these is to find out or make known what is yet unknown, often in the context of some risk.

In any event, even if there were no more risks from IVF/ET than from "normal" procreation, the moral conservative is still opposed. Part of the reason has to do with the moral status of the embryo as "human" from "conception" onward. Kass[7, 10] and Ramsey[11, 12] make informed consent a central issue here; Tiefel apparently agrees with this, but makes moral status the main one.

Kass, for instance, would require that the subject-at-risk give its consent; this is not possible; therefore, IVF/ET is ethically unjustified. For Tiefel, human life "begins at conception," and the embryo is therefore "human life"; since this gives it full human status for all moral purposes, consent would surely be required.

Edwards's quick response to this issue is worth repeating: it is "unrealistic in practice because it leads to total negation—even to denying a mother a sleeping pill, a Caesarian section, or an amniocentesis for fear of disturbing the child." For that matter, he caustically remarks, "fetuses are not asked beforehand about their own conception or even their abortion."[3] Since this is patently true regardless of the specific mode of procreation, "natural" or otherwise, insistence on consent would forbid any pregnancy whatever. It is, of course, quite pointless to demand consent from embryos, fetuses, and newborns, but it is also obvious that this is not expected. What we do expect is that others (parents, health professionals, teachers, etc.) will act responsibly on behalf of their best interests.

The same clearly applies to clinical IVF; perhaps even more stringently (although a case would have to be made for this), in view of the still tentative status of the procedures. Still, this is far short of the abstention Kass, Ramsey, and Tiefel demand and is a precaution which could reasonably be encouraged for any parent: to be more thoughtful about bringing children into the world even in "natural" ways.

Although Tiefel asserts (without argument) that life begins at conception, he later maintains that the "problem is not when life begins but when it should have human status, when it should be important and count as one of us."[1] Of course, one wants to recognize that human life is a matter of continuous development through a sequence of stages. The issue, then, concerns whether this development at any one stage is sufficient to make a difference, that is, exhibits a moral status requiring all the protections (goods, rights, etc.) which are recognized for any clearly moral human being.

One such stage is the preembryonic. Since the union of the spermatozoon and ovum is necessary to initiate the development of a new individual, this stage does not make the difference sought for. Fertilization may seem morally significant since at its completion a zygote is formed and, it would appear, a distinctively human individual is initiated. Strictly speaking, of course, this is not necessarily the case. Fertilization might result in two (or more) such individuals. It might also result in such severe chromosomal abnormalities as to preclude subsequent development. It may even result in a hydatidiform mole. Indeed, even normal development shows that fertilization results, first, in a cell mass which ultimately divides into the embryoblast and the trophoblast. While the former becomes the fetus, the latter becomes not a "child" but the extraembryonic membranes, placenta, and umbilical cord. Of course, the trophoblastic derivatives are quite as much "alive" and "human" as the embryoblast and have the same genetic composition as the fetus. Hence, this stage does not make the moral difference that Tiefel and others are seeking.

Conception, the stage initiating pregnancy marked by the implantation of the blastocyst, however, may be the difference which makes a moral difference. Throughout the entire process there is one and the same organism. However, as Eike-Henner Kluge emphasizes, "it is one and the same only in the sense that it is one continually growing aggregate of matter that develops according to a genetically fixed plan. This continuation, however, does not mean continued identity—any more than the continuation of protein molecules when ingested and assimilated by us entails that we have become the cow that we have eaten."[13] The crucial difference, then, is this "identity": at what point of development can it be said credibly that "one and the same" human individual is present? For Kluge, this point comes only with the adequate formation of the central nervous system, especially the brain, for only then is there an adequate support for the sorts of complex neural activities which can serve as the biologic foundation for distinctively human rationality, for "personhood."

Others would locate this morally significant point at "viability" (the Supreme Court), while still others would push this point further. Throughout such discussions, however, several issues tend to be obscured, issues which must give one pause at the very idea of trying to establish one or another "point" as somehow morally significant. Suppose a point were agreed on; what then? In the first place, it would be implied that *prior* to that point the developing human life would be *excluded* from "protectable humanity."[1] Presumably, then, for such stages there would be no argument against many if not all types of research manipulations. But surely this permissiveness could not be tolerated even by Tiefel. In the second place, since IVF/ET procedures occur at the *preconception* stages (and if we take Tiefel at his own words), they should be of no concern to him at all, as "human moral status" has not yet been achieved, according to him.

In the third place, supposing such a point were agreed on, we need to establish just what this implies. Here Tiefel's claim simply begs the question. Simply because the fertilized ovum (for instance) does not yet have that moral status in no way implies that it *thereby* is excluded from protectable humanity, much less *thereby* ranked with the lower animals. And even if the latter were the case (which is dubious), not even that would necessarily imply that any and all clinical or laboratory manipulations would be justified ethically.

In many respects, this anxiety about finding differences which make a moral difference itself seems suspect. What underlies it, certainly in Tiefel's case, is this "fear" about a "tendency" by the researchers and physicians to abuse and misuse their powers. Once again, that is, we are in the face of the slippery slope argument, and it is this which must be squarely confronted.

On "Slopes," "Noses," or "Wedges"

This argument has exercised many persons, including ethicists. Its appeal is familiar and seems quite powerful. It is essentially a hypothetical, conditional argument: "if . . . then. . . ." It postulates that "if" something is once done, or a course of action initiated, however innocuous this bare beginning might be, "then" certain highly unacceptable results will occur. Since these are unacceptable, the initial step is unacceptable. Or, to accept the initial step will "tend" inevitably to bring the host of horrors in its wake.

Often the argument includes one or another conditional qualifier: "tendency," "might occur," "unknown risks," and the "inevitability" of the bad results. Despite these qualifiers, however, the logical force of the argument is the appeal to necessity, otherwise there would be no compelling reason for the abstention.

Logically, of course, the argument is plainly fallacious. If the first step is accepted, the evil at the slope's bottom is inevitable. This is a version of affirming the antecedent, and from this no conclusion whatever follows. In some versions (e.g., Tiefel's), the logical fallacy of denying the consequent is also committed: the evils which will result must be rejected; therefore, not even the first step should be permitted. Again, no conclusion follows.

Even so, the argument continues to be used, and this presents a curious problem. If it is maintained merely that the initiation of a course of action might occur, then they might not occur; while this implies great caution at every stage, it hardly implies abstention. If the argument appeals to necessity, it is a clear fallacy. In either case the conclusion argued for simply does not follow. Why, then, its remarkable appeal?

At its root is a certain psychological observation, coupled with an appeal to fear: once people become accustomed to something they find it easier, perhaps even attractive, not only to do it again and again (developing a habit) but also to engage in a different but related activity which, however, is bad. Examples include welshing on a promise, not telling the truth, fudging on getting consent, etc. The focus of the "argument," then, is on the people doing the action, not on the action itself (nor the technical means required by the action).

The slippery slope, in other words, works (to the extent that it does work) primarily as a misanthropic exercise: it moves from the psychological likelihood that some persons might be tempted to engage in such actions, to the very different presumption that all persons (within a certain class, e.g., IVF/ET clinicians) will inevitably engage in such actions. That is to say, the slippery slope has its force mainly in distrust of persons—they are not able to resist the temptations to continue each step down the slippery slope all the way to the bottom. For each step down differs so little from the prior one that we are easily duped; the first was okay, so the second seems okay as well. . . .

In fact, of course, not even the psychological observation is necessarily accurate. Some people do indeed resist such temptations (for instance, I should imagine that Tiefel would). This being true, the appeal to fear loses its force as well. The move from a psychological observation (which is itself dubious in many cases) about only some persons' presumable tendency or temptability (without telling which people are that way) to the strongest possible moral prohibition does not hold up. Hence, the "argument" is not an argument at all but an illicit appeal to distrust, suspicion, and fear—and the basis for these is at least open to question.

The acceptance of the initial step, then, by no means implies that one must accept the evil consequences; it does not even mean that these particular consequences are in any way related to the initial step. But even if Tiefel were in some way correct about such potential dangers of the Pandora's box, this would hardly signify a muting of our moral awareness; it would suggest, on the contrary, a remarkable heightening and sharpening of it—as the presence of danger of any sort does. To the extent that the slippery slope is legitimate, it leads to the very opposite of what those who use it wish us to believe.

Can IVF/ET Be "Therapeutic"?

A final point remains to be considered. The moral conservative urges that the only sense in which IVF/ET can be considered therapeutic is with regard to the parents. Tiefel argues, however, that accepting the validity of this is equivalent to giving over to "dubious patient choice" and "ethical relativism." Kass argues that this procedure can be considered a "cure for infertility" (as Edwards believes)[3] only if infertility were incorporated into the "medical model" as a "disease."

However, Kass insists, infertility is precisely *not* a disease. It "is not life threatening or crippling, nor does it lead to detectable bodily damage."[7] Moreover, even if a successful pregnancy and birth are obtained, the infertility still remains. Hence, IVF/ET can be considered at most the "symptom" of a disease. In that case, however, it would have to be understood strictly as a process occurring solely within or to an individual. But infertility is not that; it is, rather, a "condition that is located in a marriage, in union of two individuals."[7]

Since infertility is not a disease, IVF/ET cannot be conceived as a therapy. What is in fact "treated" is the woman's, or the couple's, "desire" to bear a child. And, however unobjectionable in itself, to treat this desire requires a "clear medical therapeutic purpose," and infertility simply does not present such a purpose for Kass, even less so if there is a risk of damage to the would-be child (from whom, of course, no consent is possible).

On this issue, Paul Ramsey seems even more extreme. He believes that IVF/ET is focused solely on the "product" and "is therefore manufactured by biological technology, not medicine." Such technological manipulations in effect reduce the child to the status of a mere "prosthesis for his mother's condition."[11, 12]

Setting aside the questions of risk and consent, which have already been dealt with, we are left with the issue of "treating" the "desires" of the couple. Is infertility a treatable condition, and is IVF/ET a "therapeutic" procedure for it?

To this, Edwards's direct response bears repeating. There are many examples of clinical conditions which remain even after treatment, which only modifies their expression. He lists insulin, false teeth, and spectacles; patients with these conditions "want" (desire) to be nondiabetic, to eat properly, to see. Physicians quite appropriately respond to these desires by treating the symptomatic expressions. "In fact," he points out, "most medical treatment, particularly on constitutional or genetic disorders, is similarly symptomatic in nature," and infertility is precisely like those.[3] To refuse to respond to a couple's desire to have a child, when otherwise they could not, is in effect to require that they accept their childlessness. This attitude "assumes that a doctor or someone else is sufficiently authoritative to decide on the problems of the couple." On this, however, "there is no reason to believe that ethical advice from outsiders about their condition is sounder than their own judgment of it."[3]

I doubt that Kass, Ramsey, or Tiefel would disagree with Edwards about diabetes, bad eyesight, or poor teeth. I doubt indeed that they would disagree that a severely burned person's desire to have some cosmetic surgery is legitimate, even though this would leave the underlying condition as it was. In short, the argument against IVF/ET glosses over a key distinction, that between *trivial* and *nontrivial* desires.

One response to the plight of infertile persons is adoption. It need not be belabored, however, that adoption can hardly be given as the avenue for all would-be parents. This is so whatever the intrinsic values of adoption, and even if there were fewer difficulties than there now are, for many people, in finding adoptable children and being accepted as appropriate adoptive parents. In any case, even to recommend adoption to such persons, it is worth emphasizing, one has to suppose that their "desire" for a child is hardly trivial!

Unless one were prepared to argue that *every* desire to have one's own biologic child (even by "natural" means) is trivial—which seems outrageous—the point about desire is simply another straw man. To insure that no clearly trivial desire should be taken seriously by medicine is doubtless a sound point. But that is to say no more than what has been long known and practiced in medicine generally and seems particularly true of IVF/ET programs.

Of course, a fuller discussion of this issue would have to be more specific on the distinction between trivial and nontrivial desires. However difficult that may be, it seems only reasonable to believe that the desires in question are hardly, and certainly not universally, trivial. Where they are not trivial, it is perfectly acceptable (perhaps even obligatory) for physicians to utilize the means provided by clinical IVF/ET.

A Concluding Word

Tiefel, it can be supposed, would still demur, for he wants deliberately to contend that to respect even (I suppose) serious desires for such couples is to give in to ethical relativism. There is no middle road between absolute relativism and absolute paternalism. As I have suggested, this commits him to a fundamental kind of misanthropy, to being systematically suspicious of (at least) IVF/ET physicians and infertile parents. His paternalism is most stringent; "children are gifts of God to which believers have no claims, either before or after birth."[1] This means that God alone can decide the issues with which IVF/ET teams merely imagine they have to grapple. Hence, the "universal and objective" moral norms he believes lie at the heart of medicine are, in truth, God's unalterable norms. From this perspective, it must by definition be true that letting individuals decide is most "dubious" indeed.

It should also be pointed out, however, that his view presupposes a radically privileged source of knowledge, namely, of God's purported purposes. It presupposes not only that Tiefel has such access but that others of us have as well. Otherwise, the view he espouses is simply by definition unassailable: any opinion to the contrary would be merely one more "dubious" individual opinion.

That feature is troublesome enough, but not as serious as the problem his view necessarily creates: that of basic ethical disagreement and even, at times, serious ethical conflict. Must those who disagree with him (as he clearly suggests, in the case of patients) be regarded as "dubious"? Could his view tolerate even the modest admission that not every patient (e.g., Tiefel himself) is ipso facto "dubious"? I suspect that at the core of his view is a kind of moral intolerance toward any opposing view, and it is precisely for this reason that the mere presence of a dissenting view (e.g., by IVF/ET physicians) presents such harsh issues for him, even though he says nothing about the problem of moral disagreement.

In any event, a number of things seem quite evident. First, the concern about potential damage to the offspring of IVF/ET seems clearly unfounded. Second, the question of consent, while it has an obvious and significant place in many situations (e.g., for the would-be parents), cannot be legitimately required of the potential off-spring itself. Third, the attempt to assign a special, morally privileged status to one or another stage of human development is at best problematic and at worst arbitrary. Fourth, the argument that IVF/ET is not therapeutic for the couple does not stand up to analysis, as the discussion of "desire" trades on a gloss of a key distinction between desires which are genuine and those which are merely trivial. Making that distinction, however, suggests that IVF/ET is an appropriate medical response to a couple's infertility. Finally, the nub of moral conservatism turns out to be at once highly questionable, an exercise in "playing God" in far more dangerous ways than anything in the current medical armamentarium, and a viewpoint which seems incapable of accommodating moral disagreement. Hence, this viewpoint presents a kind of intolerance which the facts of human life, and of medicine, cannot support.

References

1. Tiefel, H. O. Human in vitro fertilization: a conservative view. *JAMA* 247:3235–3242, 1982.

2. Walters, L. Human in vitro fertilization: a review of the ethical literature. *Hastings Cent. Rep.* 9:23–42, 1979.

3. Edwards, R. G. Fertilization of human eggs in vitro: morals, ethics and the law. *Q. Rev. Biol.* 40:3–26, 1974.

4. Lopata, A.; Johnston, I. W.; Hoult, I. J.; and Speirs, A. L. In vitro fertilization in the treatment of human infertility. In *Bioregulators of Reproduction*, edited by G. Jagiello and H. J. Vogel. New York: Academic Press, 1981.

5. Craft, I.; McLeod, F.; Green, S.; et al. Human pregnancy following oocyte and sperm transfer to the uterus. *Lancet*, pp. 1031–1033, 1982.

6. Jones, H. W., Jr. The ethics of in vitro fertilization: 1982. *Fertil. Ster.* 37:146–149, 1982.

7. Kass, L. R. Babies by means of in vitro fertilization: unethical experiments on the unborn? *N. Engl. J. Med.* 285:1174–1179, 1971.

8. Biggers, J. D. In vitro fertilization and embryo transfer in human beings. *N. Engl. J. Med.* 304:336–342, 1981.

9. Gorovitz, S., and MacIntyre, A. Towards a theory of medical fallibility. *J. Med. Philos.* 1:51–71, 1976.

10. Kass, L. E. Making babies—the new biology and "old" morality. *Public Interest* 26:32–33, 1972.

11. Ramsey, P. Shall we "reproduce"? I. The medical ethics of in vitro fertilization. *JAMA* 220:1347, 1972.

12. Ramsey, P. Shall we "reproduce"? II. Rejoinders and future forecast. *JAMA* 220:1480–1483, 1972.

13. Kluge, E-H. *The Practices of Death*. New Haven, Conn.: Yale Univ. Press, 1975.

CHAPTER 3

Gestational Surrogacy and Surrogate Motherhood

CASES FOR
PRELIMINARY DISCUSSION

Case 3.1

The female president of a large Madison Avenue advertising company approaches the director of a prominent fertility clinic specializing in IVF. So far as she knows, she has no fertility problems, but simply has not had time in her life for childbearing. She and her husband, a prominent Manhattan stockbroker, have decided to have three children, and they would like to have them as close in age as possible to facilitate their socialization and care, as well as to shorten the demands on their parents' time during the years of childrearing. Furthermore, they have decided on having two boys and one girl.

Now that IVF is a technology that is well-proven, the executive proposes that the clinic remove a number of her ova, fertilize them with her husband's sperm in vitro, select two males and one female preimplantation embryos, and implant the resulting three preembryos in three gestational host mothers. She proposes that a battery of psychological and medical tests be given to qualify the applicants, so that the chances of behavior harmful to the fetuses be minimized, that the contract with each be drawn by one of the top contract lawyers in New York, and that the women be recruited from a Caribbean republic that has no statutory or common law impediments to gestational surrogacy contracts.

The clinic is to fly the women to Manhattan, provide all necessary medical preparations, do the implantations, confirm the pregnancies, and ensure healthful behavior on the part of the women, who, because of Governor Cuomo's bill limiting payments to surrogates to the incurred expenses, will be flown back to their country for labor and delivery. For this service, the executive is prepared to pay a $15,000 fee to each surrogate and the clinic's usual fees for each IVF, together with the charges for the travel, extra housing, and supervision; she and her husband will also, on the delivery of two healthy newborn sons and one healthy newborn daughter, donate $1 million to the not-for-profit foundation associated with the clinic.

Case 3.2

A surrogate mother was inseminated in 1981 with the sperm of one Alex Malihoff, under a contract arranged by a surrogacy broker. The child was born with a congenital disorder. Mr. Malihoff asked the hospital not to treat the child, but the hospital got a court order to provide the child with treatment. Malihoff later denied paternity and refused both to take the child and to pay the contracted fee to the surrogate. The court determined that the child was indeed sired by the surrogate's husband. The surrogate then sued Malihoff, alleging the child's disorder was caused by a virus from Mr. Malihoff's sperm.

Case 3.3

A 32-year-old woman agreed to be a surrogate for her sister and brother-in-law. She had an unknown history of intravenous drug abuse, and the baby was born with AIDS. The surrogate, her sister, and her brother-in-law each refused custody of the baby.

Case 3.4

A woman in Johannesburg, South Africa, had a hysterectomy. Before the surgery, she conceived naturally using a fertility drug, had uterine lavage performed, and had the fertilized ova implanted into her mother. Nine months later, her mother gave birth to her own three grandchildren.

REVIEW OF THE ISSUES

The questions posed by the new IVF technology did not end with the possibility of the Diaz's tragic case, nor even with the troubling issue of what was to be done with unused embryos not needed in order to achieve a couple's pregnancy. With the IVF technology, it would be possible for one woman to act as surrogate gestational mother for another's biological child, then return the newborn to its biological parents. Such embryo transfer simply employs a different uterus as the receptacle for the selected embryo than that normally intended with IVF.

Such an application of the technique could serve as a kind of therapeutic option for a couple wishing to have "their own" child but unable to do so because of, say, a surgical removal of the wife's uterus (where the ovaries were left intact). The woman's ovaries would be stimulated to produce several ova, just as in IVF; they would be harvested and fertilized with the husband's sperm in vitro, just as in IVF; but they would be implanted in the uterus of another woman, perhaps a sister or daughter or other individual contracted for the purpose, and carried to term in and by the host. The host would then go through labor and delivery and surrender the child to its "rightful" parents, receiving their thankful gratitude and any coverage of expenses or other remuneration for her trouble they had contracted to, or cared to, provide.

But this technique, as therapy, is physiologically and procedurally no different from removal of ova from a woman who is able to bear children but finds it inconvenient as interfering with other activities to which she has made major commitments of time and energy. Indeed, with careful timing she might even avoid the first surgical procedure to remove an ovum; fertilization could take place normally, with the embryo flushed from the fallopian tube or uterus before it has a chance to implant, and transferred to the host uterus. A "wet nurse" was a common enough recourse, before the advent of bottled formula, for a woman who either didn't yield sufficient breast milk or who didn't want to nurse; such a gestational host might strike some as but an extension of that old practice with a similar rationale.

The easy slide from IVF into what might properly be called "surrogate mother-hood" (but for the appropriation of that term in a less appropriate context—see below) illustrates a general point made earlier. Medical technology, invented for a clearly therapeutic purpose, may be made to serve quite different, nontherapeutic purposes. Medicine, motivated by its traditional calling to serve the concept of health, finds itself pressed by "consumers" of its "services" to adapt them to the wants, not needs, of others. Individuals, faced with the conflicting demands of career and biol-ogy, seize upon the possibilities of a piece of technology as offering a way to satisfy both. But the medical community, itself composed of individuals with a strong, tradi-tional conception of its proper role in human affairs, finds the demands of such indi-vidual consumers not to be in keeping with its traditional roles. It is not surprising that fertility clinics have generally resisted such applications.

Gestational surrogacy also raises legal and moral questions at a conceptual level. Are the surrogate gestational mother's parental rights with respect to the child to be modeled on the law of paternity, where proof of genetic parentage establishes defini-tive parentage, or are they to be predicated on the nine-month experience of preg-nancy as establishing the preponderant interest of definitive parentage? The latter has the operational superiority of establishing the identity of the legal mother at the time of birth, but it undercuts the aim of the biological parents to use a contract service to provide them with an otherwise impossible dream—that of rearing "a child of their own flesh and blood."

Interestingly, and perhaps more because of the resistance of medicine to deflec-tions from its traditional paths than the legal uncertainties just cited, the form of surrogacy cited above has not become a major social issue. Instead, another form, commonly but less properly called "surrogacy," has commanded our attention in the media, courts, and legislatures for the past several years.

William Stern, whose wife, Elizabeth, suffers from multiple sclerosis (of a kind which would most likely be seriously exacerbated by pregnancy), contracted through an intermediate agency with Mary Beth Whitehead, a married woman, to be artificially inseminated with his sperm, carry the pregnancy to term, and surrender the newborn to the Stern couple, whereupon Mrs. Stern would adopt the child. Mrs. Whitehead was to be paid a fee of $10,000 for this service; the intermediate agency was to receive $7,500.

Although she had signed the contract, Mary Beth Whitehead decided after deliver-ing the baby, whom she named Sara Elizabeth, that she did not want to surrender it for adoption by Mrs. Stern to be raised by the Sterns as their own child. A lower court awarded custody of Baby M (for "Melissa," the name given her by the Sterns) to Mr. and Mrs. Stern and approved Mrs. Stern's adoption petition on the grounds that the contract was a valid contract and that they were better potential parents for the baby than her natural mother.

The New Jersey Supreme Court overturned the decision and voided the adop-tion, declaring that no contract to surrender a child for adoption could be validly entered into before the child was even conceived, and disputing the evidence that the Sterns would be better parents than Mrs. Whitehead. The court, however, awarded custody to the Sterns on grounds that they had had effective custody throughout the many months of the appeals procedure and that Baby M's interests would now not be well served by returning her to the custody of her biological mother. The latter was awarded substantial visitation rights.

It is, first, worthwhile noting that the use of the term *surrogate mother* to describe Mary Beth Whitehead's relationship to Melissa, or to characterize any woman who has been fertilized in order to bear a child to be surrendered for adoption, is bizarre and confusing. A surrogate is one who functions in the place of another. But there is no way in which Mrs. Whitehead biologically functioned in the place of Mrs. Stern, except to bear a child fathered by Mr. Stern. *Surrogate* perhaps better describes the relationship of a woman who serves as the gestational host of an embryo developing from a fertilized ovum of another woman; here, the surrogate mother performs only the gestational functions of the biological mother.

The commodification of reproduction was very much an issue in the Baby M trial and appeal. As noted earlier, however, precedent had already been established in the practice of donors selling semen. An argument in support of the Sterns' position that the contract was a valid one would be that they had contracted for the purchase of one of Mrs. Whitehead's ova that would be fertilized by Mr. Stern's sperm; additionally, they had contracted for the use of Mrs. Whitehead's uterus to gestate the fertilized ovum. Thus, they were engaged in the purchase of a biological bodily product no more special than blood or semen, and of a service not fundamentally different than that provided by a wet nurse or child-care provider. The purchase of the ovum, since it was to be delivered in an altered state, involved a prior agreement on the part of Mrs. Whitehead to surrender the child for adoption.

The counterargument proceeds by appeal to the way in which we have legalized adoption. An adoption agreement cannot be entered into for a future, possible child, but must refer to the child by name and thus cannot be entered into before birth. Further, contracting for the use of one's uterus is perilously close to contracting for the use of one's vagina; the parallel with prostitution strikes many as compelling, and all but one of the states prohibit prostitution contracts. Finally, it becomes increasingly difficult to distinguish between a surrogacy contract and the selling of children, particularly when a part of that contract involves payment for release of one's interest in the child.

Interestingly, the New Jersey Supreme Court focused almost exclusively on the contract rather than the service. It allowed that private arrangements between consenting individuals which were not secured by contract fell out of the purview of the court's review and were, unless expressly prohibited by statute, consistent with state adoption laws.

This raises the question for lawmakers of whether to prohibit such practices as private arrangements. On the side of permitting them is the very human need to have children, and the practice as a way of enabling a couple to rear a child that is biologically related to one of them—no different than the rationale for AID. On the side of restricting or prohibiting them is our uncertainty about whether there is significant potential of psychological harm to the child in learning that he or she was conceived by and born to a woman who was perfectly willing to give her baby away.

There is also the difficult matter of maternal/child bonding that some think must begin prior to birth. We simply do not understand the role that such bonding plays in a child's developmental experience. Perhaps we can learn from the experiences of adopted children here; since we regard adoption as a desperate solution to an even more desperate situation that has befallen the child, perhaps we should be less sanguine about deliberately creating a child to face such a fate. Clearly, as in the case of AID, there is a need to study the long-term effects on children born of the new technology before comfortably standardizing these techniques, and some have called for a moratorium on this and the other form of surrogacy while such studies take place.

Since the problems faced by infertile women who are unsuccessful with the other reproductive technologies in their attempts to have their own children are powerful ones, the social likelihood is that the practice of surrogacy will continue even if elements of surrogate contracts are unenforceable. Some states are seeking to minimize this likelihood by legislating against such social arrangements. To other legislatures, it appears desirable for the practice to be regulated so that the interests of involved parties, particularly those of the offspring of such arrangements, are protected. The present tendency in a number of states is to pass regulatory legislation that will model surrogacy contracts after adoption agreements and practices.

REVIEW OF THE SELECTIONS

The debate that occurred between John Robertson and Herbert Krimmel[1] in the 1983 *Hastings Center Report* foreshadowed in some ways the enormous media event that brought surrogacy in the form of the celebrated Baby M case to the front page of every major daily paper and into the television rooms of most American households in 1987 and 1988. Yet, in the cool rationality of their arguments for and against surrogacy, one finds little hint of the passions to sweep through two families and the courts. One does sense here that American thought is widely divided on the issue—a division that was to be echoed in the New Jersey Superior and Supreme Courts within a few years.

Robertson offers a series of considerations arrayed to support the conclusion that gestational surrogacy and surrogate motherhood can and should be accommodated within the normal range of then-current contract and adoption law. He takes up and dispenses with a number of moral objections to the practices that have been advanced as reasons for banning one or both forms of surrogacy, reminding us that most human reproduction has a selfish component to it, that the risks to the parties and offspring of surrogacy arrangements are not particularly different from those of adoption and AID, that there are fundamental analogies with surrogacy for a fee and blood or semen donation for a fee and fundamental disanalogies with all of these practices and prostitution. At the same time, Robertson cautions against the many psychological and emotional factors that can attend the surrender of a baby, and concludes that "surrogate mothering for a fee is neither the evil nor the panacea that many have thought."

Krimmel (whose essay is not reproduced here) does not find any particular moral or legal difficulty with the notion of the gestational host role, for he sees here a strong analogy with assistance in education, training, or raising children. He argues, however, that the form of surrogacy in which the gestational mother provides her own ovum for AID within a surrogacy arrangement for some benefit she will receive (usually a payment) involves a change in motive for creating children that, as the philosopher Immanuel Kant might observe, involves treating them as only means and not as ends in themselves. He considers the analogy with adoption faulty, and holds the analogy with Nazi experimentation on humans to be closer. Commodifying children involves placing a value on them, and the tragic stage is set for the abnormal product of a surrogacy arrangement, unwanted by any of the parents involved in its production by virtue of genetic material or contractual agreement.

In New Jersey's Baby M case, the decisive issue was the payment of a fee to the surrogate mother for her surrender of a child conceived under a surrogacy contract and of all parental rights and interests as well. The lower court had decided the issue in favor of the biological father on grounds that he and his wife would be better parents and that the best interests of the child would thus be served by placing the infant with them, thereby enforcing the contract. The New Jersey Supreme Court carefully reviews all the possible statutory bases that might support such an action, and dismisses the validity of the original contract.

The decision was complicated by the lengthy period of time that the lower court's decision was in effect, with the child in the custody of her natural father and his wife; the judge ruled that they would retain custody as in the best interests of the child, but restored visitation rights to the natural mother.

The case here is presented not so much as an iteration of the decision in this specific case but as an exploration of the nature of the state's interest in children and their natural parents, and it details the long history of thinking that underlies our laws prohibiting the buying and selling of children.

Legal critic and essayist George Annas reviews the courts' reasoning in two other less celebrated but very important cases, one in Kentucky and one in Michigan. His reviews together with Chief Justice Wilentz's opinion represent critical insights into juridical reasoning on the behalf of society as courts struggle to reconcile the challenging opportunities and possibilities of advances in medical technology within the traditions and values that have given substance and form to our collective social history.

In the final selection for this chapter, Lori Andrews reviews the recent efforts on the part of state legislatures to come to terms with the surrogacy phenomenon. Her review is useful as well in comparing the history of legislative efforts to cope with AID with the current state of similar efforts to deal with surrogacy contracts and arrangements, since she is able to generate some predictions as to how the legislative process will ultimately cash out. It is particularly interesting to see that she expects one effect to be rethinking of the anonymity obstacles to information about semen donors contained in most AID regulatory statutes.

References

1. Herbert T. Krimmel. "The Case Against Surrogate Parenting." *Hastings Center Report* 13(5), 1983.

Surrogate Mothers:
Not So Novel After All

JOHN A. ROBERTSON

All reproduction is collaborative, for no man or woman reproduces alone. Yet the provision of sperm, egg, or uterus through artificial insemination, embryo transfer, and surrogate mothering makes reproduction collaborative in another way. A third person provides a genetic or gestational factor not present in ordinary paired reproduction. As these practices grow, we must confront the ethical issues raised and their implications for public policy.

Collaborative reproduction allows some persons who otherwise might remain childless to produce healthy children. However, its deliberate separation of genetic, gestational, and social parentage is troublesome. The offspring and participants may be harmed, and there is a risk of confusing family lineage and personal identity. In addition, the techniques intentionally manipulate a natural process that many persons want free of technical intervention. Yet many well-accepted practices, including adoption, artificial insemination by donor (AID), and blended families (families where children of different marriages are raised together) intentionally separate biologic and social parenting, and have become an accepted thread in the social fabric. Should all collaborative techniques be similarly treated? When, if ever, are they ethical? Should the law prohibit, encourage, or regulate them, or should the practice be left to private actors? Surrogate motherhood—the controversial practice by which a woman agrees to bear a child conceived by artificial insemination and to relinquish it at birth to others for rearing—illustrates the legal and ethical issues arising in collaborative reproduction generally.

An Alternative to Agency Adoptions

Infertile couples who are seeking surrogates hire attorneys and sign contracts with women recruited through newspaper ads. The practice at present probably involves at

John A. Robertson *is Marrs McLean Professor of Law at the School of Law, University of Texas in Austin.*

most a few hundred persons. But repeated attention on *Sixty Minutes* and the *Phil Donahue Show* and in the popular press is likely to engender more demand, for thousands of infertile couples might find surrogate mothers the answer to their reproductive needs. What began as an enterprise involving a few lawyers and doctors in Michigan, Kentucky, and California is now a national phenomenon. There are surrogate mother centers in Maryland, Arizona, and several other states, and even a surrogate mother newsletter.

Surrogate mother arrangements occur within a tradition of family law that gives the gestational mother (and her spouse, if any) rearing rights and obligations. (However, the presumption that the husband is the father can be challenged, and a husband's obligations to his wife's child by AID will usually require his consent.)[1] Although no state has legislation directly on the subject of surrogate motherhood, independently arranged adoptions are lawful in most states. It is no crime to agree to bear a child for another, and then relinquish it for adoption. However, paying the mother a fee for adoption beyond medical expenses is a crime in some states, and in others will prevent the adoption from being approved.[2] Whether termination and transfer of parenting rights will be legally recognized depends on the state. Some states, like Hawaii and Florida, ask few questions and approve independent adoptions very quickly. Others, like Michigan and Kentucky, won't allow surrogate mothers to terminate and assign rearing rights to another if a fee has been paid, or even allow a paternity determination in favor of the sperm donor. The enforcibility of surrogate contracts has also not been tested, and it is safe to assume that some jurisdictions will not enforce them. Legislation clarifying many of these questions has been proposed in several states, but has not yet been enacted.

Even this brief discussion highlights an important fact about surrogate motherhood and other collaborative reproductive techniques. They operate as an alternative to the nonmarket, agency system of allocating children for adoption, which has contributed to long queues for distributing healthy white babies. This form of independent adoption is controlled by the parties, planned before conception, involves a genetic link with one parent, and enables both the father and mother of the adopted child to be selected in advance.

Understood in these terms, the term "surrogate mother," which means substitute mother, is a misnomer. The natural mother, who contributes egg and uterus, is not so much a substitute mother as a substitute spouse who carries a child for a man whose wife is infertile. Indeed, it is the adoptive mother who is the surrogate mother for the child, since she parents a child borne by another. What, if anything, is wrong with this arrangement? Let us look more closely at its benefits and harms before discussing public policy.

All the Parties Can Benefit

Reproduction through surrogate mothering is a deviation from our cultural norms of reproduction, and to many persons it seems immoral or wrong. But surrogate mothering may be a good for the parties involved.

Surrogate contracts meet the desire of a husband and wife to rear a healthy child, and more particularly, a child with one partner's genes. The need could arise because the wife has an autosomal dominant or sex-linked genetic disorder, such as hemophilia. More likely, she is infertile and the couple feels a strong need to have children. For many infertile couples the inability to conceive is a major personal problem causing marital conflict and filling both partners with anguish and self-doubt. It may also involve multiple medical work-ups and possibly even surgery. If the husband and wife have sought to adopt a child, they may have been told either that they do not qualify or to join the queue of couples waiting several years for agency adoptions (the wait has grown longer due to birth control, abortion, and the greater willingness of unwed mothers to keep their children[3]). For couples exhausted and frustrated by these efforts, the surrogate arrangement seems a godsend. While the intense desire to have a child often appears selfish, we must not lose sight of the deep-seated psychosocial and biological roots of the desire to generate children.[4]

The arrangement may also benefit the surrogate. Usually women undergo pregnancy and childbirth because they want to rear children. But some women want to have the experience of bearing and birthing a child without the obligation to rear. Phillip Parker, a Michigan psychiatrist who has interviewed over 275 surrogate applicants, finds that the decision to be a surrogate springs from several motives.[5] Most women willing to be surrogates have already had children, and many are married. They choose the surrogate role primarily because the fee provides a better economic opportunity than alternative occupations, but also because they enjoy being pregnant and the respect and attention that it draws. The surrogate experience may also be a way to master, through reliving, guilt they feel from past pregnancies that ended in abortion or adoption. Some surrogates may also feel pleased, as organ donors do, that they have given the "gift of life" to another couple.[6]

The child born of a surrogate arrangement also benefits. Indeed, but for the surrogate contract, this child would not have been born at all. Unlike the ordinary agency or independent adoption, where a child is already conceived or brought to term, the conception of this child occurs solely as a result of the surrogate agreement. Thus even if the child does suffer identity problems, as adopted children often do because they are not able to know their mothers, this child has benefited, or at least has not been wronged, for without the surrogate arrangement, she would not have been born at all.[7]

But Problems Exist Too

Surrogate mothering is also troublesome. Many people think that it is wrong for a woman to conceive and bear a child that she does not intend to raise, particularly if she receives a fee for her services. There are potential costs to the surrogate and her family, the adoptive couple, the child, and even society at large from satisfying the generative needs of infertile couples in this way.

The couple must be willing to spend about $20,000-25,000, depending on lawyers' fees and the supply of and demand for surrogate mothers. (While this price tag makes the surrogate contract a consumption item for the middle classes, it is not unjust to poor couples, for it does not leave them worse off than they were.) The couple must also be prepared to experience, along with the adjustment and demands of becoming parents, the stress and anxiety of participating in a novel social relationship that many still consider immoral or deviant. What do they tell their friends or family? What do they tell the child? Will the child have contact with the mother? What is the couple's relationship with the surrogate and her family during the pregnancy and after? Without established patterns for handling these questions, the parties may experience confusion, frustration, and embarrassment.

A major source of uncertainty and stress is likely to be the surrogate herself. In most cases she will be a stranger, and may never even meet the couple. The lack of a preexisting relation between the couple and surrogate and the possibility that they live far apart enhance the possibility of mistrust. Is the surrogate taking care of herself? Is she having sex with others during her fertile period? Will she contact the child afterwards? What if she demands more money to relinquish the child? To allay these anxieties, the couple could try to establish a relationship of trust with the surrogate, yet such a relationship creates reciprocal rights and duties and might create demands for an undesired relationship after the birth. Even good lawyering that specifies every contingency in the contract is unlikely to allay uncertainty and anxiety about the surrogate's trustworthiness.

The surrogate may also find the experience less satisfying than she envisioned. Conceiving the child may require insemination efforts over several months at inconvenient locations. The pregnancy and birth may entail more pain, unpleasant side effects, and disruption than she expected. The couple may be more intrusive or more aloof than she wishes. As the pregnancy advances and the birth nears, the surrogate may find it increasingly difficult to remain detached by thinking of the child as "theirs" rather than "hers." Relinquishing the baby after birth may be considerably more disheartening and disappointing than she anticipated. Even if informed of this possibility in advance, she may be distressed for several weeks with feelings of loss, depression, and sleep disturbance.[8] She may feel angry at the couple for cutting off all contact with her once the baby is delivered, and guilty at giving up her child. Finally, she will have to face the loss of all contact with "her" child. As the reality of her situation dawns, she may regret not having bargained harder for access to "her baby."

As with the couple, the surrogate's experience will vary with the expectations, needs, and personalities of the parties, the course of the pregnancy, and an advance understanding of the problems that can arise. The surrogate should have a lawyer to protect her interests. Often, however, the couple's lawyer will end up advising the surrogate. Although he has recruited the surrogate, he is paid by and represents the couple. By disclosing his conflicting interest, he satisfies legal ethics, but he may not serve the interests of the surrogate as well as independent counsel.

Harms to the Child

Unlike embryo transfer, gene therapy, and other manipulative techniques (some of which are collaborative), surrogate arrangements do not pose the risk of physical harm to the offspring. But there is the risk of psychosocial harm. Surrogate mothering, like adoption and artificial insemination by donor (AID), deliberately separates genetic and gestational from social parentage. The mother who begets, bears, and births does not parent. This separation can pose a problem for the child who discovers it. Like adopted and AID children, the child may be strongly motivated to learn the absent parent's identity and to establish a relationship, in this case with the mother and her family. Inability to make that connection, especially inability to learn who the mother is, may affect the child's self-esteem, create feelings of rootlessness, and leave the child thinking that he had been rejected due to some personal fault.[9] While this is a serious concern, the situation is tolerated when it arises with AID and adoptive children. Intentional conception for adoption—the essence of surrogate mothering—poses no different issue.

The child can also be harmed if the adoptive husband and wife are not fit parents. After all, a willingness to spend substantial money to fulfill a desire to rear children is no guarantee of good parenting. But then neither is reproduction by paired mates who wish intensely to have a child. The nonbiologic parent may resent or reject the child, but the same possibility exists with adoption, AID, or ordinary reproduction.

There is also the fear, articulated by such commentators as Leon Kass and Paul Ramsey,[10] that collaborative reproduction confuses the lineage of children and destroys the meaning of family as we know it. In surrogate mothering, as with ovum or womb donors, the genetic and gestational mother does not rear the child, though the biologic father does. What implications does this hold for the family and the child's lineage?

The separation of the child from the genetic or biologic parent in surrogate mothering is hardly unique. It arises with adoption, but surrogate arrangements are more closely akin to AID or blended families, where at least one parent has a blood-tie to the child and the child will know at least one genetic parent. He may, as adopted children often do, have intense desires to learn his biologic mother's identity and seek contact with her and her family. Failure to connect with biologic roots may cause suffering. But the fact that adoption through surrogate mother contracts is planned before conception does not increase the chance of identity confusion, lowered self-esteem, or the blurring of lineage that occurs with adoption or AID.

The greatest chance of confusing family lines arises if the child and couple establish relations with the surrogate and the surrogate's family. If that unlikely event occurs, questions about the child's relations with the surrogate's spouse, parents, and other children can arise. But these issues are not unique. Indeed, they are increasingly common with the growth of blended families. Surrogate mothering in a few instances may lead to a new variation on blended families, but its threat to the family is trivial compared to the rapid changes in family structure now occurring for social, economic, and demographic reasons.

In many cases surrogate motherhood and other forms of collaborative reproduction may shore up, rather than undermine, the traditional family by enabling couples who would otherwise be childless to have children. The practice of employing others to assist in child rearing—including wet-nurses, neonatal ICU nurses, day-care workers, and babysitters—is widely accepted. We also tolerate assistance in the form of sperm sales and donation of egg and gestation (adoption). Surrogate mothering is another method of assisting people to undertake child rearing, and thus serves the purposes of the marital union. It is hard to see how its planned nature obstructs that contribution.

Using Birth For
Selfish Ends

A basic fear about the new reproductive technologies is that they manipulate a natural physiologic process involved in the creation of human life. When one considers the potential power that resides in our ability to manipulate the genes of embryos, the charges of playing God or arrogantly tampering with nature and the resulting dark Huxleyian vision of genetically engineered babies decanted from bottles are not surprising. While *Brave New World* is the standard text for this fear, the 1982 film *Bladerunner* also evokes it. Trycorp., a genetic engineering corporation, manufactures "replicants," who resemble human beings in most respects, including their ability to remember their childhoods, but who are programmed to die in four years. In portraying the replicants' struggle for a long life and full human status, the film raises a host of ethical issues relevant to gene manipulation, from the meaning of personhood to the duties we have in "fabricating" people to make them as whole and healthy as possible.

Such fears, however, are not a sufficient reason to stop splicing genes or relieving infertility through external fertilization.[11] In any event they have no application to surrogate mothering, which does not alter genes or even manipulate the embryo. The only technological aid is a syringe to inseminate and a thermometer to determine when ovulation occurs. Although embryo manipulation would occur if the surrogate received the fertilized egg of another woman, the qualms about surrogate mothering stem less from its potential for technical manipulation, and more from its attitude toward the body and mother-child relations. Mothers bear and give up children for adoption rather frequently when the conception is unplanned. But here the mother conceives the child for that purpose, deliberately using her body for a fee to serve the needs of others. It is the cold willingness to use her body as a baby-making machine and deny the mother-child gestational bond that bothers. (Ironically, the natural bond may turn out to be deeper and stronger than the surrogate imagined.)

Since the transfer of rearing duties from the natural gestational mother to others is widely accepted, the unwillingness of the surrogate mother to rear her child cannot in itself be wrong. As long as she transfers rearing responsibility to capable parents, she is not acting irresponsibly. Still, some persons assert that it is wrong to use the reproductive process for ends other than the good of the child.[12] But the mere presence of selfish motives does not render reproduction immoral, as long as it is carried out in a way that respects the child's interests. Otherwise most pregnancies and births would be immoral, for people have children to serve individual ends as well as the good of the child. In terms of instrumentalism, surrogate mothering cannot be distinguished from most other reproductive situations, whether AID, adoption, or simply planning a child to experience the pleasures of parenthood.

In this vein the problems that can arise when a defective child is born are cited as proof of the immorality of surrogate mothering. The fear is that neither the contracting couple nor the surrogate will want the defective child. In one recent case (*New York Times*, January 28, 1983, p. 18) a dispute arose when none of the parties wanted to take a child born with microcephaly, a condition related to mental retardation. The contracting man claimed on the basis of blood typing that the baby was not his, and thus he was not obligated under the contract to take it, or to pay the surrogate's fee. It turned out that surrogate had borne her husband's child, for she had unwittingly become pregnant by him before being artificially inseminated by the contracting man. The surrogate and her husband eventually assumed responsibility for the child.

An excessively instrumental and callous approach to reproduction when a less than perfect baby is born is not unique to surrogate mothering. Similar reactions can occur whenever married couples have a defective child, as the Baby Doe controversy, which involved the passive euthanasia of a child with Down syndrome, indicates. All surrogate mothering is not wrong because in some instances a handicapped child will be rejected. Nor is it clear that this reaction is more likely in surrogate mothering than in conventional births for it reflects common attitudes toward handicapped newborns as much as alienation in the surrogate arrangement.

As with most situations, "how" something is done is more important than the mere fact of doing it. The morality of surrogate mothering thus depends on how the duties and responsibilities of the role are carried out, rather than on the mere fact that a couple produces a child with the aid of a collaborator. Depending on the circumstances, a surrogate mother can be praised as a benefactor to a suffering couple (the money is hardly adequate compensation) or condemned as a callous user of offspring to further her selfish ends. The view that one takes of her actions will also influence the role one wants the law to play.

What Should the State's Role Be?

What stance should public policy and the law take toward surrogate mothering? As with all collaborative reproduction, a range of choices exists, from prohibition and regulation to active encouragement.

However, there may be constitutional limits to the state's power to restrict collaborative reproduction. The right not to procreate, through contraception and abortion, is now firmly established.[13] A likely implication of these cases, supported by rulings in other cases, is that married persons (and possibly single persons) have a right to bear, beget, birth, and parent children by natural coital means using such technological aids (microsurgery and in vitro fertilization, for example) as are medically available. It should follow that married persons also have a right to engage in noncoital, collaborative reproduction, at least where natural reproduction is not possible. The right of a couple to raise a child should not depend on their luck in the natural lottery, if they can obtain the missing factor of reproduction from others.[14]

If a married couple's right to procreative autonomy includes the right to contract with consenting collaborators, then the state will have a heavy burden of justification for infringing that right. The risks to surrogate, couple, and child do not seem sufficiently compelling to meet this burden, for they are no different from the harms of adoption and AID. Nor will it suffice to point to a communal feeling that such uses of the body are—aside from the consequences—immoral. Moral distaste alone does not justify interference with a fundamental right.

Although surrogate mothering is not now criminal, this discussion is not purely hypothetical. The ban in Michigan and several other states on paying fees for adoption beyond medical expenses has the same effect as an outright prohibition, for few surrogates will volunteer for altruistic reasons alone. A ban on fees is not necessary to protect the surrogate mother from coercion or exploitation, or to protect the child from abuse, the two objectives behind passage of those laws. Unlike the pregnant unmarried woman who "sells" her child, the surrogate has made a considered, knowing choice, often with the assistance of counsel, before becoming pregnant. She may of course choose to be a surrogate for financial reasons, but offering money to do unpleasant tasks is not in itself coercive.

Nor does the child's welfare support a ban on fees, for the risk is no greater than in natural paired reproduction that the parents will be unfit or abuse the child. The specter of slavery, which some opposed to surrogate mothering have raised, is unwarranted. It is quibbling to question whether the couple is "buying" a child or the mother's personal services. Quite clearly, the couple is buying the right to rear a child by paying the mother to beget and bear one for that very purpose. But the purchasers do not buy the right to treat the child or surrogate as a commodity or property. Child abuse and neglect laws still apply, with criminal and civil sanctions available for mistreatment.

The main concern with fees rests on moral and aesthetic grounds. An affront to moral sensibility arises over paying money for a traditionally noncommercial, intimate function. Even though blood and sperm are sold, and miners, professional athletes, and petrochemical workers sell some of their health and vitality, some persons think it wrong for women to bear children for money, in much the same way that paying money for sex or body organs is considered wrong. Every society excludes some exchanges from the marketplace on moral grounds. But the state's power to block exchanges that interfere with the exercise of a fundamental right is limited. Since blocking this exchange stops infertile couples from reproducing and rearing the husband's child, a harm greater than moral distaste is necessary to justify it.

Although the state cannot block collaborative reproductive exchanges on moral grounds, it need not subsidize or encourage surrogate contracts. One could argue that allowing the parties to a surrogate contract to use the courts to terminate parental rights, certify paternity, and legalize adoption is a subsidy and therefore not required of the state. Similarly, a state's refusal to enforce surrogate contracts as a matter of public policy could be taken as a refusal to subsidize rather than as interference with the right to reproduce. But given the state's monopoly of those functions and the impact its denial will have on the ability of infertile couples to find reproductive collaborators, it is more plausible to view the refusal to certify and effectuate surrogate contracts as an infringement of the right to procreate. Denying an adoption because it was agreed upon in advance for a fee interferes with the couple's procreative autonomy as much as any criminal penalty for paying a fee to or contracting with a collaborator. (The crucial distinction between interfering with and not encouraging the exercise of a right has been overlooked by the Michigan and Kentucky courts that have held constitutional the refusal to allow adoptions or paternity determinations where a fee has been paid to the surrogate mother. This error makes these cases highly questionable precedents.[15])

A conclusion that surrogate contracts must be *enforced*, however, does not require that they be specifically carried out in all instances. As long as damage remedies remain, there is no constitutional right to specific performance. For example, a court need not enjoin the surrogate who changes her mind about abortion or relinquishing the child once it is born. A surrogate who wants to breach the contract by abortion should pay damages, but not be ordered to continue the pregnancy, because of the difficulty in enforcing or monitoring the order. (Whether damages are a practical alternative in such cases will depend on the surrogate's economic situation, or whether bonding or insurance to assure her contractual obligation is possible.) On the other hand, a court could reasonably order the surrogate after birth to relinquish the child. Whether such an order should issue will depend on whether the surrogate's interest in keeping the child is deemed greater than the couple's interest in rearing (assuming that both are fit parents). A commitment to freedom of contract and the rights of parties to arrange collaborative reproduction would favor the adoptive couple, while sympathy for the gestational bond between mother and child would favor the mother. If the mother prevailed, the couple should still have other remedies, including visitation rights for the father, restitution of the surrogate's fee and other expenses, and perhaps money damages as well.

The constitutional status of a married couple's procreative choice shields collaborative arrangements from interference on moral grounds alone, but not from all regulation. While the parties may assign the rearing rights according to contract, the state need not leave the entire transaction to the vagaries of the private sector. Regulation to minimize harm and assure knowing choices would be permissible, as long as the regulation is reasonably related to promoting these goals.

For example, the state could set minimum standards for surrogate brokers, set age and health qualifications for surrogates, and structure the transaction to assure voluntary, knowing choices. The state could also define and allocate responsibilities among the parties to protect the best interests of the offspring—for example, refusing to protect the surrogate's anonymity, requiring that the contracting couple assume responsibility for a defective child, or even transferring custody to another if threats to the child's welfare justify such a move.

Not What We Do— But How We Do It

The central issue with surrogate mothering, as with other collaborative reproduction, is not the deliberate separation of biologic and social parentage, but how the separation is effected and the resulting relationship with the third party. If the third party's involvement in the reproduction is discrete and limited, collaborative reproduction is easily tolerated. Thus few people question the anonymous sperm donor's lack of rights and duties toward the offspring, except in the case where the mother and donor have expressly agreed that he would have some access to the rearing of a child.[16] The donor's claim—and possibly the child's need to connect—is less strong in such cases. Egg donations, though involving more risk and burden for the donor, should be similarly treated, for they are also discrete and limited.

Collaborative reproduction involving gestational contributors poses more difficult problems, because the nine-month gestational period creates a unique and powerful bond for both donor and offspring that seems to justify a claim in its own right. Yet in adoption we allow those claims to be nullified by the gestational mother's choice. Surrogate motherhood presents the same issue. The difference is that it is planned before conception, but that hardly seems to matter once the child is born and the mother wishes to fulfill her commitment. The issue of whether the mother should be held to a promise on which others have relied is distinct from the question of whether mothers can relinquish children deliberately conceived for others outside the agency-controlled adoption process.

Surrogate mothering casts particular light on one other collaborative technique that may soon be widely available—the transfer of the externally (or internally) fertilized egg of one woman to another woman who gestates and births it.[17] The third party in this situation is a gestational surrogate for a genetic and rearing mother, who is unable or unwilling to bear and birth her child. At first glance the gestational mother's claim to the child seems less compelling than the claim of the surrogate mother because the child is not genetically hers. Yet concerns will arise, as with surrogate mothers, over the severing or denial of the gestational bond, the degree to which the contract should be honored, and the gestational mother's relationship (if any) with the child.

The moral issues surrounding surrogate mothering also cast light on the problems with manipulative techniques such as genetic alteration of the embryo and non-uterine gestation of the fertilized egg. Since those techniques will be used primarily for paired reproduction, the main concerns will be the safety of the offspring and the morality of genetic manipulation. However, when manipulation and collaborative reproduction are combined, the relationship of the offspring to the third party contributor will come into question.

Surrogate mothering for a fee is neither the evil nor the panacea that many have thought. It is barely distinguishable from the many current practices that separate biologic and social parentage and that seek parenthood for personal satisfaction. The differences do not appear to be great enough to justify prohibition, active discouragement, or for that matter, encouragement. Like many human endeavors, in the final analysis, what matters is not *whether* but *how* it is done. In that respect public scrutiny, through regulation of the process of drawing up the contract rather than its specific terms, could help to assure that it is done well.

References

The author gratefully acknowledges the comments of Rebecca Dresser, Mark Frankel, Inga Markovits, Phillip Parker, Bruce Russell, John Sampson, and Ted Schneyer on earlier drafts.

1. People v. Sorenson, 68 Cal. 2d 280, 437 P.2d 495; Walter Wadlington, "Artificial Insemination: The Dangers of a Poorly Kept Secret," *Northwestern Law Review* 64 (1970), 777.

2. See, for example, Michigan Statutes Annotated, 27.3178 (555.54)(555.69)(1980).

3. William Landes and Eleanor Posner, "The Economics of the Baby Shortage," *Journal of Legal Studies* 7 (1978), 323.

4. See Erik Erikson, *The Life Cycle Completed* (New York: Norton, 1980), pp. 122–124.

5. Phillip Parker, "Surrogate Mother's Motivations: Initial Findings," *American Journal of Psychiatry* 140:1 (January 1983), 117–118; Phillip Parker, "The Psychology of Surrogate Motherhood: A Preliminary Report of a Longitudinal Pilot Study" (unpublished). See also Dava Sobel, "Surrogate Mothers: Why Women Volunteer," *New York Times*, June 25, 1981, p. 18.

6. Mark Frankel, "Surrogate Motherhood: An Ethical Perspective," pp. 1–2. (Paper presented at Wayne State Symposium on Surrogate Motherhood, Nov. 20, 1982.)

7. See John Robertson, "In Vitro Conception and Harm to the Unborn," *Hastings Center Report* 8 (October 1978), 13–14; Michael Bayles, "Harm to the Unconceived," *Philosophy and Public Affairs* 5 (1976), 295.

8. A small, uncontrolled study found these effects to last some four to six weeks. Statement of Nancy Reame, R.N., at Wayne State University, Symposium on Surrogate Motherhood, Nov. 20, 1982.

9. Betty Jane Lifton, *Twice Born: Memoirs of an Adopted Daughter* (New York: Penguin, 1977); L. Dusky, "Brave New Babies," *Newsweek*, Dec. 6, 1982, p. 30.

10. Leon Kass, "Making Babies—the New Biology and the Old Morality," *The Public Interest* 26 (1972), 18; "Making Babies Revisited," *The Public Interest* 54 (1979), 32; Paul Ramsey, *Fabricated Man: The Ethics of Genetic Control* (New Haven: Yale University Press, 1970).

11. The President's Commission for the Study of Ethical Problems in Medicine and Biomedical and Behavioral Research, *Splicing Life: The Social and Ethical Issues of Genetic Engineering with Human Beings* (Washington, D.C., 1982), pp. 53–60.

12. Herbert Krimmel, Testimony before California Assembly Committee on Judiciary, Surrogate Parenting Contracts (November 14, 1982), pp. 89–96.

13. Griswold v. Connecticut, 381 U.S. 479 (1964); Eisenstadt v. Baird, 405 U.S. 438 (1972); Roe v. Wade, 410 U.S. 113 (1973); Planned Parenthood v. Danforth, 428 U.S. 52 (1976); Bellotti v. Baird, 443 U.S. 622 (1979); Carey v. Population Services International, 431 U.S. 678 (1977).

14. Although this article does not address the right of single persons to contract with others for reproductive purposes, it should be noted that the right of married persons to engage in collaborative reproduction does not entail a similar right for unmarried persons. For a more detailed exposition of the arguments for the reproductive rights of married and single persons, see John Robertson, "Procreative Liberty and the Control of Conception, Pregnancy and Childbirth," *Virginia Law Review* 69 (April 1983), 405, 418–420.

15. See Doe v. Kelley, 106 Mich. App. 164, 307 N.W.2d 438 (1981); Syrkowski v. Appleyard, 9 Family Law Rptr. 2348 (April 5, 1983); In re Baby Girl, 9 Family Law Reptr. 2348 (March 8, 1983).

16. See C.M. v. C.C., 152 N.J. 160, 377 A.2d 821 (man who provided sperm for artificial insemination held to have visitation rights because of express agreement with the mother).

17. See Richard D. Lyons, "2 Women Become Pregnant With Transferred Embryos," *New York Times*, July 22, 1983, p. A1, B7.

In the Matter of Baby M, a Pseudonym for an Actual Person

Argued September 14, 1987— Decided February 3, 1988

Synopsis

Natural father and his wife brought suit seeking to enforce surrogate parenting agreement, to compel surrender of infant born to surrogate mother, to restrain any interference with their custody of infant, and to terminate surrogate mother's parental rights to allow adoption of child by wife of natural father. The Superior Court, Chancery Division/Family Part, Bergen County, 217 N.J.Super. 313, held that surrogate contract was valid, ordered that mother's parental rights be terminated and that sole custody of child be granted to natural father, and authorized adoption of child by father's wife. Mother appealed, and the Supreme Court granted direct certification. The Supreme Court, Wilentz, C.J., held that: (1) surrogate contract conflicted with laws prohibiting use of money in connection with adoptions, laws requiring proof of parental unfitness or abandonment before termination of parental rights is ordered or adoption is granted, and laws making surrender of custody and consent to adoption revocable in private placement adoptions; (2) surrogate contract conflicted with state public policy; (3) right of procreation did not entitle natural father and his wife to custody of child; (4) best interests of child justified awarding custody to father and his wife; and (5) mother was entitled to visitation with child.

Affirmed in part; reversed in part; and remanded. . . .

The opinion of the Court was delivered by

WILENTZ, C.J.

In this matter the Court is asked to determine the validity of a contract that purports to provide a new way of bringing children into a family. For a fee of $10,000, a woman agrees to be artificially inseminated with the semen of another woman's husband; she is to conceive a child, carry it to term, and after its birth surrender it to the natural father and his wife. The intent of the contract is that the child's natural mother will thereafter be forever separated from her child. The wife is to adopt the child, and she and the natural father are to be regarded as its parents for all purposes. The contract providing for this is called a "surrogacy contract," the natural mother inappropriately called the "surrogate mother."

We invalidate the surrogacy contract because it conflicts with the law and public policy of this State. While we recognize the depth of the yearning of infertile couples to have their own children, we find the payment of money to a "surrogate" mother illegal, perhaps criminal, and potentially degrading to women. Although in this case we grant custody to the natural father, the evidence having clearly proved such custody to be in the best interests of the infant, we void both the termination of the surrogate mother's parental rights and the adoption of the child by the wife/stepparent. We thus restore the "surrogate" as the mother of the child. We remand the issue of the natural mother's visitation rights to the trial court, since that issue was not reached below and the record before us is not sufficient to permit us to decide it *de novo*.

We find no offense to our present laws where a woman voluntarily and without payment agrees to act as a "surrogate" mother, provided that she is not subject to a binding agreement to surrender her child. Moreover, our holding today does not preclude the Legislature from altering the current statutory scheme, within constitutional limits, so as to permit surrogacy contracts. Under current law, however, the surrogacy agreement before us is illegal and invalid. . . .

Invalidity and Unenforceability of Surrogacy Contract

We have concluded that this surrogacy contract is invalid. Our conclusion has two bases: direct conflict with existing statutes and conflict with the public policies of this State, as expressed in its statutory and decisional law.

[2] One of the surrogacy contract's basic purposes, to achieve the adoption of a child through private placement, though permitted in New Jersey "is very much disfavored." *Sees v. Baber*, 74 *N.J.* 201, 217 (1977). Its use of money for this purpose—and we have no doubt whatsoever that the money is being paid to obtain an adoption and not, as the Sterns argue, for the personal services of Mary Beth Whitehead—is illegal and perhaps criminal. *N.J.S.A.* 9:3–54. In addition to the inducement of money, there is the coercion of contract: the natural mother's irrevocable agreement, prior to birth, even prior to conception, to surrender the child to the adoptive couple. Such an agreement is totally unenforceable in private placement adoption. *Sees*, 74 *N.J.* at 212–14. Even where the adoption is through an approved agency, the formal agreement to surrender occurs only *after* birth (as we read *N.J.S.A.* 9:2–16 and –17, and similar statutes), and then, by regulation, only after the birth mother has been counseled. *N.J.A.C.* 10:121A–5.2(a). Integral to these invalid provisions of the surrogacy contract is the related agreement, equally invalid, on the part of the natural mother to cooperate

with, and not to contest, proceedings to terminate her parental rights, as well as her contractual concession, in aid of the adoption, that the child's best interests would be served by awarding custody to the natural father and his wife—all of this before she has even conceived, and, in some cases, before she has the slightest idea of what the natural father and adoptive mother are like.

The foregoing provisions not only directly conflict with New Jersey statutes, but also offend long-established State policies. These critical terms, which are at the heart of the contract, are invalid and unenforceable; the conclusion therefore follows, without more, that the entire contract is unenforceable.

A. Conflict with Statutory Provisions

The surrogacy contract conflicts with: (1) laws prohibiting the use of money in connection with adoptions; (2) laws requiring proof of parental unfitness or abandonment before termination of parental rights is ordered or an adoption is granted; and (3) laws that make surrender of custody and consent to adoption revocable in private placement adoptions.

[3] (1) Our law prohibits paying or accepting money in connection with any placement of a child for adoption. *N.J.S.A.* 9:3–54a. Violation is a high misdemeanor. *N.J.S.A.* 9:3–54c. Excepted are fees of an approved agency (which must be a non-profit entity, *N.J.S.A.* 9:3–38a) and certain expenses in connection with childbirth. *N.J.S.A.* 9:3–54b.[1]

Considerable care was taken in this case to structure the surrogacy arrangement so as not to violate this prohibition. The arrangement was structured as follows: the adopting parent, Mrs. Stern, was not a party to the surrogacy contract; the money paid to Mrs. Whitehead was stated to be for her services—not for the adoption; the sole purpose of the contract was stated as being that "of giving a child to William Stern, its natural and biological father"; the money was purported to be "compensation for services and expenses and in no way . . . a fee for termination of parental rights or a payment in exchange for consent to surrender a child for adoption"; the fee to the Infertility Center ($7,500) was stated to be for legal representation, advice, administrative work, and other "services." Nevertheless, it seems clear that the money was paid and accepted in connection with an adoption.

---

[1]*N.J.S.A.* 9:3–54 reads as follows:

a. No person, firm, partnership, corporation, association or agency shall make, offer to make or assist or participate in any placement for adoption and in connection therewith

(1) Pay, give or agree to give any money or any valuable consideration, or assume or discharge any financial obligation; or

(2) Take, receive, accept or agree to accept any money or any valuable consideration.

b. The prohibition of subsection a. shall not apply to the fees or services of any approved agency in connection with a placement for adoption, nor shall such prohibition apply to the payment or reimbursement of medical, hospital or other similar expenses incurred in connection with the birth or any illness of the child, or to the acceptance of such reimbursement by a parent of the child.

c. Any person, firm, partnership, corporation, association or agency violating this section shall be guilty of a high misdemeanor.

The Infertility Center's major role was first as a "finder" of the surrogate mother whose child was to be adopted, and second as the arranger of all proceedings that led to the adoption. Its role as adoption finder is demonstrated by the provision requiring Mr. Stern to pay another $7,500 if he uses Mary Beth Whitehead again as a surrogate, and by ICNY's agreement to "coordinate arrangements for the adoption of the child by the wife." The surrogacy agreement requires Mrs. Whitehead to surrender Baby M for the purposes of adoption. The agreement notes that Mr. *and Mrs.* Stern wanted to have a child, and provides that the child be "placed" with Mrs. Stern in the event Mr. Stern dies before the child is born. The payment of the $10,000 occurs only on surrender of custody of the child and "completion of the duties and obligations" of Mrs. Whitehead, including termination of her parental rights to facilitate adoption by Mrs. Stern. As for the contention that the Sterns are paying only for services and not for an adoption, we need note only that they would pay nothing in the event the child died before the fourth month of pregnancy, and only $1,000 if the child were stillborn, even though the "services" had been fully rendered. Additionally, one of Mrs. Whitehead's estimated costs, to be assumed by Mr. Stern, was an "Adoption Fee," presumably for Mrs. Whitehead's incidental costs in connection with the adoption.

Mr. Stern knew he was paying for the adoption of a child; Mrs. Whitehead knew she was accepting money so that a child might be adopted; the Infertility Center knew that it was being paid for assisting in the adoption of a child. The actions of all three worked to frustrate the goals of the statute. It strains credulity to claim that these arrangements, touted by those in the surrogacy business as an attractive alternative to the usual route leading to an adoption, really amount to something other than a private placement adoption for money.

The prohibition of our statute is strong. Violation constitutes a high misdemeanor, *N.J.S.A.* 9:3–54c, a third-degree crime, *N.J.S.A.* 2C:43–1b, carrying a penalty of three to five years imprisonment. *N.J.S.A.* 2C:43–6a(3). The evils inherent in baby bartering are loathsome for a myriad of reasons. The child is sold without regard for whether the purchasers will be suitable parents. N. Baker, *Baby Selling: The Scandal of Black Market Adoption* 7 (1978). The natural mother does not receive the benefit of counseling and guidance to assist her in making a decision that may affect her for a lifetime. In fact, the monetary incentive to sell her child may, depending on her financial circumstances, make her decision less voluntary. *Id.* at 44. Furthermore, the adoptive parents[2] may not be fully informed of the natural parents' medical history.

Baby-selling potentially results in the exploitation of all parties involved. *Id.* Conversely, adoption statutes seek to further humanitarian goals, foremost among them the best interests of the child. H. Witmer, E. Herzog, E. Weinstein, & M. Sullivan, *Independent Adoptions: A Follow-Up Study* 32 (1967). The negative consequences of baby buying are potentially present in the surrogacy context, especially the potential for placing and adopting a child without regard to the interest of the child or the natural mother.

---

[2]Of course, here there are no "adoptive parents," but rather the natural father and his wife, the only adoptive parent. As noted, however, many of the dangers of using money in connection with adoption may exist in surrogacy situations.

[4, 5] (2) The termination of Mrs. Whitehead's parental rights, called for by the surrogacy contract and actually ordered by the court, 217 *N.J.Super.* at 399–400, fails to comply with the stringent requirements of New Jersey law. Our law, recognizing the finality of any termination of parental rights, provides for such termination only where there has been a voluntary surrender of a child to an approved agency or to the Division of Youth and Family Services ("DYFS"), accompanied by a formal document acknowledging termination of parental rights, *N.J.S.A.* 9:2–16, –17; *N.J.S.A.* 9:3–41; *N.J.S.A.* 30:4C–23, or where there has been a showing of parental abandonment or unfitness. A termination may ordinarily take one of three forms: an action by an approved agency, an action by DYFS, or an action in connection with a private placement adoption. The three are governed by separate statutes, but the standards for termination are substantially the same, except that whereas a written surrender is effective when made to an approved agency or to DYFS, there is no provision for it in the private placement context. *See N.J.S.A.* 9:2–14; *N.J.S.A.* 30:4C–23.

N.J.S.A. 9:2–18 to –20 governs an action by an approved agency to terminate parental rights. Such an action, whether or not in conjunction with a pending adoption, may proceed on proof of written surrender, *N.J.S.A.* 9:2–16, –17, "forsaken parental obligation," or other specific grounds such as death or insanity, *N.J.S.A.* 9:2–19. Where the parent has not executed a formal consent, termination requires a showing of "forsaken parental obligation," *i.e.*, "willful and continuous neglect or failure to perform the natural and regular obligations of care and support of a child." *N.J.S.A.* 9:2–13(d). *See also N.J.S.A.* 9:3–46a, –47c.

Where DYFS is the agency seeking termination, the requirements are similarly stringent, although at first glance they do not appear to be so. DYFS can, as can any approved agency, accept a formal voluntary surrender or writing having the effect of termination and giving DYFS the right to place the child for adoption. *N.J.S.A.* 30:4C–23. Absent such formal written surrender and consent, similar to that given to approved agencies, DYFS can terminate parental rights in an action for guardianship by proving that "the best interests of such child require that he be placed under proper guardianship." *N.J.S.A.* 30:4C–20. Despite this "best interests" language, however, this Court has recently held in *New Jersey Div. of Youth & Family Servs. v. A.W.*, 103 *N.J.* 591 (1986), that in order for DYFS to terminate parental rights it must prove, by clear and convincing evidence, that "[t]he child's health and development have been or will be seriously impaired by the parental relationship," *id.* at 604, that "[t]he parents are unable or unwilling to eliminate the harm and delaying permanent placement will add to the harm," *id.* at 605, that "[t]he court has considered alternatives to termination," *id.* at 608, and that "[t]he termination of parental rights will not do more harm than good." *Id.* at 610. This interpretation of the statutory language requires a most substantial showing of harm to the child if the parental relationship were to continue, far exceeding anything that a "best interests" test connotes.

In order to terminate parental rights under the private placement adoption statute, there must be a finding of "intentional abandonment or a very substantial neglect of parental duties without a reasonable expectation of a reversal of that conduct in the future." *N.J.S.A.* 9:3–48c(1). This requirement is similar to that of the prior law (*i.e.*, "forsaken parental obligations," *L.*1953, *c.* 264, § 2(d) (codified at *N.J.S.A.* 9:3–18(d) (repealed)), and to that of the law providing for termination through actions by approved agencies, *N.J.S.A.* 9:2–13(d). *See also In re Adoption by J.J.P.*, 175 *N.J.Super.* 420, 427 (App.Div.1980) (noting that the language of the termination provision in the present statute, *N.J.S.A.* 9:3–48c(1), derives from this Court's construction of the prior statute in *In re Adoption of Children by D*, 61 *N.J.* 89, 94–95 (1972)).

In *Sees v. Baber*, 74 *N.J.* 201 (1977) we distinguished the requirements for terminating parental rights in a private placement adoption from those required in an approved agency adoption. We stated that in an unregulated private placement, "neither consent nor voluntary surrender is singled out as a statutory factor in terminating parental rights." *Id.* at 213. *Sees* established that without proof that parental obligations had been forsaken, there would be no termination in a private placement setting.

[6] As the trial court recognized, without a valid termination there can be no adoption. *In re Adoption of Children by D., supra*, 61 *N.J.* at 95. This requirement applies to all adoptions, whether they be private placements, *ibid.*, or agency adoptions, *N.J.S.A.* 9:3–46a, –47c.

[7–10] Our statutes, and the cases interpreting them, leave no doubt that where there has been no written surrender to an approved agency or to DYFS, termination of parental rights will not be granted in this state absent a very strong showing of abandonment or neglect. *See, e.g., Sorentino v. Family & Children's Soc'y of Elizabeth*, 74 *N.J.* 313 (1977) (*Sorentino II*); *Sees v. Baber*, 74 *N.J.* 201 (1977); *Sorentino v. Family & Children's Soc'y of Elizabeth*, 72 *N.J.* 127 (1976) (*Sorentino I*); *In re Adoption of Children by D., supra*, 61 *N.J.* 89. That showing is required in every context in which termination of parental rights is sought, be it an action by an approved agency, an action by DYFS, or a private placement adoption proceeding, even where the petitioning adoptive parent is, as here, a stepparent. While the statutes make certain procedural allowances when stepparents are involved, *N.J.S.A.* 9:3–48a(2), –48a(4), –48c(4), the substantive requirement for terminating the natural parents' rights is not relaxed one iota. *N.J.S.A.* 9:3–48c(1); *In re Adoption of Children by D., supra*, 61 *N.J.* at 94–95; *In re Adoption by J.J.P., supra*, 175 *N.J.Super.* at 426–28; *In re N.*, 96 *N.J.Super.* 415, 423–27 (App.Div.1967). It is clear that a "best interests" determination is never sufficient to terminate parental rights; the statutory criteria must be proved.[3]

---

[3]Counsel for the Sterns argues that the Parentage Act empowers the court to terminate parental rights solely on the basis of the child's best interests. He cites *N.J.S.A.* 9:17–53c, which reads, in pertinent part, as follows:

> The judgment or order may contain any other provision directed against the appropriate party to the proceeding concerning the duty of support, the custody and guardianship of the child, visitation privileges with the child, the furnishing of bond or other security for the payment of the judgment, the repayment of any public assistance grant, or *any other matter in the best interests of the child.* [Emphasis supplied].

We do not interpret this section as in any way altering or diluting the statutory prerequisites to termination discussed above. Termination of parental rights differs qualitatively from the matters to which this section is expressly directed, and, in any event, we have no doubt that if the Legislature had intended a substantive change in the standards governing an area of such gravity, it would have said so explicitly.

[11] In this case a termination of parental rights was obtained not by proving the statutory prerequisites but by claiming the benefit of contractual provisions. From all that has been stated above, it is clear that a contractual agreement to abandon one's parental rights, or not to contest a termination action, will not be enforced in our courts. The Legislature would not have so carefully, so consistently, and so substantially restricted termination of parental rights if it had intended to allow termination to be achieved by one short sentence in a contract.

Since the termination was invalid,[4] it follows, as noted above, that adoption of Melissa by Mrs. Stern could not properly be granted.

[12] (3) The provision in the surrogacy contract stating that Mary Beth Whitehead agrees to "surrender custody . . . and terminate all parental rights" contains no clause giving her a right to rescind. It is intended to be an irrevocable consent to surrender the child for adoption–in other words, an irrevocable commitment by Mrs. Whitehead to turn Baby M over to the Sterns and thereafter to allow termination of her parental rights. The trial court required a "best interests" showing as a condition to granting specific performance of the surrogacy contract. 217 *N.J.Super.* at 399–400. Having decided the "best interests" issue in favor of the Sterns, that court's order included, among other things, specific performance of this agreement to surrender custody and terminate all parental rights.

Mrs. Whitehead, shortly after the child's birth, had attempted to revoke her consent and surrender by refusing, after the Sterns had allowed her to have the child "just for one week," to return Baby M to them. The trial court's award of specific performance therefore reflects its view that the consent to surrender the child was irrevocable. We accept the trial court's construction of the contract; indeed it appears quite clear that this was the parties' intent. Such a provision, however, making irrevocable the natural mother's consent to surrender custody of her child in a private placement adoption, clearly conflicts with New Jersey law.

Our analysis commences with the statute providing for surrender of custody to an approved agency and termination of parental rights on the suit of that agency. The two basic provisions of the statute are *N.J.S.A.* 9:2–14 and 9:2–16. The former provides explicitly that:

> "Except as otherwise provided by law or by order or judgment of a court of competent jurisdiction or by testamentary disposition, no surrender of the custody of a child shall be valid in this state unless made to an approved agency pursuant to the provisions of this act. . . ."

There is no exception "provided by law," and it is not clear that there could be any "order or judgment of a court of competent jurisdiction" validating a surrender of custody as a basis for adoption when that surrender was not in conformance with the statute. Requirements for a voluntary surrender to an approved agency are set forth in *N.J.S.A.* 9:2–16. This section allows an approved agency to take a voluntary surrender

---

[4]We conclude not only that the surrogacy contract is an insufficient basis for termination, but that no statutory or other basis for termination existed. *See infra* at 444–447.

of custody from the parent of a child but provides stringent requirements as a condition to its validity. The surrender must be in writing, must be in such form as is required for the recording of a deed, and, pursuant to *N.J.S.A.* 9:2–17, must

> be such as to declare that the person executing the same desires to relinquish the custody of the child, acknowledge the termination of parental rights as to such custody in favor of the approved agency, and acknowledge full understanding of the effect of such surrender as provided by this act.

If the foregoing requirements are met, the consent, the voluntary surrender of custody

> shall be valid whether or not the person giving same is a minor and shall be irrevocable except at the discretion of the approved agency taking such surrender or upon order or judgment of a court of competent jurisdiction, setting aside such surrender upon proof of fraud, duress, or misrepresentation. [*N.J.S.A.* 9:2–16.]

The importance of that irrevocability is that the surrender itself gives the agency the power to obtain termination of parental rights—in other words, permanent separation of the parent from the child, leading in the ordinary case to an adoption. *N.J.S.A.* 9:2–18 to –20.

[13] This statutory pattern, providing for a surrender in writing and for termination of parental rights by an approved agency, is generally followed in connection with adoption proceedings and proceedings by DYFS to obtain permanent custody of a child. Our adoption statute repeats the requirements necessary to accomplish an irrevocable surrender to an approved agency in both form and substance. *N.J.S.A.* 9:3–41a. It provides that the surrender "shall be valid and binding without regard to the age of the person executing the surrender," *ibid.*; and although the word "irrevocable" is not used, that seems clearly to be the intent of the provision. The statute speaks of such surrender as constituting "relinquishment of such person's parental rights in or guardianship or custody of the child *named therein* and consent by such person to adoption of the child." *Ibid.* (emphasis supplied). We emphasize "named therein," for we construe the statute to allow a surrender only after the birth of the child. The formal consent to surrender enables the approved agency to terminate parental rights.

Similarly, DYFS is empowered to "take voluntary surrenders and releases of custody and consents to adoption[s]" from parents, which surrenders, releases, or consents "when properly acknowledged . . . shall be valid and binding irrespective of the age of the person giving the same, and shall be irrevocable except at the discretion of the Bureau of Children's Services [currently DYFS] or upon order of a court of competent jurisdiction." *N.J.S.A.* 30:4C–23. Such consent to surrender of the custody of the child would presumably lead to an adoption placement by DYFS. See *N.J.S.A.* 30:4C–20.

It is clear that the Legislature so carefully circumscribed all aspects of a consent to surrender custody—its form and substance, its manner of execution, and the agency or agencies to which it may be made—in order to provide the basis for irrevocability.

It seems most unlikely that the Legislature intended that a consent not complying with these requirements would also be irrevocable, especially where, as here, that consent falls radically short of compliance. Not only do the form and substance of the consent in the surrogacy contract fail to meet statutory requirements, but the surrender of custody is made to a private party. It is not made, as the statute requires, either to an approved agency or to DYFS.

These strict prerequisites to irrevocability constitute a recognition of the most serious consequences that flow from such consents: termination of parental rights, the permanent separation of parent from child, and the ultimate adoption of the child. *See Sees v. Baber, supra,* 74 *N.J.* at 217. Because of those consequences, the Legislature severely limited the circumstances under which such consent would be irrevocable. The legislative goal is furthered by regulations requiring approved agencies, prior to accepting irrevocable consents, to provide advice and counseling to women, making it more likely that they fully understand and appreciate the consequences of their acts. *N.J. A.C.* 10:121A–5.2(a).

Contractual surrender of parental rights is not provided for in our statutes as now written. Indeed, in the Parentage Act, *N.J.S.A.* 9:17–38 to –59, there is a specific provision invalidating any agreement "between an alleged or presumed father and the mother of the child" to bar an action brought for the purpose of determining paternity "[r]egardless of [the contract's] terms." *N.J.S.A.* 9:17–45. Even a settlement agreement concerning parentage reached in a judicially-mandated consent conference is not valid unless the proposed settlement is approved beforehand by the court. *N.J.S.A.* 9:17–48c and d. There is no doubt that a contractual provision purporting to constitute an irrevocable agreement to surrender custody of a child for adoption is invalid.

In *Sees v. Baber, supra,* 74 *N.J.* 201, we noted that a natural mother's consent to surrender her child and to its subsequent adoption was no longer *required* by the statute in private placement adoptions. After tracing the statutory history from the time when such a consent had been an essential prerequisite to adoption, we concluded that such a consent was now neither necessary nor sufficient for the purpose of terminating parental rights. *Id.* at 213. The consent to surrender custody in that case was in writing, had been executed prior to physical surrender of the infant, and had been explained to the mother by an attorney. The trial court found that the consent to surrender of custody in that private placement adoption was knowing, voluntary, and deliberate. *Id.* at 216. The physical surrender of the child took place four days after its birth. Two days thereafter the natural mother changed her mind, and asked that the adoptive couple give her baby back to her. We held that she was entitled to the baby's return. The effect of our holding in that case necessarily encompassed our conclusion that "in an unsupervised private placement, since there is no statutory obligation to consent, there can be no legal barrier to its retraction." *Id.* at 215. The only possible relevance of consent in these matters, we noted, was that it *might* bear on whether there had been an abandonment of the child, or a forsaking of parental obligations. *Id.* at 216. Otherwise, consent in a private placement adoption is not only revocable but, when revoked early enough, irrelevant. *Id.* at 213–15.

[14] The provision in the surrogacy contract whereby the mother irrevocably agrees to surrender custody of her child and to terminate her parental rights conflicts

with the settled interpretation of New Jersey statutory law.[5] There is only one irrevocable consent, and that is the one explicitly provided for by statute: a consent to surrender of custody and a placement with an approved agency or with DYFS. The provision in the surrogacy contract, agreed to before conception, requiring the natural mother to surrender custody of the child without any right of revocation is one more indication of the essential nature of this transaction: the creation of a contractual system of termination and adoption designed to circumvent our statutes.

B. Public Policy Considerations

[15] The surrogacy contract's invalidity, resulting from its direct conflict with the above statutory provisions, is further underlined when its goals and means are measured against New Jersey's public policy. The contract's basic premise, that the natural parents can decide in advance of birth which one is to have custody of the child, bears no relationship to the settled law that the child's best interests shall determine custody. *See Fantony v. Fantony*, 21 *N.J.* 525, 536–37 (1956); *see also Sheehan v. Sheehan*, 38 *N.J.Super.* 120, 125 (App.Div.1955) ("Whatever the agreement of the parents, the ultimate determination of custody lies with the court in the exercise of its supervisory jurisdiction as *parens patriae*."). The fact that the trial court remedied that aspect of the contract through the "best interests" phase does not make the contractual provision any less offensive to the public policy of this State.

The surrogacy contract guarantees permanent separation of the child from one of its natural parents. Our policy, however, has long been that to the extent possible, children should remain with and be brought up by both of their natural parents. That was the first stated purpose of the previous adoption act, *L.*1953, *c.* 264, § 1, codified at *N.J.S.A.* 9:3–17 (repealed): "it is necessary and desirable (a) to protect the child from unnecessary separation from his natural parents. . . ." While not so stated in the present adoption law, this purpose remains part of the public policy of this State. *See, e.g., Wilke v. Culp*, 196 *N.J.Super.* 487, 496 (App.Div.1984), certif. den., 99 *N.J.* 243 (1985); *In re Adoption by J.J.P., supra*, 175 *N.J.Super.* at 426. This is not simply some theoretical ideal that in practice has no meaning. The impact of failure to follow that policy is nowhere better shown than in the results of this surrogacy contract. A child, instead of starting off its life with as much peace and security as possible, finds itself immediately in a tug-of-war between contending mother and father.[6]

---

[5]The surrogacy situation, of course, differs from the situation in *Sees*, in that here there is no "adoptive couple," but rather the natural father and the stepmother, who is the would-be adoptive mother. This difference, however, does not go to the basis of the *Sees* holding. In both cases, the determinative aspect is the vulnerability of the natural mother who decides to surrender her child in the absence of institutional safeguards.

[6]And the impact on the natural parents, Mr. Stern and Mrs. Whitehead, is severe and dramatic. The depth of their conflict about Baby M, about custody, visitation, about the goodness or badness of each of them, comes through in their telephone conversations, in which each tried to persuade the other to give up the child. The potential adverse consequences of surrogacy are poignantly captured here— Mrs. Whitehead threatening to kill herself and the baby, Mr. Stern begging her not to, each blaming the other. The dashed hopes of the Sterns, the agony of Mrs. Whitehead, their suffering, their hatred—all were caused by the unraveling of this arrangement.

The surrogacy contract violates the policy of this State that the rights of natural parents are equal concerning their child, the father's right no greater than the mother's. "The parent and child relationship extends equally to every child and to every parent, regardless of the marital status of the parents." *N.J.S.A.* 9:17–40. As the Assembly Judiciary Committee noted in its statement to the bill, this section establishes "the principle that regardless of the marital status of the parents, all children *and all parents* have equal rights with respect to each other." *Statement to Senate No. 888*, Assembly Judiciary, Law, Public Safety and Defense Committee (1983) (emphasis supplied). The whole purpose and effect of the surrogacy contract was to give the father the exclusive right to the child by destroying the rights of the mother.

The policies expressed in our comprehensive laws governing consent to the surrender of a child, discussed *supra* at 429–434, stand in stark contrast to the surrogacy contract and what it implies. Here there is no counseling, independent or otherwise, of the natural mother, no evaluation, no warning.

The only legal advice Mary Beth Whitehead received regarding the surrogacy contract was provided in connection with the contract that she previously entered into with another couple. Mrs. Whitehead's lawyer was referred to her by the Infertility Center, with which he had an agreement to act as counsel for surrogate candidates. His services consisted of spending one hour going through the contract with the Whiteheads, section by section, and answering their questions. Mrs. Whitehead received no further legal advice prior to signing the contract with the Sterns.

Mrs. Whitehead was examined and psychologically evaluated, but if it was for her benefit, the record does not disclose that fact. The Sterns regarded the evaluation as important, particularly in connection with the question of whether she would change her mind. Yet they never asked to see it, and were content with the assumption that the Infertility Center had made an evaluation and had concluded that there was no danger that the surrogate mother would change her mind. From Mrs. Whitehead's point of view, all that she learned from the evaluation was that "she had passed." It is apparent that the profit motive got the better of the Infertility Center. Although the evaluation was made, it was not put to any use, and understandably so, for the psychologist warned that Mrs. Whitehead demonstrated certain traits that might make surrender of the child difficult and that there should be further inquiry into this issue in connection with her surrogacy. To inquire further, however, might have jeopardized the Infertility Center's fee. The record indicates that neither Mrs. Whitehead nor the Sterns were ever told of this fact, a fact that might have ended their surrogacy arrangement.

Under the contract, the natural mother is irrevocably committed before she knows the strength of her bond with her child. She never makes a totally voluntary, informed decision, for quite clearly any decision prior to the baby's birth is, in the most important sense, uninformed, and any decision after that, compelled by a pre-existing contractual commitment, the threat of a lawsuit, and the inducement of a $10,000 payment, is less than totally voluntary. Her interests are of little concern to those who controlled this transaction.

Although the interest of the natural father and adoptive mother is certainly the predominant interest, realistically the *only* interest served, even they are left with less than what public policy requires. They know little about the natural mother, her genetic makeup, and her psychological and medical history. Moreover, not even a superficial attempt is made to determine their awareness of their responsibilities as parents.

Worst of all, however, is the contract's total disregard of the best interests of the child. There is not the slightest suggestion that any inquiry will be made at any time to determine the fitness of the Sterns as custodial parents, of Mrs. Stern as an adoptive parent, their superiority to Mrs. Whitehead, or the effect on the child of not living with her natural mother.

This is the sale of a child, or, at the very least, the sale of a mother's right to her child, the only mitigating factor being that one of the purchasers is the father. Almost every evil that prompted the prohibition of the payment of money in connection with adoptions exists here.

The differences between an adoption and a surrogacy contract should be noted, since it is asserted that the use of money in connection with surrogacy does not pose the risks found where money buys an adoption. Katz, "Surrogate Motherhood and the Baby-Selling Laws," 20 *Colum.J.L. & Soc.Probs.* 1 (1986).

First, and perhaps most important, all parties concede that it is unlikely that surrogacy will survive without money. Despite the alleged selfless motivation of surrogate mothers, if there is no payment, there will be no surrogates, or very few. That conclusion contrasts with adoption; for obvious reasons, there remains a steady supply, albeit insufficient, despite the prohibitions against payment. The adoption itself, relieving the natural mother of the financial burden of supporting an infant, is the equivalent of payment.

Second, the use of money in adoptions does not *produce* the problem—conception occurs, and usually the birth itself, before illicit funds are offered. With surrogacy, the "problem," if one views it as such, consisting of the purchase of a woman's procreative capacity, at the risk of her life, is caused by and originates with the offer of money.

Third, with the law prohibiting the use of money in connection with adoptions, the built-in financial pressure of the unwanted pregnancy and the consequent support obligation do not lead the mother to the highest paying, ill-suited, adoptive parents. She is just as well off surrendering the child to an approved agency. In surrogacy, the highest bidders will presumably become the adoptive parents regardless of suitability, so long as payment of money is permitted.

Fourth, the mother's consent to surrender her child in adoptions is revocable, even after surrender of the child, unless it be to an approved agency, where by regulation there are protections against an ill-advised surrender. In surrogacy, consent occurs so early that no amount of advice would satisfy the potential mother's need, yet the consent is irrevocable.

The main difference, that the plight of the unwanted pregnancy is unintended while the situation of the surrogate mother is voluntary and intended, is really not significant. Initially, it produces stronger reactions of sympathy for the mother whose pregnancy was unwanted than for the surrogate mother, who "went into this with her eyes wide open." On reflection, however, it appears that the essential evil is the same, taking advantage of a woman's circumstances (the unwanted pregnancy or the need for money) in order to take away her child, the difference being one of degree.

In the scheme contemplated by the surrogacy contract in this case, a middle man, propelled by profit, promotes the sale. Whatever idealism may have motivated any of the participants, the profit motive predominates, permeates, and ultimately governs the transaction. The demand for children is great and the supply small. The availability of contraception, abortion, and the greater willingness of single mothers to bring up their children has led to a shortage of babies offered for adoption. *See* N. Baker, *Baby Selling: The Scandal of Black Market Adoption, supra; Adoption and Foster Care, 1975: Hearings on Baby Selling Before the Subcomm. On Children and Youth of the Senate Comm. on Labor and Public Welfare*, 94th Cong.1st Sess. 6 (1975) (Statement of Joseph H. Reid, Executive Director, Child Welfare League of America, Inc.). The situation is ripe for the entry of the middleman who will bring some equilibrium into the market by increasing the supply through the use of money.

Intimated, but disputed, is the assertion that surrogacy will be used for the benefit of the rich at the expense of the poor. *See, e.g.,* Radin, "Market Inalienability," 100 *Harv.L.Rev.* 1849, 1930 (1987). In response it is noted that the Sterns are not rich and the Whiteheads not poor. Nevertheless, it is clear to us that it is unlikely that surrogate mothers will be as proportionately numerous among those women in the top twenty percent income bracket as among those in the bottom twenty percent. *Ibid.* Put differently, we doubt that infertile couples in the low-income bracket will find upper income surrogates.

In any event, even in this case one should not pretend that disparate wealth does not play a part simply because the contrast is not the dramatic "rich versus poor." At the time of trial, the Whiteheads' net assets were probably negative—Mrs. Whitehead's own sister was foreclosing on a second mortgage. Their income derived from Mr. Whitehead's labors. Mrs. Whitehead is a homemaker, having previously held part-time jobs. The Sterns are both professionals, she a medical doctor, he a biochemist. Their combined income when both were working was about $89,500 a year and their assets sufficient to pay for the surrogacy contract arrangements.

[16] The point is made that Mrs. Whitehead *agreed* to the surrogacy arrangement, supposedly fully understanding the consequences. Putting aside the issue of how compelling her need for money may have been, and how significant her understanding of the consequences, we suggest that her consent is irrelevant. There are, in a civilized society, some things that money cannot buy. In America, we decided long ago that merely because conduct purchased by money was "voluntary" did not mean that it was good or beyond regulation and prohibition. *West Coast Hotel Co. v. Parrish*, 300 *U.S.* 379, 57 *S.Ct.* 578, 81 *L.Ed.* 703 (1937). Employers can no longer buy labor at the lowest price they can bargain for, even though that labor is "voluntary," 29 *U.S.C.* § 206 (1982), or buy women's labor for less money than paid to men for the same job, 29 *U.S.C.* § 206(d), or purchase the agreement of children to perform oppressive labor, 29 *U.S.C.* § 212, or purchase the agreement of workers to subject themselves to unsafe or unhealthful working conditions, 29 *U.S.C.* § 651 to 678 (Occupational Health and Safety Act of 1970). There are, in short, values that society deems more important than granting to wealth whatever it can buy, be it labor, love, or life. Whether this principle recommends prohibition of surrogacy, which presumably sometimes results in great

satisfaction to all of the parties, is not for us to say. We note here only that, under existing law, the fact that Mrs. Whitehead "agreed" to the arrangement is not dispositive.

The long-term effects of surrogacy contracts are not known, but feared—the impact on the child who learns her life was bought, that she is the offspring of someone who gave birth to her only to obtain money; the impact on the natural mother as the full weight of her isolation is felt along with the full reality of the sale of her body and her child; the impact on the natural father and adoptive mother once they realize the consequences of their conduct. Literature in related areas suggests these are substantial considerations, although, given the newness of surrogacy, there is little information. *See* N. Baker, *Baby Selling: The Scandal of Black Market Adoption, supra; Adoption and Foster Care, 1975: Hearings on Baby Selling Before the Subcomm. on Children and Youth of the Senate Comm. on Labor and Public Welfare*, 94th Cong. 1st Sess. (1975).

[17] The surrogacy contract creates, it is based upon, principles that are directly contrary to the objectives of our laws.[7] It guarantees the separation of a child from its mother; it looks to adoption regardless of suitability; it totally ignores the child; it takes the child from the mother regardless of her wishes and her maternal fitness; and it does all of this, it accomplishes all of its goals, through the use of money.

Beyond that is the potential degradation of some women that may result from this arrangement. In many cases, of course, surrogacy may bring satisfaction, not only to the infertile couple, but to the surrogate mother herself. The fact, however, that many women may not perceive surrogacy negatively but rather see it as an opportunity does not diminish its potential for devastation to other women.

[7]We note the argument of the Sterns that the sperm donor section of our Parentage Act, *N.J.S.A.* 9:17–38 to –59, implies a legislative policy that would lead to approval of this surrogacy contract. Where a married woman is artificially inseminated by another with her husband's consent, the Parentage Act creates a parent-child relationship between the husband and the resulting child. *N.J.S.A.* 9:17–44. The Parentage Act's silence, however, with respect to surrogacy, rather than supporting, defeats any contention that surrogacy should receive treatment parallel to the sperm donor artificial insemination situation. In the latter case the statute expressly transfers parental rights from the biological father, *i.e.*, the sperm donor, to the mother's husband. *Ibid.* Our Legislature could not possibly have intended any other arrangement to have the consequence of transferring parental rights without legislative authorization when it had concluded that legislation was necessary to accomplish that result in the sperm donor artificial insemination context.

This sperm donor provision suggests an argument not raised by the parties, namely, that the attempted creation of a parent-child relationship through the surrogacy contract has been preempted by the Legislature. The Legislature has explicitly recognized the parent-child relationship between a child and its natural parents, married and unmarried, *N.J.S.A.* 9:17–38 to –59, between adoptive parents and their adopted child, *N.J.S.A.* 9:3–37 to –56, and between a husband and his wife's child pursuant to the sperm donor provision, *N.J.S.A.* 9:17–44. It has not recognized any others—specifically, it has never legally equated the stepparent-stepchild relationship with the parent-child relationship, and certainly it has never recognized any concept of adoption by contract. It can be contended with some force that the Legislature's statutory coverage of the creation of the parent-child relationship evinces an intent to reserve to itself the power to define what is and is not a parent-child relationship. We need not, and do not, decide this question, however.

In sum, the harmful consequences of this surrogacy arrangement appear to us all too palpable. In New Jersey the surrogate mother's agreement to sell her child is void.[8] Its irrevocability infects the entire contract, as does the money that purports to buy it.

[8]Michigan courts have also found that these arrangements conflict with various aspects of their law. *See Doe v. Kelley*, 106 *Mich.App.* 169, 307 *N.W.*2d 438 (1981), *cert.* den., 459 *U.S.* 1183, 103 *S.Ct.* 834, 74 *L.Ed.*2d 1027 (1983) (application of sections of Michigan Adoption Law prohibiting the exchange of money to surrogacy is constitutional); *Syrkowski v. Appleyard*, 122 *Mich.App.* 506, 333 *N.W.*2d 90 (1983) (court held it lacked jurisdiction to issue an "order of filiation" because surrogacy arrangements were not governed by Michigan's Paternity Act), *rev'd*, 420 *Mich.* 367, 362 *N.W.*2d 211 (1985) (court decided Paternity Act should be applied but did not reach the merits of the claim).

Most recently, a Michigan trial court in a matter similar to the case at bar held that surrogacy contracts are void as contrary to public policy and therefore are unenforceable. The court expressed concern for the potential exploitation of children resulting from surrogacy arrangements that involve the payment of money. The court also concluded that insofar as the surrogacy contract may be characterized as one for personal services, the thirteenth amendment should bar specific performance. *Yates v. Keane*, Nos. 9758, 9772, slip op. (Mich.Cir.Ct. Jan. 21, 1988).

The Supreme Court of Kentucky has taken a somewhat different approach to surrogate arrangements. In *Surrogate Parenting Assocs. v. Commonwealth ex. rel. Armstrong*, 704 *S.W.*2d 209 (Ky.1986), the court held that the "fundamental differences" between surrogate arrangements and baby selling placed the surrogate parenting agreement beyond the reach of Kentucky's baby-selling statute. *Id.* at 211. The rationale for this determination was that unlike the normal adoption situation, the surrogacy agreement is entered into before conception and is not directed at avoiding the consequences of an unwanted pregnancy. *Id.* at 211–12.

Concomitant with this pro-surrogacy conclusion, however, the court held that a "surrogate" mother has the right to void the contract if she changes her mind during pregnancy or immediately after birth. *Id.* at 212–13. The court relied on statutes providing that consent to adoption or to the termination of parental rights prior to five days after the birth of the child is invalid, and concluded that consent before conception must also be unenforceable. *Id.* at 212–13.

The adoption phase of an uncontested surrogacy arrangement was analyzed in *Matter of Adoption of Baby Girl, L.J.*, 132 *Misc.*2d 972, 505 *N.Y.S.*2d 813 (Sur. 1986). Although the court expressed strong moral and ethical reservations about surrogacy arrangements, it approved the adoption because it was in the best interests of the child. *Id.* at 815. The court went on to find that surrogate parenting agreements are not void, but are voidable if they are not in accordance with the state's adoption statutes. *Id.* at 817. The court then upheld the payment of money in connection with the surrogacy arrangement on the ground that the New York Legislature did not contemplate surrogacy when the baby selling statute was passed. *Id.* at 818. Despite the court's ethical and moral problems with surrogate arrangements, it concluded that the Legislature was the appropriate forum to address the legality of surrogacy arrangements. *Ibid.*

In contrast to the law in the United States, the law in the United Kingdom concerning surrogate parenting is fairly well-settled. Parliament passed the Surrogacy Arrangements Act, 1985, ch. 49, which made initialing or taking part in any negotiations with a view to making or arranging a surrogacy contract a criminal offense. The criminal sanction, however, does not apply to the "surrogate" mother or to the natural father, but rather applies to other persons engaged in arranging surrogacy contracts on a commercial basis. Since 1978, English courts have held surrogacy agreements unenforceable as against public policy, such agreements being deemed arrangements for the purchase and sale of children. *A. v. C.*, [1985] *F.L.R.* 445, 449 (Fam. & C.A.1978). It should be noted, however, that certain surrogacy arrangements, *i.e.*, those arranged without brokers and revocable by the natural mother are not prohibited under current law in the United Kingdom.

The Baby Broker Boom

GEORGE J. ANNAS

Should babies be treated as commodities? Should reproduction be commercialized? Should motherhood be determined by contract? A few years ago these questions seemed absurd. But the hope that surrogate motherhood would wither of its own weirdness is now beginning to seem quaint. Indeed, two recent court decisions strongly support commercial surrogate mother agreements. If surrogate mother companies were listed on the New York Stock Exchange, these cases would have sent their stock soaring.

Almost since its inception, Surrogate Parenting Associates, Inc. (SPA) was in trouble in its home state of Kentucky. In 1981, the Attorney General instituted proceedings against the corporation to revoke its charter. He charged that by entering into commercial surrogate arrangements in which a woman would be paid to be artificially inseminated, and then to bear a child for whom she would relinquish parental rights (for later step-parent adoption by the father-sperm-donor's infertile wife), the corporation violated the state's prohibition against the "purchase of any child for the purpose of adoption." The statute was amended in 1984 to add the words, "or any other purpose, including termination of parental rights" (KRS 199.950[2]).

A trial court ruled against the Attorney General, an Appeals Court in his favor, and the Supreme Court of Kentucky has now sided with the corporation (*Surrogate Parenting Associates v. Kentucky*, 704 S.W.2d 209 [1986]). The court declared that the intention of the legislature in prohibiting baby selling was solely "to keep baby brokers from overwhelming an expectant mother or the parents of a child with financial inducements to part with the child." It therefore approved of baby sales if the price was agreed to *before* conception, and the surrogate mother retained the right to cancel the contract up to the point of relinquishing her parental rights.

Surrogate motherhood is a nontechnical application of artificial insemination that requires no sophisticated medical or scientific knowledge or medical intervention. But the court saw surrogate motherhood as modern science, and did not want to interfere with "a new era of genetics," "solutions offered by science," and "new medical services."

George J. Annas, *J.D., M.P.H., is Utley Professor of Health Law, Boston University School of Medicine; and Chief, Health Law Section, Boston University School of Public Health.*

The majority's opinion thus misses the focus of the Attorney General's argument: surrogacy's essence is not science, but commerce. The only "new" development in surrogacy is the introduction of physicians and lawyers as baby brokers who, for a fee, locate women willing to bear children by AID and hand them over to the payor-sperm donor after birth. The novelty lies in treating children like commodities.

This Justice Vance, one of two dissenting justices, understood. He noted that the corporation's "primary purpose is to locate women who will readily, for a price, allow themselves to be used as human incubators and who are willing to sell, for a price, all of their parental rights in a child thus born." His rationale was that payment is made to the surrogate in two parts. The first part "of the fee is paid in advance for the use of her body as an incubator." But the second portion of the fee is not paid unless and until "her living child is delivered to the purchaser, along with the equivalent of a bill of sale, or quitclaim deed, to wit—the judgment terminating her parental rights." As the judge persuasively argues, the last payment must be for the child, since if the child is not delivered, the last payment need not be made.

The majority probably thought it was approving very *limited* baby selling: permitting a father-sperm donor to purchase the gestational mother's interest in his genetic child if the gestational mother contracted to make such a sale prior to conception and still desires to sell her child after its birth.

But limiting baby buying to fathers does not make baby buying any more tolerable than permitting a father to kidnap his biological child from its mother would make kidnapping tolerable. If mothers are to give up their parental rights to fathers, it should be *voluntarily*, and without a monetary price that converts the child into a commodity. That is what the Kentucky legislature undoubtedly had in mind when it outlawed baby selling.

The Kentucky court did not address baby selling in the case of full surrogacy: a surrogate who "gestates" an embryo to which she has made no genetic contribution. But a lower Michigan court has. Twenty-three-year-old Shannon Boff was pregnant with a child genetically unrelated to her at the time the question of her motherhood came up (*Smith & Smith v. Jones & Jones*, 85-532014 DZ, Detroit, MI, 3d Jud. Dist., March 14, 1986, Battani, J.). For the first reported time in the U.S., in vitro fertilization (IVF) had been used to fertilize an ovum from an infertile woman (who lacked a uterus), and the resulting embryo was implanted into another woman, who agreed to act as a surrogate mother by gestating the fetus.

This raised an undecided legal question: Should the genetic or the gestational mother be considered the "legal" mother? That is, which woman should have legal rearing rights and responsibilities? The genetic parents, who had paid $40,000 for this "project" ($10,000 of which went to Ms. Boff) wanted to have their own names listed on the child's birth certificate, not the names of Ms. Boff and her husband.

Unfortunately, the case was a set-up. Even though both "competing sets of parents were represented by legal counsel, they all wanted the judge to rule the same way. Since she did, there will be no appeal and no further judicial analysis of the question. Nor did the judge appoint anyone to represent the interests of the potential child. Like the Kentucky court, the Michigan judge decided to let contracts and commerce rule the day, rather than deal with any wider social issues, or consider the best interests of any child.

In so doing, the judge consistently put form over substance. For example, in determining that Ms. Boff's husband should not be presumed to be the father of his wife's child, the judge accepted the argument of their attorney that he could not be presumed the father under the AID statute because he signed a "nonconsent to any type of artificial insemination of his wife." But given his active participation in the entire project (he said he rubbed and drew faces on his wife's enlarged stomach and treated the pregnancy as if his wife was carrying their own child), his signature is hardly the "clear and convincing evidence" the statute requires. Moreover, the entire Paternity Act under which the case was brought covers only children "born out of wedlock," so the court may have had no jurisdiction at all over this case (MCLA 722.711 et. seq.).

The discussion of maternity is taken even less seriously. Like the Kentucky court, the Detroit judge saw her primary task as trying to make the law conform with and comfort modern science. Promoting private contract and personal profit were also seen as appropriate judicial strategies. To get to this point, the judge found it necessary to rule that the state's paternity statute must be applicable to women as well as men, to afford women "equal protection of laws."

This is, of course, true only if there are no significant differences between maternity and paternity. But if there are no significant differences, then the female gamete donor should logically be treated "equally" to a male gamete donor: the child would then have *two* genetic "fathers," but would have a [gestational] mother as well. Not to so recognize the gestational mother's status dehumanizes her (and all mothers?), turning her into mere breeder stock. Of course, had Ms. Boff asserted her rights and identity as the child's mother, the judge would almost certainly have upheld her claim.

In applying the paternity statute to maternity, the court concluded that the gestational mother (whom the court referred to as the "birthing mother"), is acting as a "human incubator for this embryo to develop." Where the incubator "contracted to do this" via IVF, and where subsequent tissue typing confirms the genetic links of the child to the gamete donors, then "the donor of the ovum, the biological mother, is to be deemed, in fact, the natural mother of this infant, as is the biological father to be deemed the natural father of this child."

Besides putting contract above biology, this conclusion begs the question of who the child's mother is during pregnancy, and also makes identification of the child's mother at birth impossible. It thus fails to protect either the child or its mother where decisions regarding the newborn infant's care need to be made quickly. The judge dealt with this by saying that her decree would depend upon HLA tissue-typing confirming the identity of the genetic parents, a procedure that would not resolve the issue until at least a few days after the birth.

Although commerce won out in court, Ms. Boff said she would leave the baby business herself: "I'm going into retirement; any more babies coming from me are going to be keepers."

The contrary conclusion—that the woman who gestates a child should be considered the child's legal mother for all purposes—is not based on antiscience, anachronistic, or sentimental views of motherhood. Rather, it is a recognition of the gestational mother's greater biological contribution to the child, including risks and physical contributions of the nine months of pregnancy, and the need to protect the newborn by always providing it with at least one immediately identifiable parent.

The gestational mother, for example, contributes more to the child than the ovum donor does in the same way she contributes more to the child than a sperm donor does. Other considerations also argue for this traditional view of motherhood. What if there are three "competing" mothers, as happens if the genetic ovum donor is anonymous (as most sperm donors are), the gestational mother a surrogate, and the contracting rearing mother simply someone who wants to raise the child? In this scenario the only relationship the rearing mother has is monetary: she paid the surrogate a fee to gestate the embryo and give up the child. If we *really* believe money and contracts should rule, then the identity of the child's mother will depend upon contract and payment only, and both genetics and gestation (and therefore all biological ties) will be irrelevant.

Since neither of these results seems reasonable, and since the traditional presumption would always provide the child with an identifiable mother who would be the same woman who biologically contributed the most, the traditional assumption should continue to be utilized, even in this "brave new world," and whether or not any contracts have been signed or any money changes hands. The Kentucky court's ruling, of course, is consistent with this view. The gestational mother could honor her prior contract, but could also change her mind and retain *her* child anytime before formally relinquishing parental rights.

Commercial surrogacy promotes the exploitation of women and infertile couples, and the dehumanization of babies. If the courts think this is a small price to pay to promote the "baby business," then it's time for state legislatures to define motherhood by statute.

The Aftermath of Baby M:

Proposed State Laws on Surrogate Motherhood

LORI B. ANDREWS

New Jersey's Baby M case has thrust the issue of surrogate motherhood on state legislatures throughout the country. Like artificial insemination in the 1950s and 1960s, this new reproductive technology is evoking legislative responses ranging from horrified prohibition to cautious facilitation.

Two decades ago, Sophia J. Kleegman and Sherwin A. Kaufman, in *Infertility in Women*, observed that new reproductive technologies are greeted initially with shock and must pass through several stages before they are accepted:

> Any change in custom or practice in this emotionally charged area has always elicited a response from established custom and law of horrified negation at first; then negation without horror; then slow and gradual curiosity, study, evaluation, and finally a very slow but steady acceptance.[1]

This statement, focusing on artificial insemination by donor (AID), was a valid assessment of how public policy was developing around that technology. In the 1950s and early 1960s, donor insemination was viewed with such horror that bills were introduced in state legislatures to ban the procedure. A proposed Ohio law would have criminalized AID and subjected all of the participants—the doctor, the donor, and the couple—to a fine and imprisonment.[2] No such prohibitory laws were passed, however, and in the intervening years over half the states have adopted laws that facilitate AID by declaring the consenting husband of the sperm recipient to be the legal father (even though he has not adopted the child). Nonetheless, the AID debate continues in state legislatures. In 1984, Alabama passed its first AID law. In 1986, New Mexico joined the ranks, and Ohio finally adopted a law describing the medical requirements and parenthood implications of donor insemination, bringing the total number of AID laws to thirty.[3]

Lori B. Andrews *is a project director in medical law at the American Bar Foundation, and the author of* New Conceptions: A Consumer's Guide to the Newest Infertility Treatments, Including In Vitro Fertilization, Artificial Insemination, and Surrogate Motherhood *(Ballantine, 1985).*

The 1980s have brought another vexing reproductive issue to lawmakers: surrogate motherhood. The Baby M case has provided an impetus for many legislative proposals about surrogacy. Bills in Delaware and Louisiana, for example, are prefaced by statements about how the Baby M case has raised complex legal and ethical issues. At the federal level, Ohio Congressman Tom Luken has proposed a bill that would prohibit the receipt of payment for making, engaging in, or brokering a surrogacy arrangement.[4] The bill would also prohibit advertising for a paid surrogacy arrangement.[5] The personal heartbreak and media circus of the Stern-Whitehead case led the public and legislators to call for laws to preclude similar future cases. However, less than one-third of the proposed laws have clear provisions establishing the legal parents after the birth of a baby conceived pursuant to a surrogate agreement. Under the remaining proposals, recourse to the courts is still the only way for the biological father or biological mother to gain legal custody of the child when there is conflict.

To date, only Arkansas, Nevada, and Louisiana have actually enacted laws that touch on surrogacy. In Arkansas, the statute provides simply that if a couple contracts with an unmarried surrogate, the couple are the legal parents of the child, not the surrogate.[6] The Nevada legislature passed a law that exempts surrogacy from the ban on payment in connection with an adoption. Under the Louisiana law contracts for paid surrogacy are unenforceable.[7] Another bill passed by the Arkansas lesiglature but vetoed by the governor would have provided for enforcement of all surrogacy contracts.

The majority of state legislatures are still considering the issue of surrogacy and their bills run the gamut of Kleegman's and Kaufman's typology. Will surrogate motherhood legislation, like donor insemination, evolve through the stages of horror, negation, evaluation, and acceptance ultimately toward facilitating laws? Or will the greater duration and intensity of the surrogate's involvement in collaborative reproduction lead to an alternative regulatory model? The answers to these questions will develop in state capitols as a result of legislative compromises and special interest group proddings by right-to-life groups, medical societies, adoption agencies, infertility support groups, feminists, religious organizations, and reproductive rights advocates.

Horror

Many state legislatures have reacted with horror to the issue of surrogate motherhood, often taking the issue of payment to the surrogate as their focus. Of the pending state laws, five (in Alabama, Illinois, Iowa, Maryland, and Wisconsin) would ban surrogate motherhood altogether,[8] while seven others (in Florida, Kentucky, Michigan, New Jersey, New York, Oregon, and Pennsylvania) would specifically ban only paid surrogacy.[9] Three additional bills—in the District of Columbia and alternative bills in Florida and New York—would ban paid surrogacy but allow unpaid surrogacy under an extensive regulatory scheme.[10]

The Michigan bill, an example of the prohibitory approach, states that a person entering into a surrogate parentage contract for compensation is guilty of a misdemeanor punishable by a fine of not more than $10,000 or imprisonment for not more than a year. The proposal further states that a person other than a participating party who induces, arranges, procures, or otherwise assists in the formation of a surrogate parentage contract for compensation is guilty of a felony punishable by a maximum fine of $50,000 or imprisonment for not more than five years. This bill also contains special provisions punishing those who enter, induce, or arrange a contract with an unemancipated minor female or a mentally retarded female. This sort of an arrangement would be a felony punishable by five years imprisonment or a $50,000 fine, or both.

With the exception of the Michigan law, which provides that the legal parents are the surrogate and her husband, proposed prohibitory laws generally make no provision for legal parenthood in instances when surrogacy is undertaken in violation of the law. Since the proposals in the other states do not suggest that mere participation in a surrogacy arrangement is an indication of parental unfitness (which would give the state power to take over the care and custody of the child), disputes between the biological parents over custody would require judicial intervention. In ten of the thirteen states where prohibitory bills are pending, there are also alternative bills or additional provisions that would facilitate some form of surrogacy.

Negation

Some legislators who oppose surrogacy nonetheless do not feel comfortable imposing prison sentences on parties trying to become parents in this manner. Yet they do want to discourage people from entering into surrogacy arrangements, and attempt to do so by negating the surrogate contract. Lawmakers in four states (Connecticut, Illinois, North Carolina, and Rhode Island) have proposed statutes that would make any contracts for surrogacy void and unenforceable.[11] Proposals in Alabama, Minnesota, Nebraska, and New York would void only contracts for paid surrogacy.[12] The most unusual of these statutes is that of Nebraska, which makes the contract unenforceable, but gives the biological father parental rights and obligations. The apparent intent of such a statute is to acknowledge that the man providing the sperm is the legal father but to avoid upholding other aspects of the contract, such as provisions requiring the surrogate to abort or to terminate her parental rights.

Under these proposed laws, couples and surrogates would not go to jail for participating in contractual reproduction, but if the surrogate changed her mind, the contract would not be upheld. In practical effect, such laws are similar to those that allow the surrogate to change her mind after the birth. Although they have a different symbolic weight, since laws declaring the contract void would evince societal disapproval of the arrangement while those allowing surrogacy with a mind-change option would not, such symbolism is unlikely to deter most couples who badly want a baby. As in the case of outright bans, these laws generally lack provisions for how parenthood would be decided in the instance when the surrogate changed her mind. Only the Connecticut bill specifies who the legal parents are in a surrogacy arrangement: the surrogate and her husband.[13]

Evaluation

Some legislatures have not ruled out surrogacy, but instead have proposed or authorized study commissions to assess the potential benefits and risks of surrogacy arrangements. Study commissions have been adopted by the legislatures of Delaware, Indiana, Louisiana, Rhode Island, and Texas, and at least eight other states have proposed them.[14] The bills calling for evaluation of surrogacy focus mainly on the composition of the commissions and on the issues to be considered.

The composition is likely to influence the type of proposals a commission develops. A commission of infertility specialists may conceptualize surrogacy according to a medical model, analogizing it to medical treatments for infertility such as drugs and surgery. A commission of adoption officials, however, might place surrogacy within its previous experience of adoption. These alternative interpretations may lead to different sets of policy recommendations. If surrogacy is analogized to a medical treatment, the commission might recommend that couples not undergo psychological screening to gain access to surrogacy, that surrogates be paid, and that the infertile couple be considered the legal parents. If surrogacy is analogized to adoption, it might be recommended that the couples be screened, that payment be prohibited, and that the surrogate have a certain time period after the birth of the child to assert her parental rights.

The Delaware commission is a Citizens Task Force of twelve members: a senator, a representative, three medical professionals, two clergymen, a representative of the city of Wilmington, and four public members. Members were not charged to address specific issues, but the preamble of the bill alludes to a legal question regarding privacy, and ethical issues regarding whether women should be encouraged to conceive children they will never raise and whether surrogates are mothers or manufacturers of products.

In Louisiana, the commission is composed of six legislators and one representative each from the state medical association, bar association, Catholic conference, and Interchurch Conference. The preamble of the bill establishing the commission notes that "surrogate mothering has potentially devastating problems for all the parties involved." Yet when setting forth the issues troubling the legislature that the commission is apparently to address, it makes no reference to the key problems for the parties, the potential psychological risks. (Moreover, the commission itself contains no members who are experts in such matters.) Rather, the questions revolve around

> the validity of the surrogacy contract, the question of renunciation of the contract, and other problems such as custody and visitation rights, adoption, inheritance, and other property rights.

Even though the bill is premised on the statement that the "ethics of surrogate parenting needs to be examined in this state," the actual task of the Commission is stated in terms of assessing what the law *is* rather than what it *should be*.

Under the proposed Connecticut law, the commission would be made up of people appointed by ranking legislators. The inquiry of the Connecticut commission would focus mainly on legal issues: whether contracts should be enforced, for example, and whether intermediaries should be allowed to broker and advertise.

The proposed Maine commission would consist of two senators, two representatives, a judge, the Attorney General (or a designee), the Commissioner of Human Services (or a designee), an attorney, a physician, a hospital administrator, and two members of the public. The issues identified for the commission to address are more wide-ranging than in other states, including issues involving the contract, genetic screening of the surrogate, the protocol for transfer of the infant, custody concerns, the duties of physicians to disclose risks, and authorizing a state agency to deal with surrogacy.

Massachusetts's proposed commission would be composed of two members of the senate, three members of the house of representatives, and six persons to be appointed by the governor. Those six persons must include an attorney practicing in the commonwealth and one who is a member of a bar association organized in Massachusetts, a licensed psychiatrist or psychologist, a social service worker, and a member of the general public. The purpose of the commission is to investigate the possibility of and need for regulating surrogacy.

North Carolina has two proposals for study commissions pending. One would create a Surrogate Parenting Study consisting of nine members: a senator, representative, clergyman, child psychiatrist, social service representative, doctor, lawyer, child advocate, and a chairman from the field of education. The bill specifically provides for public hearings and asks the commission to seek public opinion on such issues as the rights of potential parents to use surrogacy, whether the contract may be binding, whether screening is advisable, what the established psychological evidence is on mother-child bonding, whether it is in the child's best interest to favor either the mother or father in the surrogacy contract, and how existing laws affect surrogacy. The preamble of the North Carolina bill may, in fact, presage the future findings of the commission when it says that "no matter how the surrogacy issue is resolved, babies cannot be traded like commodities."

The second North Carolina proposal would create a twenty-five-member Adoption and Surrogate Parenthood Study Commission comprised of four senators and four representatives, two county social services directors, two private adoption agency directors, a private adoption agency worker and a county adoption worker, an adoption agency attorney, an attorney specializing in adoption, and an Attorney General's office attorney knowledgeable about adoption, a physician, two superior court clerks, a member of the clergy, an adoptive parent, a birth parent of an adopted child, an adopted person, and the Director (or a designee) of the North Carolina Division of Social Services. This commission would have a broader mandate that includes not only addressing surrogacy as such, but determining how to amend the laws to meet more adequately the needs of adopted children, adoptive parents, and birth parents. Notably lacking from the proposed study commission, however, are people with any experience in the medical, legal, psychological, or personal aspects of surrogate motherhood, who might be able to provide insight about how the process is similar to—or different from—adoption.

New Jersey's proposed commission would include two senators and two representatives, both from different political parties, the Chief Justice of the Supreme Court or a designee, two members of the Family Law Section and two from the Women's Rights Section of the New Jersey State Bar Association, as well as two members qualified by their experience in the area of domestic relations, one appointed by the President of the Senate, and one appointed by the speaker of the General Assembly. The bill charges the commission to study the policy implications raised by surrogacy, and more specifically, to consider if surrogate contracts are in accord with public policy, whether the courts have sufficient guidance to make a determination in a surrogate parenthood controversy, and whether legislative action is necessary.

Acceptance

The majority of the pending surrogacy bills incorporate the perspective that surrogacy, in some form, should be allowed. In adopting a regulatory rather than a prohibitory approach, lawmakers must grapple with such issues as whether surrogates should be paid, what type of screening participants should undergo, what safeguards are necessary to assure that participants have given voluntary, informed consent, whether the couples who are the intended parents should be recognized as the legal parents, whether the surrogate should have a certain time period after the birth in which to assert her parental rights, and whether the resulting child should, later in life, be able to obtain medical information about the surrogate or learn her identity.

In Oregon, one proposed statute takes a simplistic approach to surrogacy in that it merely exempts surrogate arrangements from the ban on babyselling.[15] Another legalizes both paid and unpaid surrogacy[16] and provides for the enforcement of the contract by either specific performance or damages.[17] A proposed Connecticut law would merely allow the Commissioner of Health Services to establish minimum standards for surrogates. Other statutes accepting surrogacy provide more elaborate regulations for the procedure. The District of Columbia bill, for example, not only sets standards for screening, recordkeeping, and other aspects of the procedure, it also requires that surrogate centers be licensed.[18] Some of the proposed statutes also list provisions that must be included in the contract, such as that the couple agree to accept the child at birth, or that the parties be medically screened.[19] The Illinois and Missouri laws further require the contract to state whether the parties have a right to meet and know each other's identity, to meet and not be identified, or not to meet and not to be identified.[20]

Paid or Unpaid Surrogacy?

Four jurisdictions (the District of Columbia, Florida, New York, and Wisconsin) would specifically allow only unpaid surrogacy,[21] while statutes proposed in at least twelve states would allow either paid or unpaid surrogacy (California, Illinois, Maryland,

Massachusetts, Michigan, Minnesota, Missouri, New Jersey, New York, Oregon, Pennsylvania, and South Carolina).[22] Some of the latter bills, such as those of California and Illinois, specify that the compensation must be "reasonable," seemingly indicating that a court would have authority to decrease compensation that it considered excessive. Under proposed Massachusetts, New York, and Pennsylvania bills, however, there is also a requirement that the fee be "just," which seems to give a court the power to increase a fee it finds too small. One of the two proposed New Jersey bills allowing surrogacy would limit payment to the surrogate to $10,000.

Even when paid surrogacy has been accepted, there has been much debate about whether payment to the surrogate is equivalent to payment for a child rather than payment for a service since in many programs the bulk of the payment is made after birth and in some the woman does not receive full payment if she miscarries. The proposed South Carolina law would codify this latter approach by providing that the surrogate will receive no compensation other than medical expenses if she miscarries before the fifth month of pregnancy and will receive only 10 percent of the agreed upon fee plus medical expenses if she miscarries during or after the fifth month. A Maryland bill specifically authorizes that "a portion of the total compensation may be withheld until the child's birth," but does not indicate whether payment is contingent on live birth. In contrast, a Michigan bill states that the surrogate agreement may not contain a payment reduction provision if the child is stillborn or born alive but impaired.

Access to Surrogacy

The proposed regulatory bills often limit who may contract with a surrogate. According to laws proposed in Florida, Illinois, New Jersey, and South Carolina, for example, the intended parents must be married. In some states surrogacy may only be used for medical reasons, as under bills in California, the District of Columbia, Illinois, Massachusetts, Michigan, New York, Pennsylvania, and New Jersey. Generally those reasons are defined as infertility or threat to the health or life of the intended mother or her child were she to conceive.[23] In most states, these medical reasons encompass the desire not to pass on a serious genetic defect to the child.[24] As their lack of attention to the issue suggests, other bills would apparently not limit the use of surrogacy to medical indications.

The proposed Missouri and South Carolina laws seem to exclude people who are disabled or in poor health from contracting with a surrogate. They require examination of the intended parents to determine if they have any medical conditions that would interfere with their capabilities as parents.

The South Carolina bill and one of the New Jersey bills require investigation of the intended parents similar to the home study done in an adoption situation. Under the South Carolina bill, the investigation must consider such factors as the intended parents' moral fitness, the stability of their family unit, and the capacity and disposition of the intended parents to give the child love, affection, guidance, permanence, education, and medical care, as well as food, clothing, and other material needs.

The surrogate's qualifications are described in detail under many of the bills, which generally focus on psychological and medical measures. Some bills, however, provide additional categories for exclusion of potential surrogates to eliminate surrogate applicants who haven't had children before[25] and to avoid incest.[26] The proposed District of Columbia law seems particularly concerned about eugenics. It prohibits any representation that a child born through surrogacy (or for that matter, embryo transfer) will possess superior genetic or physical traits.

Screening Issues

Few of the proposed laws address the issue of screening the participants. Some require a detailed medical history of the surrogate,[27] and in most instances, medical information is collected about the intended father as well.[28] In the District of Columbia this includes information about known genetically transmitted diseases (including those of blood relatives), sexually transmitted diseases, habitual use of drugs or alcohol, and exposure to radiation and toxic substances. It is unlawful for the surrogate to knowingly conceal such information. The proposed Missouri law requires certification that the providers of genetic materials and the intended parents were medically and genetically examined by a physician knowledgeable in genetics. The proposed laws usually specify that there be full disclosure of the results of medical exams and tests to the other parties to the contract.[29]

Proposed laws in at least seven states would require the surrogate and the intended father who provides the sperm to be screened for sexually transmitted diseases.[30] An Illinois bill allows the parties to contract for genetic screening, while bills in at least six states would require genetic screening of the surrogate and intended father.[31] The Michigan regulatory bill states that the surrogate mother must also, upon the request of the societal father, submit to genetic screening and authorize the release of the results to the societal father. One of the New York bills similarly provides for medical screening at the request of the intended father.

Some bills would require psychological screening or counseling of the participants in surrogacy arrangements. Under the District of Columbia bill, the surrogate (and her husband if she is married) must undergo counseling by a mental health professional about the psychological consequences of the termination of parental rights. The professional must certify that all parties are capable of consenting and that the surrogate (and spouse) received counseling. In addition, under this and one of the New York bills, the intended father may require the surrogate to undergo a psychological evaluation prior to execution of the contract. Under the Michigan bill, a mental health professional must certify that the surrogate is capable of consenting.

A proposed Illinois bill requires both the surrogate and her husband to undergo psychological screening by either a board-certified psychologist or a psychiatrist to determine that they are fit persons capable of surrendering the child upon birth. Under one of the New Jersey bills, the surrogate must undergo psychological screening, but the purpose of that screening is not identified. In contrast, bills in Massachusetts, New York, and Pennsylvania would require assessments by mental health professionals at the discretion of the judge.

The Maryland bill requires that the contract contain a provision saying that the surrogate, upon reasonable request of the biological father and his spouse, must submit to a pre-insemination psychiatric or psychological evaluation, and psychological counseling prior to and after the birth of the child if recommended as a result of the evaluation.

Bills in the District of Columbia and Michigan require that, prior to signing the contract, the intended rearing parents undergo counseling by a mental health professional on the consequences and responsibilities of parenthood under a surrogate arrangement. The proposed California statute requires psychological counseling for all involved parties beginning thirty days prior to entering the contract and ending no earlier than two months after the birth of the child. In particular, the surrogate must be counseled about the consequences of acting as a surrogate and giving her child up for adoption.

Beyond collecting medical or psychological information, some laws attempt to foster informed decisionmaking by actually requiring the participants to review that information. Under the California, District of Columbia, Illinois, Michigan, and Missouri bills, prior to entering a contract, the potential rearing couple must review the results of the medical, genetic, and psychiatric or psychological examinations of the surrogate to decide if the surrogate is acceptable. The Illinois and Missouri bills also provide that each side review the other's criminal arrest and conviction records (other than those for minor traffic offenses).

Facilitating Voluntary Informed Consent

Some proposed statutes include mechanisms intended to assure that the decision to enter a surrogacy arrangement is well-thought-out, well-informed, and uncoerced. Bills in the District of Columbia and Michigan, for example, provide a cooling-off period prior to insemination by requiring that at least thirty days pass between the execution of the contract and the artificial insemination of the surrogate. Other proposals stipulate provisions regarding legal counsel for the surrogate. Bills in at least eleven states specify that the same lawyer must not represent both the surrogate and the intended parents.[32] In at least five states, the surrogate's attorney would be paid for by the intended parents,[33] with California limiting reimbursement to $300.

Some proposals provide for court approval of the contract prior to insemination (in Illinois, Massachusetts, Missouri, New Jersey, New York, Pennsylvania, and South Carolina, for example). In Illinois and Missouri, the judge scrutinizes whether the parties "have executed the agreement knowingly and voluntarily." Similarly, bills in Massachusetts, New York, and Pennsylvania require a judicial determination regarding whether each party is freely informed and has freely and knowingly entered into the agreement. The Massachusetts judge may also determine whether the contract "protects the health and welfare of the potential child."

Decisionmaking during Pregnancy

Most of the proposed laws that touch on the surrogate's behavior during pregnancy give her the right to make health care decisions during pregnancy, including aborting or not aborting according to her own determination. Such is the case, for example, under bills in Illinois, Massachusetts, Missouri, New York, and Pennsylvania. In contrast, the District of Columbia bill limits the surrogate's control by requiring that the contract contain an agreement by the surrogate "to follow the medical instructions given to her by the physician attending her during pregnancy to protect her health and the health of the unborn child." A proposed Maryland bill includes a similar provision and additionally requires that the surrogate submit to reasonable requests by the father and his wife for prenatal medical care. A proposed New Jersey bill states that the surrogate must follow a medical examination schedule. An alternative New York bill provides that the surrogate must adhere to reasonable medical instructions and submit to "any reasonable pregnancy related medical care or treatment as provided in the contract." If she does not, the father can declare the contract null and void.

The South Carolina bill imposes the most stringent restrictions on the surrogate's behavior during pregnancy. It requires that the surrogate adhere to all medical instructions, follow a specified schedule of prenatal visits, and not abort the child unless informed by the inseminating physician that such an abortion is necessary for her physical health.

Under proposals in Illinois and Missouri, if the surrogate undergoes an abortion that is not medically necessary, the intended parents can recover the fees and expenses paid to the surrogate and reasonable attorneys' fees. If the abortion is involuntary, medically necessary, or agreed to by the parties, the surrogate is entitled to a pro rata portion of the fee, plus her medical expenses, plus attorneys' fees for enforcement of her rights. Under one of the proposed New York bills, if the surrogate refuses to comply with the father's request to abort, the father nonetheless maintains parental rights and responsibilities for the child.

Parental Rights

Under most proposals (for example, in California, the District of Columbia, Illinois, Maryland, Massachusetts, Michigan, Missouri, New Jersey, New York, Oregon, Pennsylvania, and South Carolina), the intended rearing parents have an explicit duty to assume all parental rights and responsibilities for the child upon birth, no matter what the child's condition. Under the California law, however, the couple does not have to take custody of a child who suffers from a disease or defect caused by the surrogate in violation of the contract. One pending Massachusetts bill does not give custody automatically to the intended parents, although it specifically states that the contract can be enforced. If a petition is filed concerning custody, the court shall determine what custody arrangement is in the best interest of the child. Among the factors to be considered when determining custody are the existence of fraud, duress, undue influence, or overreaching by either party to the contract or by any intermediary, the maturity and mental capacity of both parties, the home environment of the parties, the biological makeup of the child, and the consideration given by the parties to the contract.

Under both proposed New Jersey bills, in the event of a dispute over custody, the provisions of the contract shall prevail unless the court under extraordinary circumstances finds otherwise. Similarly, under the California bill and one of the Illinois bills, the agreement prevails unless that would be to the detriment of the interests of the child.

Another Illinois bill and one in Missouri provide for a court to order specific performance of the contract by either side. An action for specific performance must be sought no later than fourteen days after the intended parents learn of the birth of the child and the court hearing on the matter must be within seven days of notice to the party or parties. However, if the court finds that giving the intended parents custody is contrary to the child's best interest, or that the intended parent is not fit, or if, after the insemination, the surrogate learns that an intended parent has been convicted of a crime that the court finds indicative of the intended parent's lack of fitness as a parent, the court may award custody to the surrogate.

When the Surrogate Changes Her Mind

In a few states, the surrogate would have a certain time period during which she could change her mind after the birth of the child. One proposed regulatory law in Pennsylvania would give the surrogate twenty days after the child's birth to change her mind. The biological father's remedies in such a situation would apparently be limited to damages under the contract. Similarly, under the Michigan regulatory bill and one of the New York bills, the surrogate may revoke her consent within twenty days of the birth and bring an action for custody. A proposed Florida bill would allow the surrogate to relinquish her parental rights only after the birth and permit her to rescind her consent at any time prior to the completion of the adoption (which may be as late as six months after the birth of the child). If consent is revoked, the surrogate and her husband would be the legal parents of the child.

Under a proposed Minnesota law, the surrogate has a right to legal and physical custody of the child for two weeks after the child's birth and apparently cannot let the biological father and his wife have the child during that time period. During the fourteen-day period, she may revoke her consent. If she does so, the father must be reimbursed for the fees and expenses he spent. He will have no support obligations to the child, but may seek custody or visitation rights.

Under the proposed Florida law, if the surrogate is awarded custody of the child the intended father does not have support obligations. In contrast, in California if the surrogate is given custody of the child, the father continues to have parental responsibility. The California statute does indicate a preference for awarding joint custody or giving custody to the parent most likely to allow contact with the noncustodial parent.

Insurance and
Guardian Requirements

Regulatory bills in at least eight states require that the surrogate arrangements provide for insurance on the life of the surrogate with the beneficiary of her choice and on the life of the intended parents, generally with the resulting child as the beneficiary.[34] Most require that the minimum death benefits be around $100,000.

In addition to the financial protections for the resulting child in the case of the death of the intended parents, a number of states require that a guardian be selected for the child. Under proposed laws in California, Maryland, Michigan, Minnesota, and South Carolina, if the biological father dies before the child's birth, his wife shall assume custody of the child, unless the surrogate contract provides otherwise. Under a proposed Minnesota law, if the biological father dies, his wife has the option, within fourteen days after the birth, to claim the child, although the surrogate can renege on the agreement during that same time period.

Under bills in the District of Columbia, Illinois, and Missouri, each surrogate parenthood agreement must name a guardian for the child in case both intended rearing parents die. The California bill states that if both the intended mother and father die before the birth of the child, the surrogate may opt for custody of the child within twenty days after birth. If the surrogate mother declines, the child apparently is placed with the guardian named by the infertile couple. The Michigan and South Carolina bills award custody to the surrogate mother if both the intended mother and father die; under the South Carolina statute, the surrogate is entitled to her full compensation if the intended parents die.

Recordkeeping

Few proposals address the issue of recordkeeping. Certain bills require information about the surrogacy arrangement to be filed with a state official, such as the Secretary of the Department of Human Resources (Maryland), the Commissioner of Human Services (Minnesota), the Registrar (District of Columbia), the Office of Vital Records and Public Health Statistics (South Carolina), or the Department of Health (New York).

A proposed New Jersey bill mandates that the Department of Health must maintain records of all surrogate mothers. The records held by the department shall be kept confidential to be disclosed only to a physician and only if the information is necessary to care for a child produced by a surrogate motherhood procedure. Also, the practitioner supervising the insemination of the surrogate is required to give a copy of all medical records and the contract for surrogacy to the Department of Health. The Michigan bill requires that upon the birth of the child, the couple file the agreement with the local probate court; the probate court in turn reports to the state registrar. The District of Columbia bill requires the Registrar to report annually to the health department and the City Council the number of surrogate agreements filed.

Informational Rights of the Resulting Children

Under a proposed Maryland bill, the biological father and his spouse must make available to the child the genetic screening information acquired about the surrogate. As part of a continuing obligation to have information available to the resulting child, a New Jersey bill provides that the surrogate has a duty to disclose any genetically-related health changes to the practitioner after the birth of the child. Failure to do so renders the surrogate liable for damages.

Few bills address whether the children of surrogacy arrangements will have access to information about, or the identity of, their surrogates. Under bills in California, Illinois, Massachusetts, New Jersey, New York, and South Carolina, it appears that such records will be treated like sealed adoption records, opened only for good cause.[35] However, one of the Illinois bills and the Missouri bill would allow an emancipated person born from a surrogate contract to learn whether or not his or her prospective spouse is related to him or her.

Proposed bills in the District of Columbia and Michigan take an entirely different approach. They provide that, upon reaching age eighteen, a child born as a result of a surrogate contract may obtain copies of any documents filed. In the District of Columbia, however, the identifying information is deleted. In Minnesota, the surrogate may at any point file (or revoke) with the Commissioner of Human Services an affidavit allowing her identity to be disclosed. Unless she specifically declines disclosure, the child will be told of her identity. If the surrogate has died or has failed to file an affidavit declining disclosure and cannot be found, the child will be told of her identity. If the surrogate has kept and raised the child, the child would likewise have a right to seek the identity of the biological father.

The Future Regulation of Alternative Reproduction

Once legislators overcame their initial horror of artificial insemination by donor, the regulatory laws they passed beginning in the 1960s were unusually simple. They merely provided that the legal parents of the child were the sperm recipient and her consenting husband and that the donor had no legal bond to the child. In contrast, the majority of the proposed laws allowing surrogacy are more complex. The differences between the existing donor insemination laws and the proposed surrogacy laws may be rooted in a stereotypical perception that women are more likely than men to need the state's protection and that women are more likely to make faulty decisions if multiple safeguards are not built into the process.

Another reason may be the legitimate recognition that a pregnant woman who contracts to be a surrogate has a much greater involvement in the procreative process than does the anonymous sperm donor in traditional artificial insemination by donor. But the difference in approaches is also attributable to historical context. In the two decades since the first donor insemination laws were passed, medical practice has changed, as well as society's expectations about health care. The law of informed consent has evolved in the intervening period, so it is understandable that the circumstances surrounding the obtaining of consent are given more attention in the surrogacy bills. Genetic screening, in its infancy in the 1960s, has become an increasingly important aspect of reproductive medicine, a development likewise reflected in proposed legislation.

As legislators address the social, legal, and medical context in which surrogate motherhood is to be regulated, some are reconsidering the donor insemination laws as well. The most recent AID laws are more complex than their precursors. The 1986 Ohio law, for example, includes provisions for medical and genetic screening of the donor, recordkeeping, confidentiality, and informed consent, as well as a requirement that the sperm recipient and her husband be given access to extensive nonidentifying information about the donor's characteristics, health status, and educational background. In addition, a number of lawmakers who have introduced surrogacy bills, such as John Ray of Washington, DC and Walter Kern of New Jersey, have introduced companion bills with detailed regulatory guidelines for traditional artificial insemination by donor. Thus, the legacy of the Baby M case may not be just the passage of laws to govern surrogacy, but the reconstruction of traditional donor insemination laws as well.

References

1. Sophia J. Kleegman and Sherwin A. Kaufman, *Infertility in Women* (Philadelphia: F.A. Davis, 1966), 178.

2. Ohio S. 93 (1955).

3. These states are: Alabama, Alaska, Arkansas, California, Colorado, Connecticut, Florida, Georgia, Idaho, Illinois, Kansas, Louisiana, Maryland, Michigan, Minnesota, Montana, Nevada, New Jersey, New Mexico, New York, North Carolina, Ohio, Oklahoma, Oregon, Tennessee, Texas, Virginia, Washington, Wisconsin, and Wyoming.

4. H.R. 2443, to amend 18 U.S.C. Sec. 1822 100th Congress, 1st Session.

5. *Id.*, to amend 15 U.S.C. Sec. 52(c)(1).

6. Ark. Rev. Stat. Ann. Sec. 34-721(B) (Supp. 1985).

7. La. H.B. 327, Act No. 583 (enacted July 1987) to be codified as R.S. 9:2713; Nev. Rev. Stat. CH. 773 Sec. 6(5) (1987).

8. Alabama H. 2 Sec. 1 (by Rains); Ill. H.B. 2101 Sec. 3 (by Granberg); Iowa S.F. 358 (by Hannon); Md. H.B. 613 Sec. A (by Mitchell); Wis. proposal by Rep. Merkt.

9. Fla. S.B. 1081 Sec. 63.212(1)(i) (by Ros-Lehtinen); Ky. 88 R.S. BR 219 Sec. 3 (by Travis); Mich. S.B. 228 Sec. 9(1) (by Binsfeld *et al.*); N.J. A. 4138 Sec. 2 (by Kavanaugh *et al.*); N.Y. A.B. 5529 55-801(1) (by Schmidt); Or. S.B. 456 Sec. 2 (by Hill and Kerans) (felony); Pa. H.B. 570 Sec. 4305 (by Markosek). The following bills would also make the contract void and unenforceable: Fla. S.B. 1081 Sec. 63.212(1)(i); Ill. H.B. 2101 Sec. 4; Ky. 88 R.S. BR 219 Sec. 3; Mich. S.B. 228 Sec. 5; N.Y. A.B. 5529 Sec. 5-801(2); and Or. S.B. 456 Sec. 3.

10. D.C. Consumer Protection and Regulation of Surrogate Parenting Centers Act of 1987, Bill 7-176 Sec. 6(e) (by Ray) (unlawful to pay a fee to surrogate or her husband); Fla. S.B. 1297 Sec. 1(3)(a)

(by Frank); and N.Y. A.B. 2403 Sec. 65-a (by Halpin). These bills would allow payment for expenses: D.C. 7-176 Sec. 6(d); Fla. S.B. 1297 Sec. 1(3)(a) (this payment may not be conditioned on the termination of parental rights); and N.Y. A.B. 2403 Sec. 65-a.

11. Conn. H.B. 5398 Sec. 1(b) (by Tulisano); Ill. S.B. 499 (by Barkhausen); N.C. S.B. 305 (by Johnson); N.C. H. 1205 (by Miller); and R.I. 87-S-386 (by Carlin).

12. Ala. H. 1113 (by McKee *et al.*); Minn. S.F. 1167 (by Brandl *et al.*); Minn. H.F. 1584 (by Kelly *et al.*); Neb. L.B. 674 (by Chambers); N.Y.S.B. 4641 (by Marchi); H.B. 6277 (by Barnett *et al.*) (the New York proposals also void arrangements for I.V.F. pregnancies). An argument could be made that the North Carolina bill only covers paid surrogacy since it voids contracts "in which a woman is employed as a surrogate."

13. Conn. H.B. 5398 Sec. 2(a). The Connecticut bill provides that, if the surrogate and her husband wish to relinquish the child, the existing statutes on paternity and adoption would apply.

14. Conn. H.B. 5398 (passed through House Committee Judiciary); Ill. H.J.R. 80 (by Currie); Me. S. 239 (by Gauvreau); Mass. H.B. 5486 (by the Committee of the Judiciary); Mass. H.B. 5312 (by Clapprood); Neb. L.R. 177 (by Barrett *et al.*); N.C. S.B. 745 (by Hardison *et al.*), and N.C. S.B. 871 (by Rand); N.J. S.J.R. No. 49 (by DiFrancesco *et al.*); N.J. A.J.R. No. 76 (by Felice *et al.*); Pa. H.R. 93 (by Saloom *et al.*); Pa. H.R. 136 (by Hagarty *et al.*).

15. Or. S.B. 384 (by Hamby *et al.*).

16. Or. H.B. 3307 Sec. 2(1) (by Bunn *et al.*). The father must pay for all hospital and medical costs arising from performance of the contract. *Id.*

17. *Id.* at Sec. 2(3).

18. D.C. Consumer Protection and Regulation of Surrogate Parenting Centers Act of 1987, Bill 7-176 Sec. 3(a).

19. They include bills in California, the District of Columbia, Florida, Illinois, Maryland, Massachusetts, Michigan, Missouri, New Jersey, New York, Pennsylvania, and South Carolina.

20. Ill. S.B. 1510 Sec. 7(n); Mo. H.B. 480 Sec. 5(14).

21. D.C. Consumer Protection and Regulation of Surrogate Parenting Centers Act of 1987, Bill 7-176 Sec. 6(e) (by Ray); Fla. S.B. 1297 Sec. 1(3)(a) (by Frank); N.Y. A.B. 2403 Sec. 65-a (by Halpin); and Wis. Proposal by Magnuson. The District of Columbia bill would allow reimbursement of the surrogate's expense for health care, legal representation, food, medicine, clothing, transportation, and lodging (at Sec. 6(d)). The Florida bill also would allow for payment of pregnancy-related medical or psychological care or treatment but the subsidy cannot be conditioned upon transferring parental rights (at Sec. 1(3)(a)). The New York bill would allow medical and maternity expenses, lost wages, and reasonable attorney's fees (at Sec. 65-a), as would the Wisconsin proposal.

22. Cal. A.B. 1707 (by Duffy *et al.*); Ill. S.B. 1510 (by D'Arco); Ill. S.B. 1111 (by Marovitz); Md. H.B. 759 (by Athey); Mass. H.B. 5314 (by Morin); Mich. H.B. 4753 (by Clack *et al.*); Minn. H.F. 1647 (by Bishop *et al.*); Mo. H.B. 480 (by Committee on Children, Youth and Families); N.J. Assembly No. 3038 (by Kern); N.J. S. 767 (by DiFrancesco); N.Y. S.B. 1429 (by Dunne *et al.*); Or. H.B. 3307 (by Bunn *et al.*); Or. S.B. 384 (by Hamby); Pa. H.B. 776 (by Reber) (see also Pa. S. 742 [by Lewis], which is identical to H.B. 776 except that it does not allow the surrogate to change her mind); S.C. S. 626 (by Thomas).

23. The Illinois and New Jersey bills do not include risk to the child.

24. The Illinois and New Jersey bills do not include genetic reasons.

25. Proposals in California, Illinois, and South Carolina require that surrogates have borne at least one child before.

26. Proposed bills in Illinois and Missouri evince concerns about the potentials for incest and provide an elaborate statutory scheme to prohibit the combination of egg and sperm of blood relatives closer than cousins of the second degree.

27. These include the proposals in California, the District of Columbia, Illinois, Missouri, and South Carolina. A New Jersey bill requires evaluation of the surrogate's physical health.

28. *See*, for example, the bills in the District of Columbia, Missouri, New Jersey, and South Carolina.

29. *See*, for example, the proposals of the District of Columbia, Illinois, Maryland, Massachusetts, Missouri, New York, and Pennsylvania. The South Carolina bill requires only that the surrogate's evaluation be released to the intended father.

30. These are the proposals of the District of Columbia, Illinois, Massachusetts, Missouri, New York, Pennsylvania, and South Carolina. A New Jersey bill would require sexually transmitted disease testing for surrogates only.

31. These are the District of Columbia, Maryland, Massachusetts, Missouri, New York, and Pennsylvania. A New Jersey bill would apply to surrogates only.

32. California, Illinois (both bills), Maryland, Massachusetts, Michigan, Minnesota, Missouri, New Jersey, New York (both bills), Pennsylvania, and South Carolina.

33. California, Illinois, Massachusetts, New York, and Pennsylvania.

34. The states are California, Illinois, Massachusetts, Minnesota, Missouri, New Jersey, New York, and Pennsylvania.

35. The proposed South Carolina law does allow adoption agencies to release nonidentifying information about surrogates, however.

CHAPTER 4

Fetal Monitoring, Sex Preselection, Nonreproductive Uses of Fetuses, and Forced Medical Treatment of Pregnant Women

CASES FOR
PRELIMINARY DISCUSSION

Case 4.1

"The patient, a 40-year-old nullipara with an 18-month history of infertility, underwent genetic amniocentesis at 17 weeks' gestation for the indication of advanced maternal age. . . . An ultrasound scan before the procedure revealed a twin pregnancy with biparietal diameters of both fetuses compatible with 17.5 weeks' gestation, two clearly defined amniotic sacs, and one placenta on the posterior uterine wall. Amniotic fluid from each sac obtained separately for chromosomal studies revealed two male fetuses. Twin A had a normal male karyotype (46, XY), but chromosomal analysis of Twin B indicated trisomy-21 (47, XY + 21).

"Presented with the diagnosis of carrying one normal and one affected fetus, the parents were confronted with the difficult task of making one of two decisions: to induce abortion and lose both fetuses, or to continue the pregnancy. The mother desperately wanted to have the normal child but could not face the burden of caring for an abnormal child for the rest of her life. Having been made aware of the case report from Sweden in which selective termination of an abnormal twin had been successfully performed even though the unaffected twin was delivered prematurely, she asked if a similar procedure could be offered to her. If it had been refused she would have chosen to abort both fetuses. At that point, she was referred to us.

"Extensive medical and legal counseling and an explanation of the many risks were provided. These risks included abortion of both fetuses, premature delivery of the surviving fetus, performing the procedure on the wrong twin since markers for sac A or B were lacking, and the development of disseminated intravascular coagulation in the mother as a result of fetal death in utero. After careful consideration, the patient decided to undertake the procedure anyway. In view of the fact that the procedure had never been performed in this country, we decided, out of an abundance of caution, to obtain confirmation from a court of law of the parents' right to consent on behalf of the normal fetus."

—From Thomas D. Kerenyi and Usha Chitkara, "Selective Birth in Twin Pregnancy with Discordancy for Down's Syndrome," *New England Journal of Medicine* 304 (1981): 1525.

Case 4.2

A 33-year-old, unmarried obese white woman was admitted to the hospital in labor. She had received no prenatal care, but was thought to be near term. She was angry and uncooperative. Monitoring of the fetus suggested hypoxia and a possible breech presentation; a cesarean section delivery was recommended to the patient. She refused repeated attempts to persuade her, and requested permission to leave the hospital against medical advice. A psychiatric consultation indicated that the patient was neither delusional nor mentally incompetent. Juvenile court was consulted, appointed attorneys to represent the patient and the unborn infant, and convened a bedside hearing with the judge presiding. The court found that the unborn baby was a dependent and neglected child as defined by the Colorado Children's Code, and ordered a cesarean section to safeguard the life of the unborn child. The patient became more cooperative and agreed to a general anaesthetic, after which a successful delivery was performed of a normal female infant.

—Adapted from a case presented by Watson Bowes, Jr., and Brad Selgestad, "Fetal Versus Maternal Rights: Medical and Legal Perspectives," *Obstetrics and Gynecology* 58 (1981): 209–211.

Case 4.3

Mary and Sam married with the idea of having a family that would give them the pleasures of watching both boys and girls grow and develop. But now, after having had two girls, Sam has begun to despair of ever having a son. Although neither has a fertility problem, Sam proposes to Mary that they go to a fertility clinic to see if it can help them in preselecting for a boy.

The clinic counselor is aware of several techniques that could do anything from increase the chances of a male offspring to guarantee that their next baby will be male: induce antibodies in Mary to "female" sperm; try to separate male from female sperm through centrifuging (possible since the sperm bearing the Y chromosome have smaller heads and less mass); use IVF and select a male preembryo for implantation; sample chorionic villi or fetal amniotic cells and abort a fetus that is female. But he is reluctant to discuss any of these with Mary and Sam because the clinic exists to assist infertile couples with medical problems, and Sam and Mary's problem is not medical.

Case 4.4

Mr. R, a 28-year-old engineer, has been on dialysis for three years and is growing desperate because of the restrictions it places on his life. He cannot work regularly because of the amount of time he has to spend in a dialysis center, and he feels weak and is suffering from many of the debilitating side effects of the treatment.

Mr. R has already investigated the possibility of obtaining a transplant. However, he had been adopted as an infant and does not know his natural family. In addition, tests show that he has a rare tissue type that makes it highly unlikely that a suitable cadaver kidney can be found.

Mr. R's physical and mental state continue to deteriorate and his wife suggests a solution to the transplant surgeon. She will, she says, become pregnant, and after five or six months, have the fetus's tissue typed. If it is histocompatible with the husband's, she will have an abortion. The kidneys from the fetus could then be transplanted in her husband.

The surgeon knows that technically such a transplant could be performed, and that the graft would probably not be rejected. He also knows that Mr. R has threatened to commit suicide if he has to remain on dialysis for an indefinite period. Should he agree to transplant the kidneys of a deliberately conceived and aborted fetus?

—From "Can the Fetus Be an Organ Farm?" *Hastings Center Report* 8, no. 5 (October 1978): 23.

REVIEW OF THE ISSUES

One of the interesting questions involved in legislative attempts to regulate behavior is whether restrictive clauses of such contracts, seeking to place limitations on the behavior of the surrogate mother during pregnancy, should be enforceable, and, if so, under what mechanism. Typical provisions include prohibitions on smoking, alcohol, and illegal drugs as well as on conjugal sexual relations for up to a year before insemination; some contracts even seek to enforce limitations on exercise and diet. Possible contract law mechanisms of enforcement are: building such requirements into state contract law, provision for breach-of-contract damages, and even endorsement of a noncontractual duty of a woman to prevent harm to her fetus, not only by foregoing harmful behaviors but even by taking affirmative steps to prevent harm (such as undergoing a cesarean section). This latter strategy may evolve not only under the pressure of the intended rearing parents of the prospective child—who have typically invested a great deal of time and money in their efforts to obtain a genetically related child to rear—but also under the pressure of our growing knowledge about the technologically predictable effects of the practices and conditions of pregnant women on their offspring.

There have been enormous advances in recent years in our understanding of the development of the fetus in utero, and in developing medical techniques for monitoring that development. These techniques make a great deal of sense for a woman who has had great difficulty in carrying a baby to term, because they allow the diagnosis of treatable problems before they become critical. They also make a great deal of sense for couples who have a predisposition to children with genetic defects; where the defects are treatable in utero, they permit timely intervention, and where they are not treatable, early diagnosis provides a variety of options, from "therapeutic" abortion, to preparation for a special child or advance planning for a problematic delivery. And they make a great deal of sense in the service of social policies for a nation that has a strong welfare tradition of providing care for defective children and adults, often at great public expense.

Interestingly, some of the earliest forms of in utero diagnosis were developed prior to the historic *Roe v. Wade* Supreme Court decision that struck down all state statutes prohibiting first and second trimester abortions. Women who learned in the fifth month, for example, that they were carrying a fetus with an extra 21st chromosome (readily determined with a karyotype) could only look forward to several months of perhaps grim preparation for a child whose IQ could range anywhere from 85 to 35 (where 100 defines the midpoint of the population). On the other hand, a woman who learned that her child would be a so-called blue baby could plan to deliver at a major hospital that was set up to provide the total transfusion essential to survival of the Rh-positive neonate. The agony of parents faced with diagnosis of an untreatable defect several months before delivery, together with no legal remedy through abortion, caused many to oppose fetal diagnosis strongly as producing "useless" information. Simultaneously, it added to the pressure to liberalize abortion laws so that action could be taken on such information.

With the Supreme Court's striking down of many antiabortion statutes, impetus was added to research and development on fetal diagnostic techniques. But the original motives of early identification of fetal health problems to facilitate treatment where possible and "replacement" of the fetus where treatment was not possible are not the sole ones.

Consider the third case above. It poses questions at two levels. At the professional level, one question is whether medical technology should be used for nonmedical purposes, simply to facilitate the wishes of the consumer. At the personal level, an important question is whether preselection of one's children's sex is morally permissible. While it may not be the motive in this case, there is a preference for male children in many cultures. In India, where the preference for male children is so great that often newborn females are killed by their parents, sex preselection is seen as solving the major social problem of infanticide; it does not, of course, solve the root problem of sexism. A slippery-slope argument favored by feminists is that the use of sex preselection techniques for other than negative eugenic, medical reasons will add to the already strong bias against female children. Others see a benefit in an increase in the relative number of males; since women live longer, it would increase the supply of men available as companions to widows.

Advances in other areas of medicine as well as our understanding of fetal development have posed a new, ethically troubling set of possibilities. Our knowledge has grown in the past 20 years to the point where we can identify various behaviors on the part of the mother that are hazardous to the health of the child that the fetus will become. During this period, there were major social changes as well. There has been, in particular, an enormous increase in the use of legal and illicit drugs by women. Many of these pass through the placenta and interact with the cells of the developing fetus. Infants began to be born to women addicted to heroin who were themselves tiny heroin addicts. Terms like *fetal alcohol syndrome* have entered our vocabulary. We now know that smoking women risk low-weight, premature babies with respiratory problems and lowered IQ scores; we can even "see" the fetus respond to changes in blood gases resulting from the mother's smoking, through the use of ultrasonography. It has become clearer and clearer that certain behaviors of the pregnant woman can involve serious, lifelong damage to the child-to-be, inflicted even before that child enters the world.

But there have also been social changes in the direction of the autonomy of the woman. Chief among these was the U.S. Supreme Court decision of *Roe v. Wade*. In it, the Court affirmed the principle, rooted in its interpretation of the Fourteenth Amendment, that there is a zone of privacy extending around the reproductive decisions of the woman and her physician during the first two trimesters of a pregnancy, to the extent that the state may only regulate, for reasons of health, the conditions under which those decisions are enacted during the second trimester. This, together with the Court's decision in *Griswold v. Connecticut* striking down restrictive state laws regarding contraception, created an enormous groundswell of attitudes and expectations regarding the autonomy of the individual woman over her own lifestyle. Those attitudes have developed concurrently with an enormous and unprecedented entry of women into the professional and laboring work force, out of the relative insulation and child-centered environment of the homemaker.

The stage has thus been set for a clash between the autonomy of women and the elements of women's new lifestyle on the one hand, and the growing ability of medicine and its technology to accurately predict the prospects of fetuses given maternal decisions about lifestyle on the other. In an increasing number of cases, ranging from attempts to exercise religious beliefs in a manner potentially harmful to a near-term fetus, to cocaine addiction and alcoholism in a pregnant woman, to compelled cesarean section delivery, attempts have been made by physicians, relatives, and district attorneys to bring the force of law into the decisions of the pregnant woman. Such efforts have been made both on behalf of the health of the future child and also on behalf of the interests of the state in not having children born who, because of such maternal behavior-induced problems, become severe and long-standing health and social problems. We may thus find ourselves both pulled toward the laudable goal of working to increase the health and survival rate of our newborns and toward concern for the potentials for assault on the hard-won rights of women.

The last of the discussion cases at the start of this chapter prompts another set of questions. If the right to conceive and abort remains strictly within the control of the woman, does society have any business judging how and for what purposes those rights are exercised, provided that their exercise occurs within the temporal zone of privacy? Or, should we resist the inventiveness of humans confronted with problems of health, survival, or even convenience to bend technology, conceived for one purpose, to other ends? Legally and morally, what are the limits to the extent to which we can bend reproductive technology, and reproduction, to serve other important interests?

Again, the medical advances and technology that were supposedly developed to provide information to physicians and their female patients in pursuit of common reproductive goals begin to slide into uses quite different in motivation from those original and relatively uncontroversial ones. It is perhaps symptomatic of both the relative speed of technological innovation and the relative lack of a vision of technology's uses and limitations that we repeatedly find ourselves grappling with the unexpected twists of the social history of human power.

REVIEW OF THE SELECTIONS

Thomas Murray sets out to clarify some of the conceptual issues associated with questions about obligations to future children. He draws useful analogies between women's obligations to their fetuses and fathers' obligations to their children, noting that in both cases such obligations are not always decisive, and that the use of the police powers of the state to enforce such duties should be employed only as a last resort in extreme cases.

Lawrence Nelson and Nancy Milliken, while affirming women's ethical obligations to their future children, resist the institutionalization of fetal rights under the law on several grounds. First, they grant that medical knowledge is incomplete and that medical diagnostic and therapeutic techniques are unavoidably uncertain. Hence, it is impossible to design a consistent policy that could be uniformly applied in sanctioning force against pregnant women on behalf of their fetuses. Second, they applaud strengthening the relationship between pregnant women and the health-care system, using education and persuasion in place of "threats, lies, or physical force" in securing fetal health.

Michael Bayles discusses the uses of techniques for exercising genetic choice with respect to one's future offspring: sex preselection, screening prospective parents for potential double doses of recessive genetic diseases (such as Tay-Sachs, sickle cell anemia, beta-thalassemia), and prenatal diagnosis for fetal defects. His discussion operates at several of the levels outlined in the introduction, and, like the preceding authors, he holds for separate treatment of ethical and social policy questions.

Finally, the selection by Mary Mahowald, Jerry Silver, and Robert Ratcheson argues in favor of proceeding, on the basis of animal models, with fetal tissue transplants in humans for research and therapy. They find a number of ethical principles common to this issue and those of transplantation from live donors and cadavers and surrogate motherhood. They strive to separate transplantation-of-fetal-tissue questions from abortion issues by carefully constructing checks that would stop the feared slide down the slippery slope from ethically permissible to ethically otiose uses of fetal tissue. Their work is potentially useful for helping us cope with cases such as the last of those included for preliminary discussion in this chapter.

Works Cited

1. U.S. Supreme Court, *Roe v. Wade*, 410 U.S. 116 (1973).
2. U.S. Supreme Court, *Griswold v. Connecticut*, 381 U.S. 479 (1965).

Moral Obligations to the Not-Yet Born:

The Fetus as Patient

THOMAS H. MURRAY, Ph.D.

The health of the not-yet-born child—the fetus intended to be brought to live birth—periodically emerges as a subject of concern. From dramatic interventions such as fetal surgery through drugs and special diets on to efforts to get pregnant women to abstain from alcohol and tobacco or to bar them from workplaces possibly toxic to developing fetuses, there has been a recent surge of ideas on how to prevent, ameliorate, or remedy damage to the not-yet-born.

Many things might be done *with, by* or *to* a pregnant woman to benefit her not-yet-born child. They range from the most physically intrusive to the least, from the most technologically sophisticated to mundane efforts at education and persuasion, from those with clearly established benefit to the fetus to those of highly uncertain benefit. The ethical issues raised by interventions of all kinds designed to aid a fetus share essential features. Once some form of fetal surgery becomes established, the case of a woman who refuses it will raise many of the same moral questions as that of a woman whose alcoholism threatens her fetus's health to a point where incarceration or institutionalization are being considered. Although different in several respects, both of the cases require asking how far the state—and physicians as agents of the state—ought to go in coercively intervening in the life of a woman in order to benefit her fetus. And both presume at least a tentative answer to a difficult ethical question: What is the moral status of a fetus?

To answer such a question sensibly and with a modicum of wisdom is our ultimate goal. A burgeoning literature on fetal therapies, fetal surgery, fetal rights, and maternal-fetal conflicts has enlivened the argument. While technologically sophisticated interventions like fetal surgery are receiving the most attention, they will probably be

Professor of Ethics and Public Policy, Institute for the Medical Humanities, University of Texas Medical Branch, Galveston, Texas.

relevant to only a minute proportion of all pregnancies. Yet most of the ethical questions raised by fetal surgery are equally pertinent to a host of other, less glamorous means to the same end. Some sample questions include the following:

> How far should we go in getting diabetic women to manage their disease during pregnancy?: Should we inform them of the consequences to their fetus? Should we try to persuade them gently? Browbeat them? If they refuse to cooperate should we initiate civil or criminal proceedings to try and coerce them? Should we try to institutionalize them as has been done in some cases of drug addicted mothers, and then perhaps strip them of their children once they are born?

> What about a mother suspected of using drugs—legal or illegal—that might deleteriously affect the fetus? What of the mother who smokes or drinks? How hard do we try to discourage her smoking or drinking during pregnancy? If she continues to do either or both heavily, at what point if any do we move beyond persuasion to coercion?

> If we think that low levels of a potentially embryotoxic or fetotoxic substance are present in a workplace, should all pregnant women be kept out? What about "potentially pregnant," that is, nonsterile women? Many United States companies have "Fetal Protection Policies" that do just that.[25]

Key Issues

Given the present, chaotic state of the debate over fundamental issues of ethics, law, and public policy regarding the fetus, offering simple answers to questions such as the ones just asked would require ignoring even more important questions. It is more valuable in the long run to clarify some of the fundamental issues now. Five are discussed in this article.

1. Whether there are any moral duties to a fetus.
2. Whether viability affects those duties.
3. How the concept of duties to a fetus is frequently misused.
4. What pitfalls must be avoided in moving from moral judgments to public policy.
5. The importance of the social and historical context of the current debate.

Do We Have Moral Duties to a Fetus?

The moral status of those fetuses who will never be born alive is problematic. Right-to-life advocates claim that even the fertilized ovum is a person, entitled to all the protections and respect due every person. Many other people, including many of those with qualms about abortion, believe that the fetus, especially in its early stages of development, has a lesser moral stature than adults, infants, or even late-term fetuses. No consensus exists on such fetuses. Fortunately, we can discuss the fetus as patient without becoming bogged down in the mire of the abortion debate. All we need is a simple distinction between those fetuses destined to be brought to live birth, and those who will not know extrauterine life.

The Not-Yet-Born Child

The situation is quite different for fetuses who will be born alive. A few theorists argue that the fetus, or even the infant and young child, has no moral status, or else an inferior one.[24] Some writers, while not directly addressing the question, argue that whatever moral claims the fetus might have are always secondary to those of the woman in whose body the fetus lies.[2] Nonetheless, there is good reason to believe that we have moral obligations to the fetus destined to be born, who we will call the not-yet-born child to distinguish it from both the already-born child and from the fetus who will not be born alive. Further, this view has considerable popular support, as evidenced by the efforts aimed at preserving fetal health through antenatal medical care, public health education of pregnant women, and the like.

The Timing of a Harm
Is Irrelevant

Imagine two different cases. In the first, a man assaults a woman with the intention of inflicting grave harm on her fetus. He succeeds, causing permanent, irreparable—but not fatal—damage to the fetus's spinal cord, resulting in paralysis. In the second case, all the circumstances are identical, except that the man attacks an infant rather than a fetus, with the same result—permanent, irreparable paralysis. Was the first act any less wrong than the second? In both cases, lifelong harm was done to humans who, whatever your beliefs about when personhood begins, would eventually cross that line and attain full moral status.

My thesis, in short, is that the timing of a harm, in itself, is not morally relevant. An act resulting in harm to a not-yet-born person (who will eventually be a full-fledged person according to everyone's moral theory) is as great a harm as if it were done later. The morally relevant factors are the usual ones: the actor's intentions; excuses; mitigating circumstances, and so on. In practice, a fetus is rarely harmed intentionally; typically, harm to a fetus occurs as a result of intentional or unintentional harm to its mother. The lack of intention to harm then is what affects our judgment about the wrongness of the act, and not the fact that it was a not-yet-born person who was harmed. We would judge unintended harm to a child or adult in a similar manner. The debate over the ethics of abortion aside, then, we can talk sensibly and without inherent contradiction about moral duties to the fetus destined to become a person—to the not-yet-born person. There will be duties to avoid harm, and there may be duties to render aid.

We can discuss moral duties to not-yet-born persons without becoming hopelessly trapped in the abortion debate. Before moving on to discuss the scope of our duties to the fetus, we need to consider whether viability affects these duties.

The Moral Relevance of Viability

Viability is, at best, a slippery concept. For one thing it is a moving front. As our ability to save younger and smaller newborns improves, the so-called age of viability is reached earlier. Physicians frequently use viability as a statistical concept: the age at which some unspecified percentage of newborns will survive. Sometimes the concept is used with reference to specific infants. We could describe survival possibilities as a probabilistic function of weight or gestational age. For example, the BW or GA 10 would be the birthweight or gestational age at which 10 per cent of infants survive. The GA 50 would be the level at which 50 per cent live, and so on. These numbers would change as our ability to save these infants change.

Viability and Abortion

The central question is whether our moral obligations to the fetus change as a function of viability. Viability as a determinant of our duties to a fetus was given great importance by its inclusion in the well-known Supreme Court abortion decision, *Roe v. Wade*.[19] The complex ruling says in its summary: "For the stage subsequent to viability, the State in promoting its interest in the potentiality of human life may, if it chooses, regulate, and even proscribe, abortion except where it is necessary, in appropriate medical judgment, for the preservation of the life or health of the mother."[19]

Viability serves as a threshhold in *Roe v. Wade*. Even though the Court uses the ambiguous phrase "potentiality of human life," behind their decision must lie some notion of the fetus growing in legal and presumably moral stature as it approaches term. Otherwise, there would be no justification for linking the State's interest in protecting that potential life with viability which, at the time of that decision (1973), roughly coincided with the end of the second trimester for most fetuses.

Attempting to uncover the moral reasoning underlying a legal decision can be perilous because one may simply be wrong and because it may encourage the unfortunate tendency to see moral disapproval as a sufficient reason for taking legal action, something we will take up later. Bearing that caution in mind, we nonetheless must try to determine what moral ideas underlie the legal reasoning in *Roe v. Wade*. The court appears to believe that, prior to viability, whatever claim the fetus may have not to be killed is outweighed by a woman's right to choose whether or not to bear and give birth to a child, with all that those activities bring in their wake. After viability, the fetus's increasing nearness to actual rather than merely potential life strengthens its moral claim against being killed to the point where it overrides the mother's right to choose not to bear a child, though not so far as to force her to risk her own life in doing so.

Viability Is Irrelevant
for Nonfatal Harms

In other words, for the problem of deciding whether a woman can abort her fetus, it may be important to know what the fetus's moral status is *at that particular moment*: whether or not it is a person or how close it is to becoming a full-fledged person may be important in this context. In stark contrast, the fetus's moral standing at that moment in its development is not relevant to judging our duties to avoid or avert nonfatal harms, since, as far as we know, the fetus will some day be a full person, and the timing of such nonlethal harms is not pertinent to determining their wrongfulness. Interestingly, the law itself seems to agree.

Until 1946, a child injured prenatally then born alive but impaired rarely found a court willing to sustain a suit for damages. But in that year began what Prosser, who wrote the standard reference work on tort law, called "the most spectacular abrupt reversal of a well settled rule in the whole history of the law of torts. The child, provided that he is born alive, is permitted to maintain an action for the consequences of prenatal injuries, and if he dies of such injuries after birth an action will lie for his wrongful death."[16] Prosser believed that the earlier denials of claims on behalf of children injured while they were still fetuses were based on invalid reasoning, and he approved of the reversal.

With the concept of prenatal injuries established as a valid one, does it matter whether the fetus was viable at the time of injury? Some courts have required that the fetus have been viable, or at least "quickened" at the time of injury.[16] But many courts have rejected viability as a relevant factor in determining whether the born child may recover for prenatal injury.[9] One critic of the concept of fetal rights says pointedly: "[V]iability is a meaningless distinction in the fetal rights context because the state's interest in the health of its future citizens is equally strong throughout pregnancy."[8] Prosser himself says, "[c]ertainly the [previable] infant may be no less injured; and all logic is in favor of ignoring the stage at which it occurs." Acknowledging that proving injury early in pregnancy might be difficult, he concludes, "[t]his, however, goes to proof rather than principle; and if, as is undoubtedly the case there are injuries as to which reliable medical proof is possible, it makes no sense to deny recovery on any such arbitrary basis."[16] The moral principle, that is, does not depend on the arbitrary criterion of viability.

While most cases have focused on recovering damages for harms already done, a number of recent cases attempt to prevent harm by affecting the pregnant woman's behavior, even to the point of outright coercion. The forced caesarean cases discussed elsewhere in this volume are one sort of example.[23] In another case (reported by a newspaper) a physician accused a woman, seven months pregnant, of endangering her fetus's development by abusing drugs. The woman was ordered to enter a drug rehabilitation program and undergo regular urinalyses until the child was born.[21] Whether this is a reasonable response to the problem is the subject of the next section.

Misusing the Idea
of Duties to a Fetus

A recurrent theme in this essay is the danger of making moral judgments or public policy without sufficient regard for context. Just this sort of misuse of the concept of duties to a fetus occurs with unsettling frequency.

The Dangers of Oversimplifying
Moral Decisions

The moral world we inhabit is one marked by a multiplicity of interests and duties. We are certainly entitled to give good moral weight to our own interests. Then there are duties to those with whom we have special relationships, relationships that prescribe even strenuous moral duties in certain domains. Finally, we have duties to "strangers"—those with whom no special moral relationship exists. Most significant moral decisions have implications for many of these interests and relationships simultaneously. For example, a woman who must decide whether to place her fetus at risk of harm by working in a factory with low levels of a suspected fetotoxin must weigh her own interests in having a job with the psychological and material benefits that may bring against the risks imposed on herself as well as her fetus. She must also consider possible benefits to her fetus that the job makes possible, such as improved nutrition for herself and prenatal care facilitated by health insurance. Then there may be others dependent on her working: a spouse, other children, perhaps elderly parents. When we portray the ethical dimensions of her decision as beginning and ending with the question of whether or not she has duties to avoid exposing her fetus to risks, we rip such a complex decision out of its moral, as well as its social and political, context. Yet, this is commonly done. Or, not much better, the woman's "right" to do whatever she desires is counterposed to the fetus's right to protection from harm. Once the problem is framed this way, giving a nuanced answer becomes impossible. A more complex view of the moral life, one that encompasses a multiplicity of legitimate moral concerns, of interests and duties, of roles and relationships, allows us to frame the question in a way that can be answered, if not more easily, at least more satisfactorily.

Warnings of Fearful
Consequences

In a clash of rights, complex issues can become stripped of their nuances and turned into simplistic all-or-none contests. On either extreme, we can imagine bleak consequences. If, on the one hand, we give pre-eminence to the fetus's right to avoid being harmed, then must pregnant women structure every detail of their lives in order to avoid all suspected risks to their not-yet-born child? Such an attitude appears to have influenced some companies to adopt so-called "Fetal Protection Policies," or FPPs, that deny employment opportunities to women.[25] Fears of what would happen should fetal rights gain the upper hand generate a litany of nightmarish possibilities:

> A woman could be held civilly or criminally liable for fetal injuries caused by accidents resulting from maternal negligence, such as automobile or household accidents. She could also be held liable for any behavior during her pregnancy having potentially adverse effects on her fetus, including failure to eat properly, using prescription, nonprescription and illegal drugs, smoking, drinking alcohol, exposing herself to infectious disease or to any workplace hazards, engaging in immoderate exercise or sexual intercourse, residing at high altitudes for prolonged periods, or using a general anesthetic or drugs to induce rapid labor during delivery. If the current trend in fetal rights continues, pregnant women would live in constant fear that any accident or "error" in judgment could be deemed "unacceptable" and become the basis for a criminal prosecution by the state or a civil suit . . . "[8]

On the other hand, if we give full sway to the woman's right to control her body, can we even level moral criticism against a case such as the one of a woman who at 40 weeks gestation, in labor with abruptio placenta with fetal distress, refused a caesarean section? After the infant was delivered stillborn, she explained to a nurse that "the death of the fetus solved complicated personal problems."[12] The language of rights in conflict may not permit us to give full and weighty consideration to a host of factors that we believe are important in making moral judgments. Examining relationships, legitimate interests, and duties may give us a more adequate picture of the moral choices people face.

Obligations to the Not-Yet-Born Are Not All Or None

Take, for example, the case of the woman who must decide whether to accept a job that might pose some risk to her fetus. Let us suppose that she intends to bring the child to birth, so we do not have to worry about the ethics of abortion. As far as we know, this is a not-yet-born child; therefore the woman has some obligation to avoid harming it while it is still a fetus. What is the scope and intensity of this obligation? Must she refuse the job?

Because of the link between most discussions of the fetus's moral status and abortion, there is an unfortunate tendency to think of our obligations to the fetus as all-or-none. But there are other creatures dependent on us, to whom we have obligations, but where those duties do not unequivocally overwhelm all other considerations— our children for example. We certainly have a duty to do what is reasonable to protect our young children from harm. That requires keeping them from known and probable dangers. But we are not required to sacrifice everything else to this task. We should teach them not to play in busy streets, and offer them a protected play-area. But must we build crash-proof barriers around their playground, strong enough to stop a cement truck run wild? Obviously not. That would be beyond "reasonable" responsibility. Anytime we take them in a car, there is a risk of injury or death. Responsible parents should provide a secure carseat for their infant or toddler. But we are not forbidden from going for a drive, even though no matter how carefully we drive there is always the distinct possibility of an accident.

What is it that makes certain risks reasonable, and others the kind that responsible parents would not take? The probability of harm and its severity should it occur are certainly relevant. Also significant is the importance of the purpose for which the risk is run and the avoidability of the risk. If we want the children to see their grandparents, a long car ride may be unavoidable. And exposing our child to the considerable risks of cytotoxic drugs is clearly justifiable if and only if our purpose is to treat them for cancer.

My purpose here is to put us on more familiar ground than the exotic situations in which questions of fetal status typically arise. Two points come out of the discussion. First, whatever moral duties we might have to a fetus—a not-yet-born child—they may equal but not exceed our duties to already-born children. The circumstances of a fetus's physical enclosure within and link to its mother's body confuses many discussions. This linkage may mean that a broader range of actions might affect the fetus, and the facts of the case will be accordingly affected. But the same moral considerations apply equally to both the not-yet-born and the already-born—considerations such as intentions, probability and severity of risk, and duties to others. Second, duties to the not-yet-born, like duties to the already-born, are usually just one of many factors to be considered in judging the moral acceptability of an act.

Another advantage of discussing our obligations to the not-yet-born and already-born together is that it enables us to talk about fathers and not just mothers. To the extent that cultural blinders distort our view of a mother's responsibility to her fetus, then looking at a case with comparable morally relevant features, but one that asks about a father's responsibility to his child, may restore some moral clarity.

A Father–Child Analogy

Take the plausible case of a man who lost his job in the oil fields of west Texas. He has two children counting on him for support; his wife is also out of work. An offer comes of a job in a petrochemical plant near Houston. Taking that job will mean moving his family to a part of Texas crawling with petrochemical complexes where toxic releases into the air, ground, and water are not unknown, and where the risk of cancer is somewhat, though not drastically, higher than in their current community. There are a number of good reasons to take the job. He will be able to afford better food, clothing, and housing for his family and himself. Being unemployed threatens his sense of self-worth, which depresses him and incidentally also makes him a less thoughtful parent and spouse. Like most unemployed Americans, when he lost his job he also lost his health insurance; the new job will assure better access to health care for himself and his family. Perhaps the schools are better in the new community. Suppose he accepts the job even though he knows and regrets the increased risk that will mean for his children. Decisions such as this are all-things-considered choices: by their nature they involve weighing and balancing many things. Would we say that this man's choice was immoral? That he should not have exposed his children to the slightly increased risk of cancer whatever else was involved? It would make better sense to say that he made a responsible, morally defensible decision, even if we share his regret about the increased risk to which his children as well as his wife and himself will be exposed.

How was this man's decision any different from that of a woman who chooses to accept a job, knowing that her fetus will be exposed to some low but nonetheless increased risk of harm because of exposures there? Perhaps she too is without health insurance. Perhaps having a job is important to her sense of self-worth. Perhaps there are other children and a spouse at home who are dependent on her. The fact that she carries a fetus within her, a not-yet-born child, that she has moral duties to protect that fetus from harm, and that the workplace increases slightly the probability of harm does not make her decision immoral. Exactly the same considerations were relevant to the man's decision. To the extent that the morally relevant factors are comparable—and in this case they might well be identical—the decisions are equally justified. And if the circumstances vary, at least we know the kinds of morally significant considerations that will influence our judgments.[15] Whether it is a man or a woman is not relevant. Nor, I have argued, does it matter whether it is a not-yet-born or already-born child.

From Ethical Judgments
to Public Policy

We do not ban all conduct we regard as morally suspect, nor do we compel people to carry out every moral duty. Many things are left to personal conscience, to moral suasion, or to social pressure. For good reasons, including moral ones, we are reluctant to allow the state to force its view of correct conduct on individuals unless the harm to be avoided is grave, especially when doing so requires coercion, bodily invasion, or incarceration. These means are among the most repugnant and are reserved for extreme circumstances. If we conclude then that a woman morally ought to quit smoking during pregnancy, moderate or eliminate her consumption of alcohol, and do likewise with caffeine, this does not automatically justify heavy-handed state intervention to assure that she does these things. Some wrongs are minimally so. The state should not exercise its often great power on such things. Sometimes the effort to correct a wrong itself creates new moral problems. The moral and other costs of enforcement may outweigh the good that might be done.

The fetus becomes a "patient" when its welfare becomes the physician's concern. The obstetrician caring for a mother and not-yet-born child has two patients. In much the way that a pediatrician advises parents about their newborn's diet, monitors the infant's health, and prescribes needed medication or other therapeutic interventions, an obstetrician routinely does the same for the mother and the fetus-patient. How extensive is the obstetrician's duty to assure that the fetus-patient's welfare is being protected?

The "Child-As-Maximum" Principle

One useful guideline might be called the "child-as-maximum" principle. The principle says that our obligations to ensure the fetus's welfare can equal but not exceed our obligations to a born child. If a pediatrician would not be obliged to do more than try to persuade parents to do a certain thing—say observe a special diet—then under conditions of comparable burdens and benefits, obstetricians cannot be obliged to do more to protect a fetus, although they may be required to do less.

One inescapable difference between the obstetrician's and the pediatrician's case is of course that the former's second patient, the fetus, is encased in the body of the first patient, the mother. All interventions directed at the fetus literally must go through its mother. The burdens created, therefore, generally will be much greater, as will be the potential for morally wronging one person in the effort to aid another. This is why the child-as-maximum principle emphasizes that our duties to a born child constitute an upper-bound for our duties to a not-yet-born child rather than a strict equivalence. A drug that might benefit a fetus but that will be harmful to the mother can be refused. That same drug for that same being, now born, should probably be administered. The pediatrician in the latter instance is justified in pushing harder for consent from the parents than was the obstetrician.

A Variety of Needs, a Range of Interventions

One study shows that women who smoke a pack of cigarettes or more a day have babies on average about 180 gm smaller at birth than women who do not smoke. The same study found that women who drank twenty or more beers per month sacrificed roughly 100 gm of birthweight, while those who consumed 300 or more grams of caffeine daily (three or four cups of coffee or seven cola beverages) had babies 40 to 50 gm smaller on average.[11] What should physicians do? When the risks are small, we usually employ education and persuasion. That is the typical and appropriate response to maternal smoking, diet, nutritional supplements, and the like. These anchor one end of a continuum of possible "interventions." We can move to stronger measures, such as New York City has done, by requiring that signs be posted in public places serving alcohol warning pregnant women that alcohol may endanger their fetus's health. This is a public policy that relies as much on shame as on the educative effect of the signs.

Beyond this is a broad range of more traditionally "medical" interventions: managing maternal diabetes in pregnancy[4]; placing women with PKU on low-phenylalanine diets when they wish to become pregnant[18]; treating fetal methylmelonic acidemia by giving Vitamin B-12 to the mother[20]; treating congenital hypothyroidism by injections into the amniotic fluid[26]; drug therapy for fetal ventricular tachycardia,[10] and other possibilities.

There are surgical routes as well. In addition to the familiar exchange transfusions for erythroblastosis fetalis, a variety of still-experimental fetal surgeries are under development. They include procedures responding to urinary tract obstruction,[5] ventriculomegaly,[1] diaphragmatic hernia,[7] and hematopoietic stem cell transplantation for severe immunologic deficiencies.[22] (The law and ethics of fetal surgery have been amply discussed elsewhere.[3, 14, 17])

Our ethical analysis of any proposed interventions to benefit a fetus intended to be brought to birth should include at least the following considerations:

1. How certain is the benefit to the fetus? (Is the intervention experimental? Is it well-established? Does it carry substantial risks to the fetus?)
2. How great are the benefits? (Will a successful intervention make a large or small difference in the fetus's prognosis?)
3. How intrusive, coercive, or harmful will it be to the mother?
4. Will anything be lost or gained by waiting until after the child is born?

Even if we are convinced that the mother has a moral responsibility to agree to the intervention, the question of how far we should go in attempting to persuade or coerce her raises an entirely new set of issues at the intersection of ethics and public policy. Once we move to the level of policy, political and historical considerations become very important. At this point, a brief look at another era's concern for the health of the not-yet-born is appropriate.

Alcohol and "Race-Decay" in Edwardian England

This is not the first time that parental behavior has been held responsible for harm to the not-yet-born or the already-born. The oldest prenatal health advice of which I am aware is in the Old Testament. In Judges 13:7 the mother of Samson is told "Behold, thou shalt conceive and bear a son: and drink no wine or strong drink."

Many women today are fearful and suspicious of the movement towards ascribing moral status to the fetus. For women who aspire to compete in the economic marketplace on an equal footing with men, those fears and suspicions have substantial historical validity. Past social movements to protect helpless infants and not-yet-born children have had something less than pure and altruistic motives. One illuminating example comes from England at the turn of the century—the Edwardian era.

In the first decade of this century, England found itself losing its empire abroad and awash with immigrants at home: immigrants, moreover, whose children were more likely to survive infancy than their British neighbors. A number of laypeople and physicians believed they understood the problem—alcohol. A campaign to arouse public ire against parents who drank flourished in the first decade of the 1900s. While it was directed largely against women who drank, men came in for their share of the blame as well. Indeed, one highly influential Swiss study reported that 78 per cent of women unable to breastfeed had fathers who drank heavily. But for the most part, women were faulted.

In 1906, a British physician wrote:

Undoubtedly much of the high infant mortality is due to alcoholism, and conditions directly . . . or indirectly arising from this morbid condition. The widespread prevalence of alcoholism among women, especially during the reproductive period of life, is one of the most important factors making for racial-decay.[6]

"Race-decay" is but one of many dubious reasons given for worrying about women and drink. George Sims, a prominent journalist of the time, had a related concern: "What can be the future of our Empire, if on a falling birth rate 120,000 infants continue to die annually in the first year of their lives . . . !"[6] And he knew the cause: "Bad motherhood is the first great cause of our appalling infant mortality."[6] No less an exemplar of success than Andrew Carnegie, the American industrialist, pointed to the drunken worker as a central threat to British productivity.[6]

For the most part, this was a campaign waged by the upper classes, including a number of male physicians, against working class women. They were not doing their national duty by outreproducing the immigrants—Jews, Italians, Scots, and Irish. Theophilus Hyslop, a physician active in the anti-drink movement, referred to immigrants derogatorily and declared that if the British worker would give up alcohol, he could "drive the foreigner from our midst."[6]

Perhaps Dr. Robert Jones best expressed the sentiment feared by contemporary women: "Women are now the companions of men in . . . industrial pursuits, and the freedom to work on equal terms with men has caused . . . the same depressing physical and mental influences . . ., for which stimulants offer a temporary relief."[6] Women, that is, as vessels of reproduction, as the assurers of racial integrity, as the saviors of the empire, as the protectors of the innocent must be made to look after their offspring, and not be contaminated in the labor marketplace.

Many women understand any contemporary movement emphasizing their biologic role as bearers of children to be a threat to their economic liberty and equality—"fetal rights" being no exception. The need to control reproduction so that they could compete in the job market emerged as a major theme among pro-choice activists in Kristin Luker's study of anti- and pro-abortion activists. Conversely, having and raising children were crucial sources of self-value for many who worked against abortion.[13] Because it focuses attention on women's reproductive capacities, it is not surprising that the trend toward regarding the fetus as a patient has evoked concern and controversy. And with the long history of efforts to keep women in roles defined by and in the interests of men, it is no less surprising that women regard the current trend with suspicion. Legitimate concerns for fetal rights can also be carried along by other, questionable, motives and may carry with them other destructive social consequences.

Conclusions

Five points emerge from this analysis. First, we can discuss moral duties to the fetus destined to be born—to the not-yet-born child—without logical contradiction and without becoming hopelessly mired in debate over abortion.

Second, whether the fetus is viable may be regarded as morally significant in the context of abortion decisions, but it is not directly relevant to our duties to not-yet-born children. This is so because of the irrelevance of the timing of a harm.

Third, that we do have moral duties to fetuses, viable and previable alike, may not have the horrendous consequences for women that is typically thought. Our common error has been to focus exclusively on a pregnant woman's duty to avoid harming her fetus, without regard for the multitude of other moral considerations she ought to include in her decision. A more complex and adequate view of the moral life understands that in such decisions a host of factors may be relevant such as promises made, the woman's own interests, her obligations to other family members, and the welfare of her not-yet-born child. Seeing the mother's moral relationship to the fetus as morally analogous to a father's relationship to his child will help avoid oversimplification.

Fourth, establishing that women have moral duties to their not-yet-born children does not justify automatically coercive public policies to force them to fulfill those obligations. Again, the analogy to fathers and children may be helpful. The state must be very cautious in using its power to enforce particular notions of maternal duties. Effective enforcement might necessitate forcible invasion of a woman's body or prolonged incarceration. These are usually "last resorts" used only under very restricted circumstances. We must be careful to assure that they are not used more casually against pregnant women.

Fifth, women have ample reason to be suspicious of the growing tendency to focus on the welfare of the fetus-as-patient and, by implication, on the woman's role as bearer of children. Historically, movements allegedly directed toward aiding fetuses and children have often been motivated as much by other, less praiseworthy concerns, including racism, and especially by men's fear of women's political, social, and economic equality.

Rather than arguing over "fetal rights," let us use the less heated language of moral obligations to not-yet-born children. We must not oversimplify complex moral decisions, especially our tendency to focus on a pregnant woman's obligations to her not-yet-born child as the *only* morally important factor in her decisions. We would not tolerate such oversimplification when discussing parents' duties toward their children, and we must not tolerate it in the difficult decisions we now face regarding the welfare of the not-yet-born. History provides forceful reminders of the dangers of thinking of women as mere "vessels of reproduction." Finally, we must continue the work of clarifying our obligations toward both the fetus destined to be born and the mother who retains her full moral individuality and interests, and in whose body that developing person exists for a time.

References

1. Clewell WH, Meier PR, Manchester DK, et al: Ventriculomegaly: Evaluation and management. Sem Perinatol 9:98–102, 1985
2. Engelhardt HT: The Foundation of Bioethics. New York, Oxford, 1986
3. Fletcher JC: Ethical considerations in and beyond experimental fetal therapy. Sem Perinatol 9:130–135, 1985

4. Gabbe SG: Management of diabetes mellitus in pregnancy. Am J Obstet Gynecol 153:824–827, 1985

5. Golbus MS, Filly RA, Callen PW, et al: Fetal urinary tract obstruction: Management and selection for treatment. Sem Perinatol 9:91–97, 1985

6. Gutzke DW: "The cry of the children": The Edwardian medical campaign against maternal drinking. Br J Addiction 79:71–84, 1984

7. Harrison MR, Adzick NS, Nakayama DK, et al: Fetal diaphragmatic hernia: Fatal but fixable. Sem Perinatol 9:103–112, 1985

8. Johnsen DE: The creation of fetal rights: Conflicts with women's constitutional rights to liberty, privacy, and equal protection. Yale Law J 95:599–625, 1986

9. Keeton WP, Dobbs D, Keeton R, et al: Prosser and Keeton on the Law of Torts. Edition 5. Mineola, NY, West Publishing Co, 1984

10. Kleinman CS, Copel JA, Weinstein EM, et al: In utero diagnosis and treatment of fetal supraventricular tachycardia. Sem Perinatol 9:113–129, 1985

11. Kuzma JW, Sokol RJ: Maternal drinking behavior and decreased intrauterine growth. Alcohol Clin Exp Res 6:396–402, 1982

12. Leiberman JR, Mazor M, Chaim W, et al: The fetal right to live. Obstet Gynecol 53:515–517, 1979

13. Luker K: Abortion and the Politics of Motherhood. University of California, Berkeley, 1984

14. Murray TH: Ethical issues in fetal surgery. Bull Am Col Surg 70(6):6–10, 1985

15. Murray TH: Who do fetal protection policies really protect? Tech Rev 88(7):12–13, 20, 1985

16. Prosser WL: Handbook of the Law of Torts. Edition 3. St Paul, MN, West Publishing Co, 1964

17. Robertson JA: Legal issues in fetal therapy. Sem Perinatol 9:136–142, 1985

18. Robertson JA, Schulman JD: PKU women and pregnancy: The limits of reproductive autonomy. Unpublished manuscript

19. Roe v Wade, 410 U.S. 113, 1973

20. Schulman JD: Prenatal treatment of biochemical disorders. Sem Perinatol 9:75–78, 1985

21. Shaw MW: Conditional prospective rights of the fetus. J Leg Med 5:63–116, 1984

22. Simpson TJ, Golbus MS: In utero fetal hematopoietic stem cell transplantation. Sem Perinatol 9:68–74, 1985

23. Strong C: Ethical conflicts between mother and fetus in obstetrics. Clin Perinatol 14(2)

24. Tooley M: Abortion and Infanticide. New York, Oxford University Press, 1983

25. US Congress, Office of Technology Assessment: Reproductive Health Hazards in the Workplace. US Government Printing Office: Washington, DC, 1985

26. Weiner S, Scharf JF, Bolognese PJ, et al: Antenatal diagnosis and treatment of fetal goiter. J Reprod Med 24:39–42, 1980

Institute for the Medical Humanities
The University of Texas Medical Branch
Galveston, Texas 77550

Compelled Medical Treatment of Pregnant Women

Life, Liberty, and Law in Conflict

LAWRENCE J. NELSON, Ph.D., J.D., NANCY MILLIKEN, M.D.

As recently stated by the ethics committee of the American College of Obstetricians and Gynecologists, the maternal-fetal relationship is a "unique one" as it involves "two patients with access to one through the other."[1] In no other situation is the physician faced with one patient literally inside the body of another patient. Conceptually, the medical care of each can be approached independently, but practically, neither can be treated without affecting the other. Because of this unique relationship, conflicts between the interests of the woman and the fetus can arise if the former refuses treatment recommended for the benefit of the latter (eg, refusing cesarean section for documented fetal distress and anoxia) or if she is unwilling or unable to change behaviors that potentially could harm her fetus, such as smoking, consuming alcohol, eating inadequately, or engaging in certain job-related or recreational activities.

Kolder et al[2] recently documented a substantial number of court-ordered obstetric procedures performed despite a woman's refusal of treatment considered necessary to preserve the life or health of the fetus. As the survey included only obstetricians directing fellowship and residency programs in maternal-fetal medicine, there certainly are instances of compelled treatment not included in their report. Other recent reports seem to confirm this.[3-5] Perhaps most important, the report by Kolder et al documented that almost half of the fellowship directors thought that judicial force should be used to impose treatment thought to be lifesaving, including surgery, on unconsenting pregnant women for the sake of the fetus. Court-ordered obstetric treatment raises a host of fundamental ethical and legal questions for physicians, pregnant women, and society—questions that have not been adequately explored in the medical literature.

From the Bioethics Consultation Group, Berkeley, Calif. (Dr. Nelson), and the Department of Medicine, Division of Medical Ethics (Dr. Nelson), and Obstetrics, Gynecology, and Reproductive Sciences (Dr. Milliken), University of California, San Francisco.

Reprint requests to the Bioethics Consultation Group, 1400 Shattuck Ave, Suite 6 (PO Box 10145), Berkeley, CA 94709 (Dr. Nelson).

In this article, we will first discuss the ethical basis of the physician-patient relationship during pregnancy and present our perspective on the ethical reconciliation of maternal-fetal conflict. Next, we will analyze the legal aspects of physician management of pregnant women who refuse medically indicated treatment. Finally, we will present the policy reasons why neither the medical profession nor society should support judicially compelled treatment of pregnant women. We conclude that the pregnant woman's ethical obligation to care for her fetus should not be legally enforced.

Obstetrics, Ethics, and the Physician-Patient Relationship

As a result of the rapid development of obstetric knowledge and technology, the physician's relationship to the fetus has changed dramatically. In part because the fetus has become the subject of many direct medical interventions, it has emerged as the obstetrician's second patient. The preface to the most recent edition of *Williams Textbook of Obstetrics* reflects this view: "Quality of life for the mother and her infant is our most important concern. Happily, we live and work in an era in which the fetus is established as our second patient with many rights and privileges comparable to those previously achieved only after birth."[6] Although this excerpt is not a description of a fetus' legal rights, it does suggest that obstetricians commonly conceptualize the fetus as a patient to whom they owe ethical duties as they would to any other patient.

The fetus has not become a patient in its own right because the goal of obstetrics has changed; that goal has always been the birth of a healthy baby to a healthy mother. Rather, medicine's means to achieve this goal have changed significantly during the past few decades. Formerly, the physician was able to treat only the mother and had to assume that in maintaining her health, the health of the fetus would be enhanced. The fetus itself was largely beyond the diagnostic and therapeutic reach of the physician. Advances in knowledge of fetal physiology and the development of new technology have enabled physicians to see the fetus in detail with ultrasound, to assess its condition with amniocentesis and fetal heart rate monitoring, and to operate on it in utero. In short, medicine's enhanced ability to treat the fetus directly has profoundly affected, perhaps even created, physicians' perception of the fetus as a separate patient. Such a perception is reinforced by clinical experience of the fetus as a technically interesting and challenging patient.

One might infer from the foregoing that it is only the new emphasis on the fetus as patient that determines the physician's ethical obligation to promote its well-being. This is not true. The physician's obligation to promote fetal health is firmly rooted in his or her ethical obligations to the pregnant woman. In seeking prenatal care, a pregnant woman is at least implicitly demonstrating that she has freely chosen to pursue a successful pregnancy. Regardless of an individual physician's conceptualization of the fetus as a separate patient, he or she is required to monitor the fetus and recommend appropriate treatment in accordance with the standard of care because of the woman's choice to bring her pregnancy to term. The failure to do so would be both ethically wrong and medical malpractice. Therefore, the fetus does not need to be seen as a second or separate obstetric patient to create a duty on the part of a physician to render it excellent care.

While the physician's relationship to the fetus has undergone significant expansion and qualitative change, the physician's relationship to a pregnant woman has a venerable history. The pregnant woman who presents for prenatal care is clearly the obstetrician's patient. Their interaction is governed by the fiduciary nature of any physician-patient relationship in which an individual patient voluntarily entrusts the physician with her medical concerns, and the physician reciprocates with the skillful application of medical knowledge to serve the patient's interests faithfully. The ethical principle of beneficence requires a physician to implement the therapy that best promotes the patient's health while minimizing potential harm. In the context of obstetrics, the physician has the responsibility to monitor the health of both the woman and the fetus and to advocate treatment intended to enhance the health of both.

In addition to the principle of beneficence, the physician is ethically obliged to recognize the principle of respect for individual autonomy. In keeping with this latter principle, all adult patients traditionally are deemed to have the right to accept or reject medical recommendations based on their personal priorities and values,[7] a right respected and protected by the law.[8–11] Like other adults, a pregnant woman must make decisions about medical care within the broader context of her life. Her responsibility to her fetus will sometimes be weighed against responsibilities to her children, husband, and others with whom she has a special relationship. Her decisions also may be influenced by a religious faith or commitments to strongly held personal values, and she may not always agree with her physician's advice.

Usually it is frustrating for physicians when patients do not follow their advice. Often it is painful when the patient's medically foolish decision results in serious damage or death. Perhaps nowhere are the physician's frustration and pain with a patient's noncompliance more excruciating than in obstetrics, where the decisions of the pregnant woman affect not only her own health but also that of her fetus. However, these feelings alone do not ethically justify ignoring or circumventing a pregnant woman's refusal to follow medical advice.

Because she is an autonomous adult, a competent pregnant woman has the same prerogative as other adults to control her own life and what will happen to her body. In addition, because conceiving and bearing a child is a highly personal and private matter, others (including physicians) should be very reluctant to substitute their value judgments in such a matter for those of the woman herself. Therefore, due to respect for an individual's autonomy and privacy, physicians should recognize and honor a competent pregnant woman's informed decision to reject medical advice about her care.

This view surely can be criticized for ignoring the value of the fetus as a being with interests separate from those of its mother. Factually, a fetus is a human life with a distinct genetic constitution that develops and possesses an organ system distinct from its mother's. However, the ethical evaluation of fetal life varies dramatically within our society. Some contend that a fertilized human ovum is a human life with the same rights as any live-born man or woman.[12] Others see the fetus as at most a potential human life that receives the protection of the ethical principle forbidding harm to persons only after it lives outside of the mother's body. Still others have claimed that a fetus achieves protectable ethical status at quickening or when it reaches the point of viability.[4] A more recent view argues that the fetus gains ethical status when it has developed neurologically to the point where it has consciousness.[13] Not only is there a lack of agreement on how to value fetal life, particularly when it comes into conflict with the interests of the mother, but this disagreement is violently expressed both literally in abortion clinic bombings and figuratively in slogan slinging on both sides of the issue.

In light of this seemingly intractable controversy, it is arbitrary for a physician to resolve maternal-fetal conflict by claiming that his or her ethical evaluation of the fetus is the "right" one while the woman's is "wrong." When there is such profound disagreement, we believe that the ethically preferable course of action is to leave the determination of the weight of the fetus' interests to the mother in conflict situations. Nonetheless, it is certainly ethically permissible (perhaps even mandatory) for a physician to try to persuade a pregnant woman refusing medically indicated treatment to change her mind. Neither patient autonomy nor the doctrine of informed consent requires physicians to accept patient refusal passively and without inquiry, protest, or argument. However, the purposeful use of threats or deception to "convince" a patient to change her mind is ethically unacceptable.

Legal Analysis

Law and Ethics

The study by Kolder et al[2] showed that a number of physicians have been willing to seek court orders compelling pregnant women to undergo treatment for the sake of their fetuses. While judicial sanction may reduce a physician's exposure to legal liability, it does not eliminate the ethical issues involved. In fact, the very decision to pursue a court order implicates important ethical values. Judicial involvement inevitably invades a woman's privacy, entails the disclosure of confidential medical and personal information, and thrusts the woman into the adversarial system, where she must defend her choices on a highly personal matter at a time when she is psychologically and physically ill-disposed to do so. Moreover, the request for a court order demonstrates the physician's willingness to use physical force against a competent adult to effect treatment, an ethically perilous course of action for a physician to adopt under any circumstances.

Furthermore, physicians cannot legitimately claim that they are compelled by the law to seek such orders. There is no affirmative legal duty on the part of the clinician to seek a court order in these circumstances.[4] Also, there is no reported case of a court imposing civil damages on any physician for failing to seek judicial review of any competent adult's refusal of treatment,[4] a finding corroborated by the study of Kolder et al.[2] Finally, the fact that a child may be able to sue his mother for prenatal injuries caused by her conduct[14,15] does not mean that the state would have the power to force her to forsake such conduct,[5] much less that a physician could be held liable for failing to force her similarly.

Persuasive arguments can be made that a pregnant woman not intending to have an abortion has an ethical obligation to accept reasonable, nonexperimental medical treatment and to behave otherwise in a manner that will benefit and not harm her fetus. Indeed, we are convinced that such an ethical obligation exists and that women should behave accordingly. Also, physicians should generally act toward their pregnant patients under the assumption that such an obligation exists and that the woman will fulfill it. Nevertheless, it is quite another matter to transform this ethical obligation into a legal duty by enforcing it with the coercive power of the law.

The Controversy Regarding Compulsory Treatment

Several articles in the medical literature address the subject of compulsory treatment of pregnant women.[16–26] Many contain incorrect and misleading statements about the law applicable to maternal refusal of treatment and about a physician's potential legal liability for either honoring or disregarding the pregnant woman's wishes. The following discussion will present and analyze what we consider to be the major legal arguments surrounding maternal-fetal conflict.

The Significance of *Roe vs Wade*   Many commentators[16,18,23,26] and one court[27] have asserted that the Supreme Court's landmark decision on abortion, *Roe vs Wade*, supports compulsory medical treatment of pregnant women by the state and its courts for the sake of the fetus. This assertion is based on the Court's ruling that the state has a compelling interest in protecting the potentiality of human life at the point of viability (ie, the time when the fetus has the capability of "meaningful life outside the mother's womb") and can forbid abortions after that point—except when abortion is "necessary to preserve the life or health of the mother."[28] This "compelling interest" in the fetus can then be vindicated by the state's forcing a pregnant woman to undergo treatment intended to benefit a viable fetus. A corollary of this argument is that because the woman has "waived" her right to an abortion after carrying the pregnancy beyond the point of viability, the state can force her to accept treatment for the benefit of the fetus.[15]

This misinterpretation of the law set forth in *Roe* is probably the most common and serious oversight made in the debate about maternal-fetal conflict. While it is true that *Roe* acknowledged the state's compelling interest in the fetus at viability, it placed an essential limit on the exercise of this interest by expressly permitting a woman to obtain an abortion even after fetal viability if "it is necessary to preserve [her] life or health." Thus, it is incorrect to assert that *Roe* grants the state unrestricted authority to protect the viable fetus or to prohibit abortions after viability.[4] Furthermore, *Roe* simply permits, but does not compel, states to forbid abortion after viability when the mother's life or health is not thereby compromised. In addition, *Roe* says nothing about whether the state may force treatment on a woman to promote fetal health.[5]

Two other Supreme Court decisions that upheld abortion statutes have made clear that the "health" of the pregnant woman must be broadly defined.[29,30] The Court found the statutes challenged in these cases constitutional because they allowed the physician to make his determination about the woman's need for an abortion "in the light of all attendant circumstances—psychological and emotional as well as physical—that might be relevant to the well-being of the [mother]."[31] In short, abortions after fetal viability cannot be totally forbidden by the state because the woman's interest in the preservation of her life and health is superior to the state's "compelling interest" in the preservation of viable fetal life.[4]

More to the point of the subject at hand, the Supreme Court has ruled on two occasions that the state is constitutionally forbidden from requiring a woman to undergo an abortion procedure that would require her to bear *any* increased risk to her health to enhance the health or to save the life of her viable fetus. In *Colautti vs Franklin*, the Court struck down a Pennsylvania statute requiring the use of the abortion technique providing "the best opportunity for the fetus to be aborted alive" because it did not "clearly specify . . . that the woman's health must always prevail over the fetus' life and health when they conflict."[31] In its latest ruling on abortion, the Court struck down a similar Pennsylvania statute because it required the woman to bear an increased medical risk to save her viable fetus and violated the ruling of *Colautti* that statutes that require a trade-off between the woman's health and fetal survival are unconstitutional.[32] (In his dissent in this case, Justice White interpreted the majority as holding that the state's compelling interest in preserving the life of a viable fetus "cannot justify *any* regulation that imposes a quantifiable medical risk upon the pregnant woman who seeks to abort a viable fetus; if attempting to save the fetus imposes any additional risk of injury to the woman, she must be permitted to kill it.")

Consequently, when the health interests of a woman and her fetus conflict, the state appears to be constitutionally bound to place the woman's interests above the fetus'.[2,5] As many courts have held that the right to privacy implicated in the abortion decision entitles competent adults to refuse recommended medical treatment,[8,33] it should follow that a state and the courts are constitutionally barred from forcing a pregnant woman to undergo medical treatment for the sake of the fetus if that treatment endangers her life or health in any way. As almost all medical interventions that could benefit the fetus entail at least some risk to the woman's life or health (particularly a procedure like cesarean section), the courts should not be able to force a competent woman to undergo those interventions against her will.

Child Neglect Law Some commentators have claimed that existing state law prohibiting child neglect authorizes the courts to compel a pregnant woman to undergo treatment.[26,34] They argue that just as the law prohibits parents from refusing to provide necessary medical treatment to their children, it also prohibits a woman from refusing treatment necessary to protect the fetus' health.

The most fundamental problem with this view is that it facilely equates live-born children and fetuses. One proponent of intervention for the fetus' sake has acknowledged that child neglect laws were not originally intended to include fetuses and has identified only one such law that specifically includes a fetus within the definition of "child."[35] One trial court has concluded that a viable fetus is a child under Ohio's child abuse law and that a mother's prenatal use of heroin was child abuse.[36] However, a trial court decision does not establish judicial precedent as do appellate court decisions. Two appellate courts have ruled that fetuses are not "children" over whom a court can assert control due to parental neglect or abuse.[37,38]

As Rhoden[5] has pointed out, the law has never imposed duties on pregnant women in the same manner as it imposed duties on parents toward their children. Moreover, it is far from clear whether the law should treat fetuses, which are still inside a woman's body, in the same way as it treats children, who are physically separate from their parents.[5] Ordering treatment of a pregnant woman invades her body, while ordering treatment of a child does not. "Because there are no correlative physical burdens involved in providing medical treatment for one's child, child neglect law is far less relevant than it initially appears."[6]

Also, as shown above, *Roe* does not establish that women have a legal duty to expose themselves to any medical risk for the sake of their fetuses. In light of *Roe* and its progeny, even the explicit inclusion of the fetus within the purview of child abuse and neglect statutes should not be constitutionally sufficient to empower the state to force a pregnant woman to undergo unwanted and risky treatment for the sake of the fetus. Furthermore, as shown below, there are many compelling medical and social reasons for not equating fetuses and children and for not forcing competent pregnant women to undergo treatment they do not want.

The Legal Status of the Fetus   Many proponents of intervention on behalf of the fetus base their position on the legal status of the fetus and perceive it as having rights and receiving protection from the law like any other human being. Bowes and Selgestad,[16] for example, claim that the full-term viable fetus clearly has protectable rights. To be sure, the law has in the past afforded and continues to afford the fetus certain legal rights and protections.[34,29] For example, a fetus can be named an heir to an estate, although this property right is vested only on live birth. In addition, the majority of jurisdictions permit parents of a stillborn viable fetus to sue the negligent party for wrongful death, although some states permit this only if the fetus is live born.[4] However, it is not at all clear that such legal actions are meant to protect fetal "rights" rather than parental rights to dispose of their property as they wish or to produce offspring born without wrongfully inflicted injury.[4,28]

The criminal law historically did not recognize the killing of an unborn fetus as a homicide unless it was born alive.[40–42] But in some states, a fetus now can be the victim of manslaughter[40] or vehicular homicide.[43] In fact, in California it is first-degree murder to kill a viable fetus with malice aforethought.[44] Curiously, the law provides that the death of a viable fetus is not murder if the act of killing is "solicited, aided, abetted, or consented to by the mother of the fetus."[44] This unique provision departs dramatically from the usual legal rule that consent is not a defense to a murder charge[4] and indicates that the fetus lacks the same legal status as live-born persons.

A number of commentators have cited the words of the *Smith* case stating that "justice requires that the principle be recognized that a child has a legal right to begin life with a sound mind and body"[46] as a basis for a fetus' legal right to gestation without injury and as a justification of compulsory treatment of its mother.[26,34] Nonetheless, the *Smith* case plainly does not establish such a right or justify compelled treatment.[4] This case decided that a child after birth has a right to recover damages for injuries wrongfully inflicted by a third party prior to birth; it did not establish that a fetus has any rights. *Smith* expressly did not rule on the legal status of the fetus when it observed that its decision applied to an injured, live-born child and thus it was "immaterial whether before birth the child is considered a person in being" that would have legal rights that could be violated.[46] In their review of reproductive genetics and the law, Elias and Annas[47] have concluded that there is no such thing in the law as a "right to be born physically and mentally sound." One appellate court has reached the same conclusion.[48]

The precise legal status of the fetus is both controversial and difficult to interpret. In any event, the grant of some legal protection does not give a fetus full legal rights, just as the limited legal protections granted to animals and corpses do not bestow rights on them.[49] The variable and unsettled legal status of the fetus described above can perhaps best be explained and justified by the social policies that ground different aspects of the law. A fetus may or may not possess legal protections and "rights," depending on the legal context and the social values at stake.[50] Like other commentators,[2-5,51] the social policies and values at stake in resolving maternal-fetal conflict lead us to believe that it is best to avoid maternal coercion.

Legal Precedent for Intervention   Articles in the medical literature have either implied[25,26] or stated outright that there is extensive and reliable judicial precedent for subjugating the rights of the pregnant woman to those of her fetus and providing treatment over maternal objections.[16] Jurow and Paul,[17] citing the *Georgetown* case as an example (as did Bowes and Selgestad), have stated that there are many legal precedents that have ordered medical procedures to protect the unborn child. These statements are not accurate.

First, the *Georgetown* case has nothing to do with the legal status of fetuses. In that case, a judge ordered that a blood transfusion be given to a mentally incapacitated 25-year-old woman who could not speak for herself but who was reported to be a member of the Jehovah's Witness church, a religion that prohibits the receipt of blood transfusions.[52] She happened to be the mother of a young child, but she was not pregnant when her case was decided. Second, while there are a number of trial court decisions regarding compelled treatment of pregnant women,[2-5] only two reported appellate court decisions (*Jefferson* and *Raleigh Fitkin*) exist that directly support judicial intervention on behalf of the fetus,[27,58] and neither rests on a strong legal foundation.[2,4,5]

Elias[47] and Annas[47,54] have extensively criticized the New Jersey Supreme Court's decision in *Raleigh Fitkin* because it dealt with a moot matter (the woman left the hospital and was never forced to do anything), the court's opinion was brief and devoid of policy discussion, and it was decided before *Roe* established the right of privacy regarding abortion and before this same court recognized the right of privacy as applicable to decisions to refuse treatment. The court's opinion in *Jefferson* relied on the misinterpretation of *Roe vs Wade* discussed above as authority for compulsory treatment of pregnant women and adopted a novel interpretation of the applicability of the child neglect law.[47] Even one of the justices who concurred in the result observed that he believed "the legislature intended that the juvenile courts exercise jurisdiction only where a child has seen the light of day. I am aware of no 'child deprivation' proceeding wherein the 'child' was unborn."[27] Consequently, there is not strong legal precedent for overriding a pregnant woman's informed refusal of medical care.

Liability of Physicians and Court Action

Bowes and Selgestad,[16] as well as others,[56] have stated that a physician may well be held criminally or civilly liable for either honoring or disregarding a competent woman's refusal of medical treatment intended to benefit her fetus. The former article proposes that court action is the only clear way to protect physicians and hospitals from these potential liabilities. Such concern over liability for following a competent woman's wishes is largely misplaced, although treating her over her objections in the absence of a court order is certainly legally perilous.

If a physician were to diagnose a pregnant woman's medical condition properly, to inform her accurately and completely of the risks and benefits of refusal and acceptance of the recommended treatment (including that of fetal harm or demise), and to make a reasonable assessment of her mental capacity, he or she should not be subject to any legal liability for honoring the woman's refusal of treatment. The courts have flatly rejected the notion that a physician can be held criminally or civilly liable for honoring a competent, informed adult's refusal of even lifesaving medical treatment.[8,9,56] If the woman had been properly informed of the consequences of her choice and had been nonnegligently determined to have proper mental capacity, she should be legally unable to complain against those who simply followed her wishes and respected her legal rights in the matter. Due to the protection afforded by the exercise of the woman's constitutional right of privacy and common law rights to self-determination and bodily integrity, civil lawsuits brought postpartum by the child's father or the child against the attending obstetrician, the hospital, or the mother herself should also fail.

The same standards of competency to give or withhold informed consent will apply to the pregnant woman as to any other adult patient. The fact that a patient disagrees with the advice of the attending physician does not demonstrate that she is incompetent.[57] Also, the fact that the woman may be in labor does not per se affect her competence. If mentally ill or psychotic patients are not automatically considered legally incompetent to make treatment decisions by virtue of their diagnosis,[57,58] surely a pregnant woman cannot be automatically considered incompetent simply because she is in labor. In any event, it is certainly advisable for a physician carefully and thoroughly to inform a pregnant woman refusing medically indicated treatment of the risks to her and her fetus and to have this discussion properly witnessed and documented.

On the other hand, a physician who forces a pregnant woman to undergo treatment unwillingly in the absence of a court order potentially faces very serious legal consequences. Forced treatment would be a civilly actionable battery (ie, an offensive or harmful unconsented touching). Because battery is an intentional wrong, the physician and anyone else who treated the woman could be held liable for all harm to the woman proximately caused by their actions, regardless of whether they intended the harm or performed the treatment in a nonnegligent manner. They would also face the possibility of paying punitive damages as well. Furthermore, the physician's medical malpractice insurer may not be obligated to defend him or her or pay any monetary damages assessed, because battery is an intentional rather than a negligent wrong.[4] In addition, the obstetrician could be subject to other legal actions for breach of confidentiality, invasion of privacy, or the infliction of emotional distress.

Some physicians apparently believe that they are better off legally if they perform unauthorized treatment than if they honor the mother's refusal. They reason that it is better to face a battery suit having rendered treatment that probably will produce a healthy baby than to face a lawsuit based on the occurrence of damage to the baby caused by the refusal. The soundness of this belief is suspect for a number of reasons. First, as stated above, if a competent woman refuses treatment with accurate and complete knowledge of the material consequences of her choice for her and her fetus, the law should not permit her to escape responsibility for her own decision by attempting to hold the physician or hospital liable for respecting her legal rights. The law should never place physicians in a position where they may be liable no matter what they do.

Second, there is no assurance that the judge and jury will be aware of the child's good outcome (if such in fact occurs). The facts about the child's outcome may well not be admissible into evidence in the mother's lawsuit because they are irrelevant to the wrong allegedly done to her. If the judge and jury do not know of the child's outcome, they cannot possibly take it into account when deciding the outcome of the mother's suit. Finally, because the fetus' legal status is unsettled and controversial, the courts may not recognize a defense to a woman's battery action based on the good to the child resulting from the physician's ignoring the woman's refusal of the recommended treatment. Indeed, if our interpretation of *Roe* and its progeny is correct, it might be a violation of the woman's constitutional rights for a court or a legislature to take any action that permits the fetus' interests to take precedence over hers.

Medical and Social Policy

In our view, there is no compelling ethical or legal justification for requiring competent pregnant women to undergo medical treatment against their will. Others disagee and advocate the use of coercion against pregnant women in certain situations.[55,59,60]

Commenting on the Kolder study, Annas[61] detected the beginning of an alliance between physicians and the courts to force pregnant women to accept medical treatment for the sake of their fetuses. Before such an alliance becomes entrenched, its assumptions, its terms, and what its operation would entail must be carefully examined.

The most plausible case for compelling a pregnant woman to undergo treatment for the sake of her fetus can be made in those situations when either the failure to provide the indicated treatment puts the fetus at great risk of serious physical harm or the treatment promises to be of significant benefit to the fetus, and the risks of the treatment itself to the mother and fetus are low or minimal. For example, Chervenak and McCullough[59] have proposed guidelines that would permit fetal diagnosis and treatment, presumably even against the mother's wishes, when "the risks [of treatment] to the fetus are minimal, the potential benefit to the fetus is substantial, and the risks to the woman are those she should reasonably accept on behalf of the fetus." In short, forced maternal treatment would be sanctioned if treatment presented substantial benefit to the fetus and low risk to the mother. This is a simple, appealing, and reasonable-sounding proposal until one tries to define its terms or apply it to clinical situations.

It is extremely difficult to identify clearly the clinical situations in which the failure to provide treatment poses a risk of harm to the fetus serious enough to warrant forcible intervention. Would only the certainty of fetal demise without intervention warrant compelled treatment, or would the risk of fetal harm be sufficient? If the risk of harm would be the relevant criterion, the degree of severity of harm sufficient to justify the undeniably serious act of forcing treatment on an unconsenting adult woman would have to be identified. The standard could be articulated as "serious harm," "grave harm," or "significant harm." However phrased, such a standard is ripe for idiosyncratic and arbitrary interpretation. Forcing women to undergo medical treatment against their wills is too weighty a matter to be left to the vagaries of personal interpretation by physicians and judges. Moreover, such an inherently vague standard contains the risk of unequal treatment of women in similar medical situations.

Attempts to devise precise criteria encounter the problem of medical uncertainty. In many obstetric situations, the medical knowledge may not be available to make the correct diagnosis or to describe accurately the likelihood of occurrence of fetal harm.[5,47] For example, abnormalities on the fetal heart rate tracing may not be indicative of true fetal distress or predictive of fetal damage in the absence of medical intervention. As Kolder et al[2] rightly noted, while physicians are quick to embrace uncertainty as a justification for their errors, they are less quick to recognize its effect on patient self-determination. Furthermore, reported cases of court-ordered cesarean sections in which the woman delivered vaginally without incident despite medical predictions that she could not do so[5,62,63] illustrate that if physicians' medical recommendations are legally enforceable, they will be allowed to be wrong, while the woman involved will never be allowed to be right or wrong. As Elias and Annas[47] have observed, "It seems wrong to say that patients have the right to be wrong in all cases except pregnancy."

In addition to these difficult problems in identifying the fetal risk that would purportedly justify a decision to force medical treatment on a woman, there are similar problems in judging what constitutes an "acceptable" level of risk of harm to the mother. Using Chervenak and McCullough's term, one can justifiably be puzzled about the ability to identify those risks that a woman should "reasonably" accept for the benefit of her fetus. This formulation also fails to mention who is to decide what is "reasonable" in this context, a substantial problem given the elasticity of the term. What is one person's "serious harm" could well be "minor" to another person.

Furthermore, whoever makes this judgment will invariably have to make tricky assessments regarding maternal factors that may significantly increase the risk of the proposed intervention. For example, there is an undeniably greater risk of morbidity and mortality associated with cesarean delivery as compared with vaginal delivery.[6] These risks may significantly increase in the presence of maternal thrombocytopenia, a recent myocardial infarction, or pulmonary conditions that would complicate the administration of general anesthesia, which might be necessary in an emergency. We suggest that no one has the wisdom or ethical authority to declare what is an "acceptable" or "reasonable" risk for a woman to take if she herself is unwilling to face it.

In addition, some women refuse treatment for religious reasons.[27] For example, pregnant Jehovah's Witnesses have been known to refuse blood transfusions.[10,53,64] To force such a woman to receive blood may, in her own mind, expose her to eternal damnation as well as cause her to suffer psychological stress or rejection within her earthly community. It is important to distinguish between this situation and the routine practice of having neonates or children receive transfusions over the religious objections of their parents. A live-born child can be given a transfusion without forcibly invading the mother's body, although it does "invade" her wishes, while a transfusion done for the sake of the fetus must necessarily invade the mother's body and ignore her wishes.

Because our society values bodily integrity highly, the "geographical" difference between a live-born child and a fetus is a very significant one. Our society and its legal system go to great lengths to protect the right of persons to preserve their bodily integrity.[4] For example, the legal system does not force persons to donate organs involuntarily to others, even if they are relatives in desperate need. In *McFall vs Shimp*, a man terminally ill with aplastic anemia sued to compel his cousin to donate bone marrow in a late effort to save his life.[65] The judge refused to compel the donation and stated that legal compulsion of such a bodily intrusion, even though it entailed little risk of harm, "would change every concept and principle upon which our society is founded."[65] Another judge refused to order a woman to undergo a cesarean section after acknowledging that he lacked the right to force her to donate an organ to a child of hers, even if that child were dying.[66]

Furthermore, our society refuses to force the donation of organs or tissue from cadavers to benefit or save the lives of the thousands in need of them. (The American Council on Transplantation estimates that of more than 23,000 potential cadaver organ donors available yearly, only 3000 [about 13%] actually become donors.) We see no good reason why pregnant women should be treated with less respect than corpses. In fact, it seems bizarre that many persons should die for want of a vital organ that could be taken from a corpse, while a living pregnant woman can be forced to undergo major surgery that exposes her to a not insubstantial risk of harm or death.

A policy that would permit the courts or the police to intervene in the activities of pregnant women that arguably placed their fetuses at some risk of harm must be considered in light of its potential effectiveness and what its enforcement would require. Every action a pregnant woman takes has a potential impact on her fetus, including the simplest and most common activities of daily living: eating, drinking, sexual intercourse, and physical activity (whether too much in the case of a woman at risk of preterm labor or too little in the case of women with clearly excessive weight gain). In addition, women may expose their fetuses to potential harm when they work, due to occupational hazards. Consequently, an effective public policy designed to prevent fetal harm would require extensive monitoring of and possible interference with each of these activities. This would entail an unprecedented social intrusion into the homes and private lives of pregnant women and their families.

The only plausible justification for a policy with such tremendous impact on the lives and civil liberties of pregnant women would be overwhelming need. However, it is far from clear that such need exists. Common clinical experience shows that it is an unusual woman who does not do everything within reason for the best interests of her fetus. In fact, clinicians are often impressed with the medical risks and lifestyle restrictions voluntarily assumed by pregnant women to ensure a good outcome for their pregnancies. In short, situations in which fetuses may die or be born damaged as a direct result of maternal behavior are likely to be rare.[47] This being so, the price of intervention to women's liberty and privacy seems too high.

We recognize that the behavior of women who are abusers of alcohol or drugs poses significant potential for fetal harm. However, there are solid reasons to doubt that a system of legal punishment or intervention would decrease the incidence of this behavior, as it is usually an addiction over which these women have little control. If anything, a system of legal coercion and punishment might drive these women away from the prenatal care that they and their fetuses especially need.

The enactment of a public policy that would compel women to avoid certain behaviors for the sake of the fetus would also drastically change the nature of the physician–pregnant woman relationship. While many physicians probably can recall a case in which they might have welcomed legal sanction to force a pregnant woman to prevent fetal harm, they may underestimate the impact of such a precedent on their relationship to all patients. The relationship between a physician and a pregnant woman would become much less one of a partnership dedicated to a common goal and more a relationship of adversaries, like police officer and criminal suspect. The ability of a pregnant woman and her physician to negotiate a better course of care when the optimal course is not chosen by the patient would become severely compromised if she could be forced to do whatever the physician recommended.[47] In addition, some pregnant women undoubtedly would refrain from seeking prenatal care or lie about their behaviors or symptoms if they knew their physicians could use the truth to force treatment on them. This, of course, would severely restrict physicians' ability to diagnose correctly and treat adequately both pregnant women and their fetuses.

The philosophical question confronting society is whether it wishes to enforce a policy that would entail on an unprecedented scale serious invasions of a woman's privacy, restriction of her civil liberties, and interference with her religious and per-sonal beliefs. In a secular society such as ours that embraces no particular moral point of view and that attempts to encompass groups with widely divergent views on how persons should live their own lives, individuals are required to forgo "the temptation to impose by state force [their] own view of proper private morality."[67] Given the heated and intractable controversy surrounding the ethical evaluation of the fetus and the well-established interests of all adult persons in bodily integrity and self-deter-mination, we conclude that the decision of a competent pregnant woman to forgo medical treatment likely to benefit her fetus should remain hers, even if others see her choice as unethical.

Conclusion

There are many troublesome questions surrounding the use of judicial force to com-pel pregnant women to undergo medical treatment or behavior change for the bene-fit of their fetuses. We believe that it is unwise, in the last analysis, to recognize fetal rights that would create an adversarial relationship between a pregnant woman and her fetus. Incompleteness of medical knowledge and the unavoidable uncertainty of medical diagnostic and therapeutic techniques make it impossible to define a clear, precise, and accurate medical model on which society could base a fair and uniformly applied legal policy that would sanction the use of force against pregnant women. There is also insufficient reason to undermine the ethical principle of patient auton-omy and the legal right to self-determination and bodily integrity for a subset of our society, namely, pregnant women.

Ultimately, it is not feasible to determine in a just and fair manner which actions or inactions of a pregnant woman should warrant interventions as drastic as involuntary treatment or surgery. It is also not possible to enforce such a policy effectively without extensive and probably distasteful intrusion into the private lives of pregnant women and their families. Furthermore, it is speculative at best whether these changes would cause improvement in the relationship between prenatal care givers and pregnant women and in the effectiveness of prenatal care. We suspect it would in fact do quite the contrary.

We conclude that a pregnant woman who does not intend to have a legal abortion has an affirmative ethical obligation to accept reasonable, nonexperimental medical treatment for the sake of her fetus and to behave otherwise in a manner intended to benefit and not harm her fetus. This obligation is rooted in her unique and significant influence on the health and development of the human entity she voluntarily carries, an entity that will ultimately develop into a person with human rights. Nevertheless, we do not believe that this ethical obligation should be legally enforced. The attempt to do so would not itself be ethical, practically effective, or advantageous for society or the individual. In fact, such legal enforcement would create more harm that it could prevent. Thus, the interventionist "solution" to the problem of maternal-fetal conflict is worse than the original problem.

Finally, we endorse the goal of enhancing fetal health. Physicians will play an essential role in achieving this goal by fulfilling their ethical obligations to pregnant women. This will include monitoring the health of pregnant women and their fetuses and recommending treatment to maximize the prospects of both. While physicians have an ethical obligation to respect the decisions of an informed, competent pregnant woman, they may ethically be an advocate for the fetus when the pregnant woman is making her choices. This advocacy may include the use of persuasion to try to influence the woman to do the "right" thing, but not the use of threats, lies, or physical force. Because most prenatal care relationships between physicians and pregnant women last several months, there is an opportunity to anticipate conflicts and spend additional time to ensure that a pregnant woman's fears or misinformation, which may prevent her from doing what is best for her pregnancy, can be addressed and corrected.

If society and the medical profession are truly interested in enhancing fetal health, their efforts should be directed toward increasing the availability and quality of voluntary prenatal care for all pregnant women and the availability of drug and alcohol rehabilitation programs and other social services for those pregnant women who need them and discouraging physicians from running to the courthouse for an order forcing a woman to accept treatment she does not want. John Stuart Mill has said, "Mankind are greater gainers by suffering each other to live as seems good to themselves, than by compelling each to live as seems good to the rest."[68] We agree: society will, in the end, gain far more by allowing each pregnant woman to live as seems good to her, rather than by compelling each to live as seems good to the rest of us.

The preparation on this article was assisted in part by a grant from the Robert Wood Johnson Foundation, Princeton, NJ. The opinions expressed herein are those of the authors and do not necessarily represent the views of the Foundation.

References

1. Gianelli DM: ACOG issues guidelines on maternal, fetal rights. *American Medical News*, Aug 28, 1987, p 7.

2. Kolder VE, Gallagher J, Parsons MT: Court-ordered obstetrical interventions. *N Engl J Med* 1987;316:1192–1196.

3. Gallagher J: Prenatal invasions and interventions: What's wrong with fetal rights. *Harv Women's Law J* 1987;10:9–58.

4. Nelson LJ, Buggy BP, Weil CJ: Forced medical treatment of pregnant women: 'Compelling each to live as seems good to the rest.' *Hastings Law J* 1986;37:703–763.

5. Rhoden N: The judge in the delivery room: The emergence of court-ordered cesareans. *Calif Law Rev* 1986;74:1951–2030.

6. Pritchard JA, MacDonald PC, Gant NF: *Williams Obstetrics*. East Norwalk, Conn, Appleton-Century-Crofts, 1985, pp xi, 867–871.

7. Jonsen AR, Siegler M, Winslade WJ: *Clinical Ethics*. New York, Macmillan Publishing Co Inc, 1986, pp 47–51.

8. *Bouvia vs Superior Court*, 179 Cal App 3d 1127 (Cal App 1986).

9. *Bartling vs Superior Court*, 163 Cal App 3d 186 (Cal App 1984).

10. *Mercy Hospital vs Jackson*, 510 A 2d 562 (Md 1986).

11. *Satz vs Perlmutter*, 379 So 2d 359 (Fla 1980).

12. Congregation for the Doctrine of the Faith. *Instruction on Respect for Human Life in Its Origin and on the Dignity of Procreation*. Vatican City, Vatican Polyglot Press, 1987.

13. Gertler GB: Brain birth: A proposal for defining when a fetus is entitled to human life status. *South Calif Law Rev* 1986;59:1061–1078.

14. *Grodin vs Grodin*, 301 NW 2d 869 (Mich App 1980).

15. *Stallman vs Youngquist*, 504 NE 2d 920 (Ill App 1987).

16. Bowes WA Jr, Selgestad B: Fetal vs maternal rights: Medical and legal perspectives. *Obstet Gynecol* 1981;58:209–214.

17. Jurow R, Paul RH: Cesarean delivery for fetal distress without maternal consent. *Obstet Gynecol* 1984;63:596–598.

18. Bross DC, Meredyth A: Neglect of the unborn child: An analysis based on law in the United States. *Child Abuse Negl* 1979;3:643–650.

19. Lieberman JR, Mazor M, Chaim W, et al: The fetal right to live. *Obstet Gynecol* 1979;53:515–517.

20. Englehardt HT Jr: Current controversies in obstetrics: Wrongful life and forced fetal surgical procedures. *Am J Obstet Gynecol* 1985;151:313–318.

21. Bross DC: Court-ordered intervention on behalf of unborn children, in Hoffenberg EI (ed): *Quality Child Advocacy*. Denver, National Association of Counsel for Children, 1983, pp 70–76.

22. Raines E: Editorial comment. *Obstet Gynecol* 1984;63:598–599.

23. Robertson J: The right to procreate and in utero fetal therapy. *J Legal Med* 1982;3:333–366.

24. Soloff PH, Jewell S, Roth LH: Civil commitment and the rights of the unborn. *Am J Psychiatry* 1979;136:114–115.

25. Dal Pozzo EE, Marsh FH: Psychosis and pregnancy: Some new ethical and legal dilemmas for the physician. *Am J Obstet Gynecol* 1987;156:425–427.

26. Landwirth J: Fetal abuse and neglect: An emerging controversy. *Pediatrics* 1987;79:508–514.

27. *Jefferson vs Griffin Spalding County Hospital Authority*, 274 SE 2d 457 (Ga 1981).

28. *Roe vs Wade*, 410 US 113 (1973).

29. *Doe vs Bolton*, 410 US 179 (1973).

30. *United States vs Vuitch*, 402 US 62 (1971).

31. *Colautti vs Franklin*, 439 US 379 (1979).

32. *Thornburgh vs American College of Obstetricians and Gynecologists*, 106 S Ct 2101 (1986).

33. *Superintendent of Belchertown State School vs Saikewicz*, 370 NE 2d 417 (Mass 1977).

34. Myers JE: Abuse and neglect of the unborn: Can the state intervene? *Duquesne Law Rev* 1984;23:1–76.

35. NJ Stat Ann Sec 30:4C-11 (West 1981).

36. *In re Ruiz*, 500 NE 2d 935 (Ohio Ct Com Pleas Wood Cty 1986).

37. *In re Steven S.*, 126 Cal App 3d 23 (Cal App 1981).

38. *In re Dittrick Infant*, 263 NW 2d 37 (Mich App 1977).

39. Lenow JL: The fetus as a patient: Emerging rights as a person? *Am J Law Med* 1983;9:1–29.

40. *Commonwealth vs Cass*, 467 NE 2d 1324 (Mass 1984).

41. *People vs Greer*, 402 NE 2d 203 (Ill 1980).

42. *Hollis vs Commonwealth*, 652 SW 2d 61 (Ky Ct App 1983).

43. *State vs Willis*, 457 So 2d 959 (Miss 1984).

44. *People vs Smith*, 59 Cal App 3d 751 (Cal App 1976).

45. Cal Penal Code §187(b)(3).

46. *Smith vs Brennan*, 157 A 2d 497 (NJ 1960).

47. Elias E, Annas GJ: *Reproductive Genetics and the Law*. Chicago, Year Book Medical Publishers Inc, 1987, pp 118–120, 253–262.

48. *Becker vs Schwartz*, 386 NE 2d 807 (NY 1978).

49. Glantz L: Is the fetus a person? A lawyer's view, in Bondeson W, Englehardt HT, Spicker S, et al (eds): *Abortion and the Status of the Fetus*. Dordrecht, the Netherlands, D Reidel Publishing Co, 1983, pp 107–117.

50. Baron CH: 'If you prick us, do we not bleed?': Of Shylock, fetuses, and the concept of person in the law. *Law Med Health Care* 1983;11:52–63, 81.

51. Johnsen DE: The creation of fetal rights: Conflicts with women's constitutional rights to liberty, privacy, and equal protection. *Yale Law J* 1986;95:599–625.

52. *Application of the President and Directors of Georgetown College Hospital*, 331 F 2d 1000 (1964).

53. *Raleigh Fitkin–Paul Morgan Memorial Hospital vs Anderson*, 201 A 2d 537 (NJ 1964), cert denied, 377 US 984.

54. Annas GJ: Forced cesareans: The most unkindest cut of all. *Hastings Cent Rep* 1982;12:16–17, 45.

55. Robertson JA: Legal issues in fetal therapy. *Semin Perinatol* 1985;9:136–142.

56. *In the Matter of Storar*, 420 NE 2d 64 (NY 1981).

57. *Conservatorship of Waltz*, 180 Cal App 3d 722 (Cal App 1986).

58. *Rivers vs Katz*, 504 NYS 2d 74 (NY 1986).

59. Chervenak FA, McCullough LB: Perinatal ethics: A practical analysis of obligations to mother and fetus. *Obstet Gynecol* 1985;66:442–446.

60. Mathieu D: Respecting liberty and preventing harm: Limits of state intervention in prenatal choice. *Harv J Law Public Policy* 1985;8:19–52.

61. Annas GJ: Protecting the liberty of pregnant patients. *N Engl J Med* 1987;316:1213–1214.

62. *In re Baby Jeffries*, No. 14004 (Jackson Cty P Ct Mich, May 24, 1982).

63. Fletcher JC: Ethical considerations in and beyond experimental fetal therapy. *Semin Perinatol* 1985;9:130–135.

64. *In re Application of Jamaica Hospital*, 491 NYS 2d 898 (NY Sup Ct 1985).

65. *McFall vs Shimp*, No. 78-17711 (C P Allegheny Cty Penn, July 26, 1978).

66. Unpublished opinion, No. 84-7-50006-D (Super Ct Benton Cty Wash, April 20, 1984).

67. Engelhardt HT Jr: Introduction, in Bondeson W, Englehardt HT, Spicker S, et al (eds): *Abortion and the Status of the Fetus*. Dordrecht, the Netherlands, D Reidel Publishing Co, 1983, pp xi–xxxii.

68. Mill JS: On liberty, in Warnock M (ed): *Utilitarianism and Other Writings*. New York, World Publishers, 1962, pp 126–250.

Genetic Choice

MICHAEL D. BAYLES

The last chapter outlined methods by which individuals and couples can have children genetically related to them. This chapter considers issues raised by methods developed in the last two decades that provide people some choice of the genetic features of their children. For the most part, these methods enable people to choose not to have children with certain features.

Three types of methods of genetic choice are available. One type enables people to increase the chances of having a child of a specific sex. Another type, carrier screening, enables people to determine whether they are likely to transmit deleterious genetic features to offspring. The third type, prenatal diagnosis, can be used to determine whether a fetus has some specific characteristic and then abort it if that is desirable. Not all the conditions that can be detected by prenatal diagnosis are genetic; some of them result from drugs, maternal illness, or other causes.

Sex Preselection

Case 2.1 Jeremiah and Katharine have two daughters, ages six and nine. Katharine is thirty-four years old. Jeremiah would like to have a son; indeed, he wants one very much. Katharine would like another child but does not especially care whether it is a boy or girl. However, she does not want to have more than one more child, and plans to be sterilized after the birth of the next child, whether Jeremiah likes it or not. The risks of having a child with Down syndrome are increasing as Katharine gets older; besides, she would like to go back to nursing, which she gave up when their older daughter was born.

Jeremiah reads a newspaper story describing a patented process that makes it possible to select with considerable accuracy the sex of a child at conception. The process involves taking semen from the husband and separating the male-determining sperm from the female-determining sperm. The process destroys most of the female-determining sperm. Physicians at the clinic then artificially inseminate the woman with the male sperm. This process cannot be used to produce females, but Jeremiah is only interested in having a boy. Katharine agrees to the treatment; after the

Chapter references in this selection are to the original work from which it is taken.

Department of Philosophy, Florida State University, Tallahassee, Florida

third month, she is pregnant. Jeremiah is joyous, because he is sure that this time he will have a son. Now and then, though, Katharine notices him sitting quietly with a worried look. She finally asks him what is wrong, and he says that he sometimes has doubts that this child will be a son, and he does not know what he will do if it is not.

In recent years, several methods in addition to the one just described have been developed to increase the chances of conceiving a child of a particular sex.[1] One technique involves injecting the woman with antibodies against male- or female-determining sperm. Animal sperm have been separated by using a medium of varying viscosity. Two methods that do not involve medical intervention have been suggested. One is to time intercourse to occur two days before ovulation in order to have a girl, or at ovulation for a boy. Another technique recommends a different timing, a vinegar douche, shallow penetration, and no female orgasm in order to have a girl; and opposite conditions for a boy. These two methods have not been well established; indeed, they recommend contrary timing of intercourse. A more accurate method, which is not yet possible, would be to ascertain the sex of embryos in IVF before transfer. Existing methods are not as accurate as IVF would be; at best, they increase the probability of a child being of one sex or another.

One rather different method for reliably determining the sex of the fetus now exists: prenatal diagnosis. At about sixteen weeks, amniotic fluid is withdrawn from the womb, fetal cells are cultured, and the sex is determined by chromosomal analysis. Some new techniques of recovering fetal cells may allow this procedure to be performed at an earlier date. To ensure the desired sex of the child, a woman must abort a fetus of the unwanted sex.

Sex Preference

Considerable evidence exists that many men and women, like Jeremiah, desire male children. Indeed, many prefer to have a male child first, and then a female. But is it rational to desire a child of a particular sex? A preference for one sex over the other, for its own sake, is simply sexism: It implies that one sex is intrinsically more valuable than another, but good reasons can be and have been given against this view by many authors, so such a desire is irrational.

Most people would not admit to such a pure sex preference but claim that the desire for a child of a particular sex is instrumental to fulfilling other desires. However, there are strong reasons for believing that many of the most common instrumental reasons are unsound and probably mask an irrational sexism. Reasons often given in the past for instrumentally preferring children of one sex (particularly males) are to inherit, to carry on the family name, and to have workers. But none of these reasons

[1]For more details, see M. Ruth Netwig, "Technical Aspects of Sex Preselection," in *The Custom-Made Child? Women-Centered Perspectives*, ed. Helen B. Holmes, Betty B. Hoskins, and Michael Gross (Clifton, N.J.: The Humana Press, Inc., 1981), pp. 181–86.

are relevant in the modern Western world. Today, male and female children inherit equally. Females can carry on the family name if they want; they need not change their names when they marry. Few jobs exist that women cannot fulfill as well as men (and of course they are generally better than men at some jobs).

One might reply that someone like Jeremiah need not be sexist or irrational to want a boy. He has two daughters, and he would simply like to have a boy as well. Had he had two boys, he might have wanted a girl. But why would two daughters and one son be preferable to three daughters? Someone like Jeremiah might respond that he would like a son so that he could have certain pleasures in child rearing—such as fishing and playing ball with him. But that too is probably a sexist assumption. As the father of two daughters, I have fished and played ball with them, watched my daughter play on a ball team, and gone camping and hiking with them, as well as cooked, cleaned house, done laundry, and engaged in various other so-called women's activities with them.

There may be some activities that are strongly sex-related in that members of one sex are generally better at them than members of the other sex. For example, perhaps most women have a greater aptitude for ballet than men. Recognition of such differences in role aptitude is not sexist, but the assumption that no members of the other sex can perform the same roles well or that one set of such roles is preferable to the other is sexist. Thus, a desire to have a male (female) child because of a preference for one set of "sex-linked" roles is sexist. Nor can one argue that variety is desired. Were children allowed to develop freely their own interests and talents, children of the same sex would probably exhibit as much diversity as children of opposite sexes.

Consequently, an instrumental preference for a child of one sex or the other is also often irrational. However, in some cases it is reasonable to desire a child of one sex rather than another for instrumental reasons. Undoubtedly, the most serious reason concerns X-linked genetic diseases, such as hemophilia. Only males exhibit the disease; females can only be carriers. Thus, if a woman is a carrier of such a disease, it would be rational to desire female children. Ironically, this is not the sex preference most people express. In this case, sexism is not involved. The preference here is not for a female child, but for a healthy child, and a female has a significantly better chance of being healthy.

Ethical Analysis

We can assume that sexism is wrong. Arguments to this effect have been offered by many authors, and the history of sexism clearly shows the misery and unfortunate consequences it has wrought. Nonetheless, sexism is still prevalent in society. That sex preselection on the basis of intrinsic and most instrumental sex preference expresses an unethical sexist attitude is sufficient for holding that it is wrong. Its practice would probably reinforce sexist attitudes both in those who practice it and in others.

Two other general social consequences are often thought likely to result from sex preselection. First, evidence exists that most people who want a child of each sex prefer to have a male first, and that first-born children are apt to achieve more than later-born children.[2] If couples used sex preselection to have a male child first, and males were thus on average better social achievers than females, this would tend to reinforce sexist attitudes. Second, if sex preselection resulted in more males than females, the sex imbalance could have undesirable social consequences, such as insufficient mates. There might be good results as well. Population growth might decrease, because people often have more children in an attempt to have some of each sex. A better balance of male/female companionship among the elderly might result. The elderly population is now disproportionately female since women live longer than men; were there considerably more males than females born, the elderly population would be more evenly balanced between the sexes. Younger women would be in short supply and might have more social opportunities. (Of course, more younger men might then lack mates and be lonely.) However, most of these projections about the consequences of a sex imbalance are mere speculation. They are not well enough founded to support an ethical principle.

In sum, sex preselection on the basis of intrinsic sex preference is always wrong, and so is most sex preselection on the basis of instrumental sex preference. One should accept an ethical principle condemning sex preselection as the expression of irrational desires and as reinforcing sexism in society. Unlike the irrational desire for genetic offspring, these irrational desires might have further untoward consequences if people act on them. However, sex preselection for clearly rational instrumental reasons, for example, to avoid offspring with sex-linked genetic diseases, constitutes an ethically permissible and desirable exception. Jeremiah's intrinsic desire for a son is the expression of a sexist attitude, and he and Katharine are ethically wrong to try to have a son.

Policy Analysis

Although most sex preselection is ethically wrong, policies to prevent its practice are not acceptable. Laws to prohibit sexism are justifiable in many areas, but sex preselection presents special problems. It would be impossible to enforce such a prohibition in practice if timing methods were effective. Any effort to prevent the use of timing methods would involve an unacceptable governmental intrusion into people's private lives. The best that could be done would be to prohibit the use of artificial insemination techniques for sex preselection by fertility clinics and others. Such a step would not effectively prevent such sex preselection, because people would lie about their reasons or an underground business would develop, so it would be pointless to restrict fertility clinics.

Should a sex imbalance result and the consequences be highly undesirable, then some social policy might be necessary and possible. The policy would not consist in prohibiting sex preselection, but in encouraging it! Incentives, such as extra tax deductions, could be offered for having children of a particular sex, or for having them first. Such policies might also reinforce sexism and would be acceptable only if the

---

[2]Roberta Steinbacher, "Futuristic Implications of Sex Preselection," in *The Custom-Made Child? Women-Centered Perspectives*, ed. Helen B. Holmes, Betty B. Hoskins, and Michael Gross (Clifton, N.J.: The Humana Press, Inc., 1981), p. 188.

consequences of unfettered sex preselection were quite bad. Indeed, it might be wise not to accept them even then but merely to increase efforts at educating people not to be sexists.

Regardless of the ethics of abortion, the use of prenatal diagnosis and abortion for most sex selection is ethically wrong simply as sex preselection. However, that does not provide a reason for a policy against its use or withholding information about the sex of the fetus after amniocentesis. People may also simply be curious about the fetus's sex.

Carrier Screening

Case 2.2   Louis and Miriam are in their early twenties. They have been married about a year but have not yet had any children. Both want to have their life together fairly well-adjusted before taking on parental responsibilities. They hear about a program at a clinic in their city to screen Jewish couples for carrier status of the recessive gene for Tay-Sachs disease. Miriam is especially concerned about it, because a friend of hers has recently given birth to a child with Tay-Sachs. The child faces a general neurological deterioration and almost certain death before school age. Her friend is going through emotional turmoil. Louis is less enthusiastic about having the tests. "After all," he says, "the disease results from recessive genes, so there is no chance of a child of ours having the defect unless both of us are carriers. Even then, the odds are only one in four. Why not simply have prenatal diagnosis done during pregnancy to determine whether the fetus has the disease? Even if both of us are carriers, we could go ahead and conceive and use prenatal diagnosis to find out if the baby is normal."

This case concerns one of the usual forms of carrier screening, that for a recessive autosomal (non-sex chromosomal) gene which is rare but more frequently found in a specific population. For recessive conditions, both parents must be carriers before there is a chance a child will have the condition. That is, to have a recessive disease, a child must inherit an affected gene from each parent. In this case, Tay-Sachs is found with a much higher frequency among Ashkenazi Jews—those from Eastern Europe— than others. A slightly more prevalent form of carrier screening is for defects in blood—sickle cell anemia among blacks, and beta-thalassemia among people of Mediterranean origin. Most carrier screening is relatively inexpensive and accurate and involves analysis of a small blood sample. Carrier testing is possible for a few other genetic conditions, and the number continues to grow. A few conditions are caused by dominant genes; with them, only one parent need be a carrier, but that parent will also suffer from the defect or disease. Most dominant disorders are detected in spontaneous mutants.

Value Analysis

Louis's and Miriam's differing attitudes towards carrier screening center on the value of the knowledge that will be gained. The primary outcome of genetic testing is knowledge—knowing whether a person is a carrier or has a condition. Knowledge can be desired either intrinsically or instrumentally. When knowledge is intrinsically valued, a person simply wants to know something for its own sake, out of curiosity. When knowledge is desired instrumentally, it is valued because of its consequences, usually because it enables one to take some action.

Information obtainable from genetic screening is primarily of instrumental value. Some people may simply be curious about their genetic constitution, but that is not the usual reason for having the tests. People desire knowledge about carrier status in order to relieve their anxiety about having a child with a defect, and to enable them to take action to avoid having such a child. When tests are done to find out whether a newborn or adult actually has a disease, the people involved desire the knowledge in order to treat or ameliorate the condition. Sometimes the fear of finding out about a disease may be greater than any alleviation of anxiety. For example, Huntington disease results from a dominant gene and does not become manifest until later in life, usually between the ages of thirty and fifty. The disease involves progressive mental deterioration and uncontrollable physical movements. Woody Guthrie, the musician, died of it. The worry and anxiety of knowing that one has such a disease can be overwhelming, and the suicide rate amongst people who have it is high. Many people would rather not know whether or not they have it. The same may be true of some carrier screening, for some people have a lower self-image when they discover they are carriers. Thus, the bad consequences of genetic information can sometimes outweigh the good ones, and the information is not then instrumentally valuable.

The desire for genetic information is rational because it is surely rational to want to avoid having a child with a defect. One aspect of that desire is to avoid begetting (conceiving) a child with a significant handicap. Generally, a significant handicap is one that decreases the value of life to the person who lives it. The life of a child with a handicap can be of value but it is still rational to desire not to conceive such a child. Handicaps are by definition undesirable characteristics, and it is rational to avoid them. One might object that one also avoids the existence of the person, not merely the handicap. Yet, it is precisely the fact that no person exists that makes it quite rational to avoid begetting such a person. One would not, except under the most unusual circumstances, make a radio using a defective speaker even if that radio would have some value. Another aspect of the desire to avoid begetting a child with a significant handicap is to avoid the suffering of oneself and others. Handicapped children place greater burdens on their parents and siblings in terms of time, effort, and financial resources than do normal children.

Another relevant value pertains to risk taking. With recessive traits, one out of four children will have the deleterious disease. With dominant traits, one out of two children of an affected parent will have it. Other conditions have varying degrees of risk. Thus, attitudes about risk are important for making decisions. Unfortunately, no known method exists for showing that an attitude toward risk is rational or irrational. Some people are gamblers and risk-takers while others are cautious. No evidence exists that people would generally adopt one attitude rather than another were they fully informed of the facts. However, even if attitudes towards risk can rationally vary, they are not equally acceptable when the well-being of others depends on the decision. It may be reasonable to take significant risks with one's own life, for example, by riding a motorcycle, but it is unreasonable or ethically inappropriate to take significant risks with another person's life.

Ethical Analysis

Suppose Miriam talks Louis into going to the clinic to find out more about the test for Tay-Sachs. What information should Louis obtain and evaluate in order to give his informed consent to the procedure? This question is quite important in programs that involve mass screening; large-scale programs are apt to process people routinely without adequately explaining matters to them.

The point of having the test is to gain information. If Louis is to decide whether that information is worthwhile, he needs to be informed of all the relevant facts. How much will the tests cost? Sometimes the information obtainable is not worth the expense of obtaining it. Another important question is, What precisely does the procedure entail? Louis also needs to know what he can do with the test results. As such knowledge is only instrumentally valuable, he needs to know what options the information gives him. In the case of Tay-Sachs, as Louis already knows, if both he and Miriam are carriers, prenatal diagnosis can be performed to determine whether a fetus actually has the disease. Another option would be to use artificial insemination by a noncarrier donor or to use a noncarrier surrogate mother. Louis should also want to know how bad the disease is, as well as the chances that someone of his background is a carrier. In short, Louis needs to be advised of the chances that he is a carrier, the nature of the test, the nature of the disease, and all the available options for action should both he and Miriam be carriers. With less than this information, he could not make a rational decision whether or not to have the test.

It might be argued that Louis has a duty to undergo the test, that he has a duty to discover whether he is at risk of having a child with a severe genetic disease or defect. After all, his ignorance could result in the birth of a child with a serious handicap; the child would suffer the consequences of Louis's action more than Louis.

Whether Louis has a duty to have the test depends on whether he and Miriam would have a duty not to have an affected child if it were revealed that both are carriers. If they would not have such a duty, they do not have a duty to find out that they are carriers and at risk of having such a child. Two factors are relevant to whether carriers have a duty to avoid having an affected child—the value of the life to the child and the effects of its life on others. Both of these factors must then be considered in light of variable risks of having an affected child.

The principle of avoiding risk to the unborn is that it is prima facie wrong to take a substantial risk of a significant defect or handicap to an unborn child. A number of reasons support this principle. First, since the child does not exist, failure to reproduce does not harm it, and as we saw in the previous chapter, there is no duty to reproduce. Second, such a handicapped individual would lack an equal opportunity with others in society. For their own interests, parents would have deliberately brought into existence a person lacking equality of opportunity. Third, if the handicap would be so severe that life would not be of value to the individual, misery would have been inflicted on that person. Consequently, while other considerations might outweigh the prima facie wrongness of risking a significant handicap that would still leave life of value, nothing short of averting a large-scale disaster could justify bringing into existence someone whose life was of no value to that person.

The principle regarding risk to the unborn deliberately does not specify degrees of risk and handicap, only that they be substantial and significant. The two considerations must be balanced against one another. The greater the handicap, the less the risk should be; and vice versa. At this point, what makes life valuable, and thus what constitutes a significant handicap, is not fully specified. As we shall see in Chapter 5 where that issue is considered in detail, the crucial elements of a valuable life are pleasant experiences and the fulfillment of interests, both of which can be detrimentally affected by pain or lack of physical or mental abilities.

The principle regarding risk to the unborn has been justified solely by consequences for the child. However, effects on others, primarily the parents and siblings, are also relevant. The principle regarding burdens to others states that the burdens a child's life will place on others constitute an ethically relevant reason not to bring an unborn child into existence. In deciding whether to reproduce, couples should consider whether they would enjoy raising a child, as well as possible harmful effects on existing siblings. Since there is no duty to reproduce and the unborn child does not exist, it would not be harmed by not being brought into existence; but existing people might be. Thus, even if the child's life might be of value to it, the burden to others is a relevant reason for not reproducing.

Case 2.3   Nathaniel and Olive are very much in love. A year or so after their marriage, they consider having a child. However, in their situation, they think it best to talk to a genetic counselor first. Both have mildly expressed sickle cell disease, but they lead reasonably normal lives and their few attacks are under control.

The counselor tells them that pregnancy for a woman with sickle cell disease is rather risky. About half of such pregnancies result in spontaneous abortion or stillbirth, and the maternal death rate is very high.[3] Nathaniel and Olive are quite lucky that their sickle cell anemia is not severe. Ten percent of people born with the disease die by the age of ten, and many others live with great pain and are severely handicapped. Given that both of them have the disease, each of their children is also certain to have it.

This case presents an issue of risk taking. Unlike the problem of Louis and Miriam where the risk is whether a child will have the disease, in this case the risk pertains to the severity of the disease. For carriers of recessive conditions (like Louis and Miriam), the risk is one in four that their children will have the disease, and often this cannot be determined by prenatal diagnosis. The ethical questions in all of these cases are whether the principle regarding risk to the unborn applies, and whether other reasons for having a child outweigh it if it does.

[3]Robert M. Veatch, *Case Studies in Medical Ethics* (Cambridge, Mass.: Harvard University Press, 1977), p. 182.

In the case of Nathaniel and Olive, the principle clearly applies; a child of theirs is certain to have a life-threatening disease. The question is whether good reasons exist that outweigh the prima facie wrongness of their begetting a child together. Couples like Nathaniel and Olive may consider taking such a risk to have a child. One must here distinguish the desires to have genetic offspring, to bear offspring, and to rear them. As we have seen, the desire to beget offspring for its own sake is not rational. It is the only desire that need be frustrated if Nathaniel and Olive are to have a child without this risk of defect. If Olive were artificially inseminated with the sperm of a noncarrier donor, she could bear a child and they could both rear it. She would even have begotten the child, but not with Nathaniel. Similarly, Nathaniel could beget a child by a noncarrier surrogate mother without risk of sickle cell disease. He could even beget by a noncarrier ovum and have the embryo transferred to Olive. Consequently, only the couple's desire to beget a child with each other supports reproduction in the usual manner. As a subclass of the desire to have genetic offspring, the desire to have genetic offspring with a specific person is also irrational. It surely does not override the principle of avoiding risk to the unborn. Thus, the risk is not one that may ethically be taken.

In general, then, the desire for genetic offspring cannot override the principle of avoiding risk to the unborn. It is not, however, always clear that the principle of risk applies. Suppose a couple is at risk of having a child with a disease like galactosemia, which can result in cataracts, mental retardation, and digestive disorders. The effects of galactosemia can be controlled by diet, primarily by avoiding milk and milk products, but this can cause considerable difficulty for parents, especially in preparing meals for a large family. With treatment, such a disease does not result in significant handicap to the individual, although it is a significant bother. Thus, the principle of risk to the unborn does not pertain, or at least has little weight. However, couples might decide not to risk such a child because of the burdens to them.

Another ethical issue that arises in carrier screening concerns confidentiality. Suppose Louis were tested and found to be a carrier of Tay-Sachs. Then each of his siblings has a 50 percent chance of being a carrier as well. Ethically, it seems clear, Louis should inform his brothers and sisters that they should also be tested. Suppose, though, he refuses to do so. May a physician suggest screening to the siblings without Louis's consent? One might suggest that his brothers and sisters need never know that Louis is a carrier; Louis's physician could simply tell them that they should be screened. But that would not work. Either Louis's siblings would know it was his doctor or they would ask why the doctor thought they should be screened. The same problem would arise were the information given to their family physicians, supposing the testing center could find out who the doctors were.

The ethical conflict is between Louis's claim to confidentiality and his siblings' claim to have information important to them. The two values must be weighed. To do so, one must clarify the situation and consider the two values or desires as affecting oneself. Louis's fear of disclosure is irrational; being a carrier does not significantly affect his health, and he is not at fault for being a carrier. Even if the claim of confidentiality is weighted heavily, in this situation the value of the information is greater than that of confidentiality. Consequently, an acceptable principle of confidentiality would allow an exception for such a case. But the exception would extend only to Louis's siblings, who should ethically keep the information confidential.

A final difficulty that arises from carrier screening pertains to truth telling. Sometimes carrier screening is not performed until after the birth of an affected child. In that case, carrier screening might indicate that the putative father is not the genetic father. Should the counselor tell the man that he is not a carrier and so there is no risk in a subsequent conception? This would clearly indicate that he was not the father. Some counselors confronted with this situation lie and say that the defect was due to a spontaneous mutation so that there is no risk in a subsequent pregnancy.[4]

Although this type of situation cannot be avoided, the ethical situation can be clarified in advance. The purpose of screening is to obtain information, and prior to the screening the putative father should be told what types of information might be obtained. Prior to consent, he should be advised that information of nonpaternity might be discovered. At that point, he can decide whether he wishes to risk finding out that information. Although a child might suffer should a putative father discover he was not the biological father and legally contest his paternity and obligation to support, this consideration is not stronger for handicapped than for normal children. Granted, the burden on a handicapped child may be greater than on a normal one, but the burden on the putative father is also greater, both emotionally and financially. Securing the putative father's consent beforehand will not make the discovery any easier for him or the child, and will probably make his decision to be tested more difficult, but it clarifies the duty of the physician to inform.

Policy Analysis

The primary policy issue in carrier screening concerns legally compulsory screening. Most mandatory screening is for treatable diseases in infants, but in the early 1970s a number of states enacted laws requiring all blacks to be screened for carrier status for sickle cell disease. Sometimes the legislatures were probably confused as to what they were requiring, thinking that the tests were for the disease rather than the carrier state. Are there circumstances in which mandatory screening is acceptable?

Two related reasons might support compulsory screening for carrier status. (1) Screening might decrease the number of children born with handicapping diseases. (2) This decrease might save public funds for the care of handicapped individuals. Mandatory carrier screening will not contribute significantly to either goal. Both of these possible benefits depend on people avoiding birth of handicapped children. Screening itself only provides information enabling people to avoid giving birth to such children. At a minimum, one would also have to ensure that most couples at risk were counseled as to how they could avoid such births. For the policy to be effective, the couples would then have to act to avoid such births.

The question is whether a compulsory screening program would be more effective than a voluntary one. Little reason exists to think that it would be. Although coun-

[4]"Genetic Screening," *Encyclopedia of Bioethics* (1978), 2, 571.

seling does have some effect in decreasing the number of children couples have, depending on the severity of the disease anywhere from 35 to 75 percent have the same number they planned to have before counselling.[5] Since most of these people were voluntarily counseled, it is unlikely the success rate would be as high among people screened involuntarily. If no significant reduction in births of defective children is achieved, there will be little or no financial savings either. Because of this, and because a mandatory program is an infringement of people's freedom, compulsory screening is not acceptable. Nonetheless, a voluntary program is supportable. Such a program is likely to be more effective because participants will be motivated to avoid the birth of children with defects (the primary reason for coming), and it will increase their freedom to control their reproductive activity.

One might ask at what age such screening should be offered. Many of the mandatory carrier programs screened newborn children. However, the main purpose of carrier screening is to provide information for reproductive decisions—decisions that newborn children do not confront. In a voluntary program, there is no reason for age restrictions. Voluntary programs should, however, be aimed at people before their reproductive attitudes are set. This means that, at the least, general education about genetics and reproduction should begin in elementary school. Actual screening and information about contraception and parenting should occur before reproductive years—in junior high school.

Prenatal Diagnosis

Prenatal diagnosis includes a variety of techniques designed to provide information about whether a fetus has a defect. The following techniques are currently used. (1) Maternal blood serum can be tested. Such tests for alpha-fetoprotein can determine whether the fetus is likely to have neural tube defects (those in the spine or brain). (2) Ultrasound can be used to picture the fetus. (3) Fetoscopy, which involves inserting a needle-like instrument into the womb, enables physicians to visualize the fetus. (4) Amniocentesis, the most frequent type of prenatal diagnosis, involves using a needle to withdraw some of the amniotic fluid in the womb; the fluid can then be used for a variety of tests. Fetal cells in the fluid are often cultured and the chromosomes examined for defects. Amniocentesis is not usually performed until the fourteenth to sixteenth week of pregnancy, and culturing fetal cells then takes several weeks. Amniocentesis enables tests to be performed to discover most chromosomal anomalies, the most common being Down syndrome, as well as an increasing number of rare metabolic errors. One can also use amniocentesis with fetoscopy to obtain samples of fetal blood to test for sickle-cell anemia and other blood disorders.

So far as is known, all of these techniques are reasonably safe when performed by experienced physicians. At first, there was much concern about the safety of amniocentesis, but subsequent study has shown that the primary risk is inducing a sponta-

---

[5]"Genetic Diagnosis and Counseling," *Encyclopedia of Bioethics* (1978), 2, 563.

neous abortion in about 0.5 to 1.0 percent of the cases. The type of amniocentesis which involves drawing samples of fetal blood from the placenta has a somewhat higher risk of spontaneous abortion than drawing amniotic fluid. Ethically, these spontaneous abortions differ even from abortions for medical indications; there is no desire or intent to cause fetal death or knowledge that the fetus will die. Ultrasound, a relatively new technique, has been shown to be safe at the levels used, although it is so new that no information exists about its possible long-term effects. Safety is not currently a major issue in prenatal diagnosis.

People undergo prenatal diagnosis for basically the same reasons as carrier screening—to relieve anxiety about defects of the fetus, and to avoid the birth of a significantly handicapped child. In 95 percent or more of the instances of amniocentesis, the fetus is discovered not to have the defect in question. If a defect is found, then avoiding the birth of a child involves a second trimester abortion, around twenty weeks' gestation.

Much of the concern and ethical argument about prenatal diagnosis has centered around the abortion issue, which is discussed in the next chapter. It should be noted, however, that prenatal diagnosis decreases rather than increases the number of abortions.[6] Some women at risk would have an abortion rather than continue the pregnancy. Prenatal diagnosis usually shows that no defect is present, so these women are able to continue the pregnancy without fear of the specific defect. Other women have an abortion because the fetus is discovered to have a defect. However, as the number of those who would have had an abortion but are reassured is greater than the number who have an abortion, prenatal diagnosis decreases the number of abortions. Also, some women at risk of having children with defects will become pregnant only if amniocentesis is available.

Case 2.4 Paula is in her late twenties and her husband Quincy is a year or two older. Paula is pregnant for the first time and goes to the genetics clinic to request prenatal diagnosis for Down syndrome, a chromosomal abnormality causing mental retardation. She works in an institution for mentally retarded persons and is anxious about having a child with Down syndrome. The general incidence of Down syndrome is low for someone Paula's age, less than one-half of one percent, although it increases rapidly for women over thirty-five years old and is about two percent for women over forty. Nor is there a history of the condition in her family. Consequently, the genetics clinic denies her request because there is no medical indication for prenatal diagnosis. After a normal pregnancy, Paula delivers a child with Down syndrome.

Ethical Analysis

This case raises the issue of access to prenatal diagnosis. The primary medical indications for it are advanced maternal age (where the risk of a number of chromosomal anomalies is higher), previous spontaneous abortion or birth of a child with a defect,

---

[6]See Aubrey Milunsky, ed., *Genetic Disorders and the Fetus* (New York: Plenum Press, 1979), Chapters 5–7.

family history of defects, or carrier screening indicating that there is a higher than normal risk of a child with a defect. Should prenatal diagnosis be denied to women who, like Paula, want it even though there is no medical indication? The arguments for offering the service in these cases are that the normal risk of a defect is about one in two hundred, so there is always some risk of a defective fetus. If no defect is found, anxiety is relieved. In Paula's case, because she works with retarded persons, the anxiety was probably greater than for many other women without medical indications.

The arguments against offering prenatal diagnosis in such cases are these: First, a small risk of spontaneous abortion exists and that risk is not worth taking unless there is an above average risk of defect. However, should the genetics unit make this decision about risk, or should Paula? Paula bears the consequences—either a defective child or the loss of a normal one if a spontaneous abortion occurs. The difference between the risk of a defect in her case and the so-called risk cases is certainly less than two percent. That does not seem like a great enough difference simply to take the decision out of Paula's hands.

Second, there are considerations of cost. If Paula is paying, it is her decision to spend her money on the screening. Cost considerations primarily apply if the government is paying for the procedure. The government might conclude that performing the tests on someone in Paula's situation is not cost-effective; that is, the costs of the test will be greater than money saved by not having to provide for defective children whose birth would be averted. One might reply that many other medical procedures do not save money, and the costs of Paula's anxiety and worry as well as the suffering of any defective children should also be taken into account. Nevertheless, given finite resources, the government might reasonably decide not to fund prenatal diagnosis unless patients are in a class for which it is cost-effective; it simply cannot afford to provide all possible medical tests for everyone who wants them.

A third reason against offering Paula the test is a shortage of resources. This point concerns a lack of facilities, usually laboratories, to perform the tests. If there is a shortage, then tests should be reserved for the high risk patients most apt to benefit by avoiding the birth of a defective child. This concern has been a real one in Canada, where some centers have had to consider raising the maternal age indication from thirty-five to thirty-seven because of lack of facilities for providing tests for all women thirty-five years of age or more who requested them. Even so, if there is laboratory room and Paula is not depriving anyone else of access, this reason has no force.

Another reason has been offered for denying prenatal diagnosis even for women at risk. The suggestion is that if adequate treatment exists for the condition, then prenatal diagnosis should not be offered. An example would be galactosemia. The objection to providing the test for this condition is basically the objection against the use of abortion for this reason. Its soundness therefore depends on the ethics of abortion. If abortion at this stage is not prima facie morally wrong, then the principle of burdens to others supports a decision to abort an affected infant. Even if abortion is a prima facie wrong, consideration of burdens to others might outweigh its wrongness. Consequently, prenatal diagnosis can be denied due to the availability of treatment only if abortion for the proffered reason is ethically wrong. As we shall see in Chapter 3, abortion for such reasons is not ethically wrong, so there is no basis for denying prenatal diagnosis.

Another issue that arises in prenatal diagnosis is withholding information. One example has already been broached earlier, namely, withholding the sex of the fetus to prevent a woman aborting for sex preselection. However, other reasons also arise. For example, whenever a chromosomal analysis is performed from amniocentesis, most other major chromosomal anomalies are discovered. Thus, the fetus might be found to have XYY chromosomes. Some evidence indicates that males with an extra Y chromosome (which determines male sex) are more likely to be violent and to become inmates of prisons or institutions for the insane. However, the vast majority of XYY men are not violent or insane, and the evidence of greater risk is uncertain. If parents are told of this characteristic, it might adversely alter the way they raise the child if they decide to continue the pregnancy. Yet the purpose of prenatal diagnosis is to discover information; this is why the woman wants the diagnosis. To withhold information seems contrary to the very purpose of prenatal diagnosis.

As in carrier screening, these difficulties can be clarified by advance agreement. Before prenatal diagnosis is performed, a woman can be advised that all sorts of information might be gained, that the significance of some of it is ambiguous, and that she can have all information gained or only selected parts. In short, it can be agreed in advance what type of information will be imparted. It is up to the woman to decide what information is worth having and what is not. Even if it would be ethically wrong for her to have an abortion for sex preselection or an XYY condition, that is a matter for ethical and policy conditions for abortion, not for information from prenatal diagnosis. Not all women want the information in order to decide about abortion; some of them are simply curious about the sex of the fetus.

Another aspect of agreements prior to prenatal diagnosis should be considered. When prenatal diagnosis began, a number of centers refused to provide it unless the woman agreed to have an abortion should a defect be found. Otherwise, it was claimed, the risks were not worth taking. Today, major centers do not have that requirement. For one reason, the risks of amniocentesis are simply not that great. For another, more than 95 percent of the time no defect is found, and anxiety is relieved; this relief would be denied to women who would not agree in advance to an abortion. Also, the abortion decision, it is claimed, is one which a woman should make without pressure or requirements set by others. Nonetheless, a few private doctors or hospitals may still require such an agreement.[7] For the reasons given, that practice is not ethically acceptable.

These last two issues point out a fallacy in much thinking about prenatal diagnosis, namely, that its sole purpose is to discover fetuses with defects or diseases so that they can be aborted. Probably most medical practices still operate on that assumption, but it is not correct. First, some people may want to be better prepared to care for a child should it be damaged. Major psychological, economic, and living adjustments may be necessary. Second, sometimes steps can be taken to ameliorate the child's condition (see Chapter 6). For example, cesarean section delivery might be advisable to reduce chances of birth injury to particularly susceptible fetuses. Intrauterine treatment is

---

[7]Joe Rubin, "Malpractice Board Urged by MD/Lawyer," *The Medical Post*, December 1, 1981, p. 17.

also possible for some defects or diseases. So even people opposed to abortion have reasons for prenatal diagnosis.

Another ethical issue that pertains to carrier screening as well as prenatal diagnosis concerns whether counseling should be directive or nondirective. The pure idea of nondirective counseling is that a counselor provides people with information and assists them in thinking through their decisions, but does not advise, recommend, or influence decisions. In directive counseling, by contrast, a counselor does recommend courses of action to clients.

Nondirective counseling is generally accepted as the ethically appropriate model. The primary reason for this view is to preserve clients' freedom to control their lives. Directive counseling is likely to impose the counselor's or society's values on the client. It logically need not do so; a counselor could always frame recommendations solely in terms of a client's values, but in practice that would rarely occur. Few counselors are trained to recognize or analyze the cultural views of others.

The ideal of nondirective counseling is ethically inappropriate. People want and should be free to make important decisions affecting their lives on the basis of their values. Nonetheless, clients are not always the only people involved. If a pregnancy occurs and proceeds to term, then an affected child is also involved. The principle regarding risk to the unborn provides one reason not to leave decisions completely up to clients.

But the fundamental flaws in the nondirective ideal of genetic counseling are that it is unattainable and ignores features of a model appropriate for other medical situations[8] (perhaps because reproductive decisions are considered more a matter of life-style than medicine). It is not the mere making of recommendations that deprives clients of freedom, and one can do so without making recommendations. For instance, one can withhold information; nondirective counselors do not always—or perhaps even usually—present all the available options. Nondirective counseling influences clients in a nonexplicit way to conform to the counselor's bias. The tone of voice, body movements, and the language in which information is given can strongly influence clients. Since these aspects are not brought into the open, clients are not likely to recognize their influence. Of course, directive counseling can take a strong, authoritarian, and dogmatic position which also deprives clients of freedom of choice, but then clients can clearly recognize the counselor's intention.

In other medical situations, clients usually ask physicians for recommendations and advice. Clients often ask nondirective counselors for recommendations or what they would do. Many counselors try to avoid answering, thus depriving clients of one of the chief benefits they seek. In short, clients often want more than information; they also want advice and recommendations based on a counselor's experience with the outcomes of other patients. To offer such advice openly in a nonthreatening and explicit manner does not deprive clients of freedom to accept or reject such advice or recommendations. Clients frequently ignore or act contrary to medical advice. How-

---

[8]See Michael D. Bayles, *Professional Ethics* (Belmont, Calif.: Wadsworth Publishing Company, 1981), pp. 69–70.

ever, counselors should make clear that they will assist and support clients whatever they decide, or else they should withdraw from the case.

Policy Analysis

Few policy issues of prenatal diagnosis need to be examined. For the most part, the policies that govern medical practice also adequately deal with prenatal diagnosis, including malpractice based on negligent performance of tests and failure to obtain informed consent. Actual practice in this area may be more deficient (due to failure to offer all options) than in other areas of medicine, but this merely indicates a deficiency in the enforcement of the policies, not in the policies themselves. However, a few specific questions deserve some consideration.

One such issue concerns civil suits by parents against physicians or counselors who have not provided specific information or informed them of the availability of tests. Failure to inform women of the availability of tests when they have medical indications for prenatal diagnosis constitutes negligence, even if such failure is still common practice. Whether failure to provide information constitutes negligence is more complex; it is unclear what information is to be provided, and consent documents do not spell it out.

If parents incur extra expense when a defective child is born due to such negligence, then they should be compensated as in other cases of negligence. The usual legal standard for damages is that plaintiffs should receive compensation to place them in the position they would have been in but for the negligent conduct of the defendant. Thus, one might argue that women or couples in such cases should receive the entire costs of raising the child, because had they been informed, they would have had an abortion and the child would not have been born. (In Canada, abortions are legal only for the physical or mental health of the woman, not merely because of possible defect of the fetus, but in practice, abortion is available in these cases.) However, damage awards might plausibly be restricted to the extra expenses over and above those of a normal child, because the woman or couple was willing and expected to incur those expenses. Moreover, in prenatal diagnosis, one can contend that after aborting an affected child the woman would probably proceed to become pregnant again to have a normal child. In short, had she been adequately informed, it is likely she would have eventually had a normal child. Consequently, the difference between the position she would have been in and the one she actually is in, is that between the costs of a normal and of an affected child.

A more complicated situation arises if an affected child sues a physician, clinic, laboratory, or its parents for damages in what is called a "wrongful life" case. The child claims that it should be compensated for the suffering and extra costs incurred as a result of the negligence. Until a few years ago, children lost all such cases.[9] The central argument used in those cases was that one cannot compare the life of a child with

---

[9]See, for example, Gleitman v. Cosgrove, 49 N.J. 22, 227 A.2d 689 (1967); Gildiner v. Thomas Jefferson Univ. Hosp., 451 F. Supp. 692 (E.D. Pa. 1978); Becker v. Schwartz, 46 N.Y.2d 401, 386 N.E.2d 807 (1978).

defects to a state of nonexistence, which is the condition that would have prevailed had an abortion been performed or had the child not been conceived. However, that argument is unsound.[10] One can consider the value of that life and compare it to nonexistence, which has a zero value. The child will, however, only be worse off and have suffered damages should its life be worse than nonexistence. Consequently, the child would be entitled only to damages that would bring its life to the level of nonexistence, and to punitive damages if the defendant was grossly negligent. With this basis for compensation, few children would qualify for damages, and the damages to which they would be entitled are probably so slight as not to make it worth suing.

In 1980, a California appellate court did hold that a child born with Tay-Sachs could sue a laboratory that negligently screened its parents for carrier status.[11] As to damages, the court claimed that the inability to calculate damages does not bar recovery for wrongdoing. The child, the court held, was entitled to damages as if it had been injured after conception, but based on its actual life expectancy (four years) rather than that of a normal person (seventy-plus years).

However, this solution has a logical difficulty. Had the parents been informed of their carrier status, this child would not have been born. They would have had amniocentesis and aborted this child. Consequently, it is not possible to square the damages granted with traditional standards.

In a subsequent case the California Supreme Court held that a child could not recover for pain and suffering or other general damages, because that would have to be offset by the incidental benefit the child received, namely, life.[12] Juries do not have adequate experience to make such judgments. However, the court held that a child could recover special damages for medical expense, special training, and so forth. The court rested its argument on the traditional standard for damages, but essentially deleted considerations of the value of life versus nonexistence. We indicated above that such evaluations are technically possible, but that they would not usually contribute much in damages. Consequently, the court's omission of this factor is acceptable for legal purposes.

A final policy consideration concerns funding. Most genetic screening and counseling is at least partially funded by governments. In Canada, with its national health insurance system, carrier screening, prenatal diagnosis, and legal abortions are funded. In the United States, prenatal diagnosis is not often covered by government programs such as Medicaid, or by private insurance. Private insurance companies might find it financially beneficial to include prenatal diagnosis for some women at risk because the tests might be less expensive than the cost of medical care for children born with defects. This depends, in part, on how many births of defective children are avoided and how much of the cost of care for defective children the com-

---

[10]Michael D. Bayles, "Harm to the Unconceived," *Philosophy and Public Affairs*, 5, no. 3 (1976), 295; Clifton Perry, "Wrongful Life and the Comparison of Harms," *Westminster Institute Review*, 1, no. 4 (1982), 7–9.

[11]Curlender v. Bio-Science Laboratories, 106 Cal. App. 3d 811, 165 Cal. Rptr. 477 (1980).

[12]Turpin v. Sortini, 31 Cal. 3d 220, 182 Cal. Rptr. 337, 643 P.2d 954 (1982).

panies would pay. Even were it not financially beneficial, the cost of adding such coverage would often be willingly borne by subscribers.

In Medicaid, of course, the government has refused to fund abortions except to save the life of a woman and occasionally in cases of rape. (This policy is considered in the next chapter.) Given that the government is funding carrier screening for Tay-Sachs, sickle cell, and thalassemia, it is anomalous not to fund prenatal diagnosis and elective abortion under Medicaid.[13] A generally accepted purpose of carrier screening is to enable couples to avoid the conception or birth of infants with defects, and for these diseases this can be accomplished by prenatal diagnosis and elective abortion. The government has simply made this widely accepted approach less available to the poor, implicitly encouraging them instead to avoid conception, use artificial insemination or some other technique, or give birth to defective children who will be cared for at government expense. This policy is acceptable only if abortion of defective fetuses should be prohibited.

Bibliography

1. Bergsma, Daniel; Lappe, Marc; Roblin, Richard O.; and Gustafson, James M., eds. *Ethical, Social and Legal Dimensions of Screening for Human Genetic Disease*. Birth Defects: Original Article Series; The National Foundation March of Dimes, vol. X, no. 6. New York: Symposia Specialists, Stratton Intercontinental Medical Book Corporation, 1974.

2. Fletcher, John C. "Ethical Issues in Genetic Screening and Antenatal Diagnosis," *Clinical Obstetrics and Gynecology*, 24, no. 4 (1981), 1151–68.

3. "Genetic Diagnosis and Counseling," *Encyclopedia of Bioethics* (1978), 2, 555–66.

4. "Genetic Screening," *Encyclopedia of Bioethics* (1978), 2, 567–72.

5. Holmes, Helen B.; Hoskins, Betty B.; and Gross, Michael, eds. *The Custom-Made Child? Women-Centered Perspectives*. Clifton, N.J.: The Humana Press, Inc., 1981.

6. Milunsky, Aubrey; and Annas, George J., eds. *Genetics and the Law II*. New York: Plenum Press, 1980.

7. Powledge, Tabitha M.; and Fletcher, John. "Guidelines for the Ethical, Social and Legal Issues in Prenatal Diagnosis," *New England Journal of Medicine*, 300, no. 4 (Jan. 25, 1979), 168–72.

8. "Prenatal Diagnosis," *Encyclopedia of Bioethics* (1978), 3, 1332–46.

9. Reilly, Philip. *Genetics, Law, and Social Policy*. Cambridge: Harvard University Press, 1977.

10. Research Group, Institute of Society, Ethics and the Life Sciences. "Ethical and Social Issues in Screening for Genetic Disease," *New England Journal of Medicine*, 286, no. 21 (May 25, 1972), 1129–32.

11. Williamson, Nancy E. "Boys or Girls? Parents' Preferences and Sex Control," *Population Bulletin*, 33, no. 1 (January 1978), 3–35.

[13]See John C. Fletcher, "The Morality and Ethics of Prenatal Diagnosis," in *Genetic Disorders and the Fetus*, ed. Aubrey Milunsky (New York: Plenum Press, 1979), p. 633.

The Ethical Options in Transplanting Fetal Tissue

MARY B. MAHOWALD, JERRY SILVER, AND ROBERT A. RATCHESON

Fetal tissue transplants have now been successful in primates, raising the possibility of treatment for Parkinson's disease and other chronic illnesses. Whether or not abortion is morally justified, use of human fetal tissue for research or therapy is justified in certain circumstances. The rationale, both for permitting transplantation of fetal tissue and for limitations in exercising the technology, is based on the same set of ethical principles that supported restrictive legislation in the past: respect for autonomy and a balancing of harms and benefits that gives priority to those most affected.

As if the ongoing abortion controversy were not complex enough, recent developments in neuroscience have exacerbated the situation. At this point, the following scenario may be anticipated:

A fifty-year-old patient, debilitated from Parkinson's disease, is unable to work or live independently. He and his family have suffered from the economic and emotional effects of the disease. Physically, he experiences rigidity of his arms and legs; he has lost facial expression; his extremities shake; he walks with a shuffling gait; he has difficulty swallowing and speaking. As the disease progresses, these symptoms are becoming more pronounced. Although some symptoms can be alleviated by medication, successively larger doses are required, to a point where the doses may actually trigger symptoms. Since no cure is presently available, the patient can only look forward to further deterioration and premature death.

An experimental treatment has recently been demonstrated to be effective in relieving symptoms of parkinsonism induced in primates. The technique involves obtaining neural tissue from viable or nonviable fetal primates and transplanting this tissue into the

Mary B. Mahowald *is associate professor of medical ethics and co-director of the Center for Biomedical Ethics, Case Western Reserve University School of Medicine and University Hospitals of Cleveland.* Jerry Silver *is associate professor of developmental genetics and anatomy, Case Western Reserve University School of Medicine.* Robert A. Ratcheson *is professor of neurology and director of neurological surgery, Case Western Reserve University School of Medicine and University Hospitals of Cleveland.*

brain of an afflicted adult animal. It is unlikely that American neurobiologists who developed the technique will be able to pursue the work with humans—unless legal restrictions on the use of fetal tissue are modified. Whether the same results can be obtained through use of neural tissue from dead fetuses is as yet unknown.

This scenario describes the situation that now faces a number of American researchers.[1] Impressive advances during the past year have made it impossible to avoid the thorny ethical questions surrounding potential use of fetal transplantation in human beings. The issue exemplifies what William James terms a genuine option—a choice between alternatives that are live, momentous, and unavoidable.[2]

Rationale and Method

The new technique is based on the relatively old idea that specific fetal tissue transplants can replace or repair adult tissue. Fetal tissue can be transplanted with greater success than adult tissue because it is less immunologically reactive, thereby reducing the incidence of rejection. Fetal tissue also has a greater capacity to develop than adult tissue. This may be attributed to the relative lack of differentiation and rapid growth of fetal tissue, which develops both physically and functionally after transplantation.

The age of the fetus may be critical to success: mid-gestation or earlier has thus far produced the best results in rodents,[3] while transplantation in primates has produced survival and growth from both viable and nonviable donors. A nonviable fetus may survive for a short time before death occurs. During that time, and for several hours after, the tissue is still living, and is thus capable of further development and function if transplanted to a viable organism. This is comparable to the viability of organs or tissue obtained from cadaver donors, except that the fetal brain may not yet be dead.

The process is straightforward. Abortion is induced and performed through a method intended to preserve the desired fetal tissue. A specific segment of brain tissue is then removed from the fetus and placed in a strategic area of the recipient's brain. Within weeks, the healthy tissue begins to function as part of the organism into which it was transplanted, and symptoms of the disease decline.

Current Status
of the Research

During the past year neuroscientists have accelerated and modified their experimental use of the technique with animals. Swedish scientists Lars Olson and Ake Seiger extended their earlier work involving intraocular grafts in rats. Olson considered the eye an ideal site for brain tissue research "since it is actually a protrusion of the brain, and the progress of the transplant could be easily observed there."[4] Use of this technique has provided a way of learning how brain cells grow and develop: which cells can be transplanted well, what steps are likely to lead to survival and nerve fiber production, when the cells will make connections and when they will not, and at which stage of fetal development cells are optimal for grafting.

In the United States, Raymond Lund (University of Maryland)[5] and Carl Cotman (University of California—Irvine)[6] have shown in separate experiments with rats a tendency for implanted tissue to find its way to the brain site appropriate to its physiologic function. Cotman has also studied the hippocampus (an area of the brain typically affected by Alzheimer's disease), and found that undamaged nerve fibers start to sprout again. In Cleveland, Jerry Silver has developed a technique for regenerating nerve pathways in mice.[7] In Rochester, New York, John Sladek has dealt with the problem of replacing neurons in primates. At a meeting of transplant researchers in New York in April 1986, he showed evidence that the fetal transplantation method had been successful in treating symptoms of Parkinson's induced in monkeys.[8] Several other laboratories throughout the country are also working on these techniques.

In Sweden, four patients suffering from Parkinson's disease have been treated through implantation of tissue from their own adrenal glands into precise areas of the brain. These tissues supply dopamine, a natural chemical that can reduce symptoms of parkinsonism. Olson is reported to have said that "all improved dramatically for a while."[9] Although patients eventually reverted to their previous disease symptoms, no harmful effects were evident. Human adrenal transplants provide a way of bypassing the ethical problems associated with use of fetal tissue. It is improbable, however, that use of the adrenal tissue will be as successful therapeutically, because the greater developmental capability of fetal tissue provides an advantage not found in grafts from mature individuals.

The success of the Swedish experiments, coupled with the recent success in primates suggests that Parkinson's may be the first human disease to be successfully treated through transplantation of fetal brain tissue. Other degenerative diseases such as Alzheimer's, and congenital anomalies such as hypogonadism (a condition in which growth and sexual development are retarded) are also potentially reparable through the technique, as are neural tube defects, whether genetic or traumatic in origin (spina bifida and spinal cord injury, for example).[10] Some scientists even believe that the technology will someday be used to reverse brain damage, a goal previously considered impossible. Although most researchers are optimistic about its eventual therapeutic effectiveness, they differ in their expectations of when the technique will be sufficiently developed for clinical applications to humans. Even if access to fetal tissue is restricted, research and therapeutic applications are likely to proceed, but less expeditiously than otherwise.

Current Restrictions

Between 1969 and 1973, all fifty states passed the Uniform Anatomical Gift Act (UAGA), which allows for the gift of "all or part of the body" of a dead fetus for research or therapeutic purposes.[11] Either or both of these purposes may be served by using human fetal tissue for transplantation. Retrieving viable brain tissue from a dead fetus could be viewed as violating the UAGA requirement of "respectful treatment of the decedent's remains." This is unlikely, however, unless a special case is made for retrieval of brain tissue as distinct from retrieval of other tissue or organs provided by human cadavers. According to Charles Baron,[12] nine states permit research on dead fetuses under the terms of the UAGA, eight more do the same with very slight modifications, and six totally prohibit research on dead fetuses obtained from elective abortions.

Twenty-five states have enacted enabling provisions of the UAGA, but have no further restrictions on fetal research. In the last mentioned group, it is apparently legal for researchers to use tissue obtained from fetal remains for transplantation, so long as either parent grants permission, and the other does not object. As far as we know, however, no use of human fetal tissue for transplantation has yet been reported, and none has been funded through government grants.

In July 1974, the year after the *Roe v. Wade* decision legalized abortion during the first two trimesters of pregnancy, a congressional moratorium was imposed upon federal funding of fetal research. The following summer, the National Commission for the Protection of Human Subjects of Biomedical and Behavioral Research published guidelines applicable to research conducted or funded by the Department of Health and Human Services.[13] These guidelines recommend federal support of certain categories of fetal research, conditional on the approval of local institutional review boards (IRBs), informed consent of the mother, and the nonobjection of the father.

Experimentation with an abortus determined to be viable after delivery is not permitted; such an abortus or "viable fetus *ex utero*" is defined as a premature infant. The term "viable" means the ability "after either spontaneous or induced delivery, to survive (given the benefit of available medical therapy) to the point of independently maintaining heart beat and respiration." A fetus *ex utero* whose viability is still in question may not be involved in research unless the project imposes no added risk, or its purpose is to enhance the possibility of survival.

If the fetus is nonviable, nontherapeutic research is permitted only if the following conditions are present: (a) vital functions are not artificially maintained; (b) procedures that would terminate the heartbeat or respiration of the fetus are not employed; (c) the purpose of the research is the acquisition of important biomedical knowledge that cannot be obtained by other means. In the procedure required for successful fetal brain tissue transplantation, condition (b) cannot be satisfied, and condition (a) may not be satisfied.

Clearly, the restrictions on research with living fetuses, whether viable or nonviable, are more stringent than those involving dead fetuses, which are defined in the regulations as "exhibit[ing] neither heartbeat, spontaneous respiratory activity, spontaneous movement of voluntary muscles, nor pulsation of the umbilical cord (if still attached)."

Possibilities for therapeutic use of fetal tissue were unknown to the Commissioners or state and city lawmakers who developed legislation and guidelines governing fetal research. They were concerned about exploitation and commercialization of fetuses in the wake of an abundance of fetuses available after *Roe v. Wade*. Even where the link between research and therapeutic applications might have been recognized, no immediate therapeutic goal was evident at that time. If the clinical significance of current transplantation techniques had been anticipated, different solutions to the problem might have been proposed.

New Knowledge, Old Questions

Despite the significant therapeutic possibilities of fetal neural tissue transplants, the process raises enormous ethical problems. Old questions must now be reexamined in light of new knowledge: What are our moral obligations (if any) to a fetus that has been or may be aborted? What are our obligations to the pregnant woman who undergoes abortion, whether spontaneously or electively? What are our obligations to an individual whose health can be restored through transplantation? What are our obligations to the larger society, in which many may benefit through research support and therapeutic applications?

In the interest of informed critical discussion, let us consider more familiar procedures that have raised some of the same ethical questions: transplantation from live donors; transplantation from cadavers; and "surrogate motherhood." To the extent that common issues are raised, common resolutions may be suggested.

Transplantation from Live Donors   Although some still oppose this technique on moral grounds, it has become generally acceptable, even morally commendable, so long as three conditions are satisfied: (1) the donor or the donor's proxy has provided free and informed consent; (2) the burden to the donor (including loss of an organ or tissue, risk, and possible pain of the procedure) is proportionate to its expected benefit to another or others; (3) other means of obtaining the expected benefit are not available. Although proponents of active euthanasia might argue otherwise, we believe that the second condition is not met if the procedure entails direct termination of the donor's life, as would occur in whole brain or heart transplantation from a living donor.

However, if it were possible to remove a small portion of brain without sacrificing the donor's life, then this condition could be met in transplantation of brain tissue. While removing vital organs from a living donor may be defended on grounds of beneficence toward a dying patient, this is clearly a more difficult position to support than removing nonvital organs or tissues from living donors.[14] The less invasive, painful, or life-threatening the procedure is to the donor, the easier it is to defend. Condition (2) also suggests that the use of anesthesia to reduce the donor's pain, or possible pain, may be morally required for transplantation.

A comparable rationale applies to transplantation of tissue from living fetuses, whether viable or nonviable. So long as the removal of a specific organ or tissue would not directly terminate the life of the donor, the above three conditions are applicable. However, the following caveats are also pertinent to fetal tissue transplantation: (a) a woman who elects abortion may thus forfeit the role of proxy for the abortus, and (b) the personhood of the donor (the abortus) is a subject of moral dispute. With regard to (a), another proxy could be selected if the woman's proxy status were denied; with regard to (b), we have obligations to an abortus even if it is not a person, as the UAGA recognizes. Nonetheless, if the fetus *ex utero* is not a person, obligations to the abortus are less binding than those we have toward donors who are persons. Because of its closer approximation to uncontroversial personhood, a viable abortus is more likely to be counted as a person than is a nonviable fetus *ex utero* or a viable fetus *in utero*.

Transplantation from Cadavers   Organ and tissue donation is encouraged from ca-daver donors so long as free and informed consent has been previously indicated or obtained from the family. These donors are no longer capable of suffering pain be-cause brain activity has ceased. Although technological supports or surgical pro-cedures maintain vital functions so as to insure successful organ retrieval, these do-nors are in fact dead. Arguments favoring donation are based on therapeutic results for recipients, as well as on the claim that donation assuages the grief of donor fami-lies. The procedure is sometimes seen as a way of honoring and "extending the life" of the loved one through the "gift of life" to others.[15]

Transplantation of certain organs has evoked more serious psychosocial concerns than others, and raised more serious philosophical issues. The heart is an obvious example in this regard, since it is seen not only as crucial to vital function, but as a symbol of the individual's emotional life and ability to love. In the hypothetical case of whole brain transplantation, the organ is not only a symbol but the actual source of the donor's cognitive and conscious function. The problem of personal identity, which to a lesser extent is raised in other organ transplants also, is then most signifi-cantly posed: *who* is the person whose brain used to belong to *A* if and when that entire brain is transplanted into the body of *B*? Although whole brain transplants are not feasible, it is theoretically possible to transplant viable brain tissue from (brain-dead) cadavers. Whether, or to what extent, this would alter the identity of the recip-ient is a question that cannot be adequately addressed here. Among other considera-tions, it requires thorough analysis of the literature on personal identity.[16]

Surrogate Motherhood   Unlike transplantation of vital organs from cadavers or transplantation of spare organs from living donors, the technical option of surrogate motherhood has not evoked broad support. Surrogate motherhood is commonly construed as a situation in which a woman becomes pregnant through insemination with the sperm of a man who wishes (usually with his infertile wife) to have a child; it more accurately defines a situation in which a woman gestates an embryo formed through fertilization of another woman's ovum. Either situation is comparable to that of fetal tissue transplantation, because in both cases women's bodies are used for the sake of another, and there is risk of demeaning human life through commercialization.

Other features are also applicable to both surrogacy and fetal tissue transplanta-tion: there may be compelling medical reasons for undertaking the procedure; the pregnant woman may (and should) provide free and informed consent; and a good effect is intended and expected. With fetal tissue transplantation (as with transplantation generally), a bad effect (loss of an organ or tissue) is suffered for the sake of the recipient, and there is no similarly bad effect in surrogacy. Whether the possible good effects of the two types of procedure are comparable depends on whether the value of providing biologically related offspring to an infertile couple is greater or less than the value of curing a seriously debilitating disease for someone already born. We are not ourselves sure which counts as the greater good.

The preceding comparisons suggest the following conditions as moral requirements for fetal tissue transplantation: consent of a proxy; a significant research or therapeutic goal, and ascertainment that other (less problematic) means of obtaining the goal are not available. They also suggest that retrieval of essential organs or tissue from dead fetuses is more acceptable than their retrieval from nonviable living abortuses. We believe, however, that use of essential organs or tissue from nonviable fetuses is morally defensible if dead fetuses are not available or are not conducive to successful transplants.

We have added concerns regarding the use of nonviable living fetuses because of their possible sensitivity to pain, and the fact that such donors are not legally "brain-dead." The first concern may be satisfactorily addressed on a practical level by using anesthesia. The second is more troublesome and complicated, and applies also to organ donation from anencephalic infants. Michael Harrison has recently proposed "brain absence" as a categorization permitting transplantation from anencephalics.[17] Although the term corresponds to the literal meaning of anencephaly, it does not accurately reflect the status of some infants who are diagnosed as anencephalic but who have not yet died; although most of the organ is "absent," some brain and/or brain function remains so long as the infant maintains a degree of vital function. "Nonviability" is a more accurate description; this term would apply not only to anencephalic infants, but also to fetuses or individuals whose imminent death is unavoidable.

The Problem of Access:
Abortion and Intent

Despite the similarities between fetal tissue transplantation and other procedures, significant differences remain. Central among these is the way in which fetal tissue becomes available—through abortion. Spontaneous abortions (noninduced pregnancy loss occurring before twenty completed weeks of gestation) are less problematic than induced abortions because they are analogous to the circumstances through which life-saving organs ordinarily become available—the cessation of brain function in trauma victims. But the number of spontaneously aborted second-trimester fetuses is relatively small, and many of these lack sufficiently healthy tissue for successful transplantation.[18]

Induced abortions during any stage of pregnancy are legally permissible if the procedure is undertaken for the sake of the pregnant woman's life or health. Although 1.3 million fetuses are aborted yearly in the United States,[19] the number of healthy fetuses that might thus be obtained is again quite small. The more advanced the gestation, the less likely abortion is to occur, whether spontaneously or electively. Some second trimester abortions are induced after prenatal monitoring has indicated fetal defects; the defects themselves tend to reduce the probability of successful transplant.

Clearly, electively aborted, healthy fetuses are the primary source for transplantation of fetal tissue. But these abortions, unlike situations in which transplantation is made possible because of trauma or spontaneous abortion, carry the onus of deliberateness—i.e., fetal death appears to be intended. If intent is morally relevant, this feature is problematic. Accordingly, those states that have proscribed research with fetuses obtained through elective abortions, while sanctioning research with fetuses obtained through spontaneous abortion, have argued that a woman who chooses abortion thereby forfeits the right to make further decisions relevant to the abortus. By not choosing abortion, she retains the right to make such decisions—even as a parent may give permission for research involving his or her child.

However, the fact that abortion is "induced" or "elected" (terms often used synonymously in the clinical setting) does not imply that fetal death is directly intended. In some cases, abortions are induced because the continuation of the pregnancy poses a serious threat to the woman's life or health. What is intended then is to restore the woman's health or save her life by interrupting the pregnancy, severing the tie between the woman and her fetus. If the tie could be severed without terminating fetal life, this would be the preferred outcome. Fetal death may thus be a foreseen but unintended consequence of an abortion that is therapeutic for the pregnant woman.[20]

Even where fetal death is intended, one could argue that the pregnant woman should determine the fate of her fetus—whether living or dead, viable or nonviable, *in utero* or *ex utero*. As we have already suggested (in remarking about closer approximation to "uncontroversial personhood"), this argument is least persuasive if the fetus is living and viable, or possibly viable. Court orders and legal decisions have maintained the obligation of practitioners to provide care for these fetuses or abortuses.

The UAGA allows use of tissue obtained from dead fetuses so long as one parent consents, and the other does not object. Several possible requirements of the technique make it even more important to respect the autonomy of the pregnant woman: gestation may need to be prolonged, and the method of abortion may need to be altered, in either case in order to increase the chances of therapeutic success for the recipient. If midgestation is the optimal time for human transplantation (a possibility that has not been established), a woman who would otherwise undergo abortion during the first trimester might be asked to continue her pregnancy until the second trimester. Maintaining the pregnancy is comparable to maintaining vital functions of a cadaver donor through mechanical support. However, while the latter practice is legally permissible, prolonging vital functions of a living fetus for research purposes is prohibited by federal guidelines.

Among alternative methods of abortion, the procedure used in the primate experiments (hysterotomy) is least directly damaging to the fetus but entails greater risk for the pregnant woman. In contrast, the method which is most directly damaging to the fetus (dilatation and evacuation, or D&E) is statistically safest for the pregnant woman if performed at the appropriate stage of gestation.[21] Other abortion procedures (e.g., prostaglandin or saline infusion) may be both medically indicated and productive of viable fetal tissue. In light of the different effects of different methods, however, the pregnant woman's free and informed consent is morally appropriate not only with regard to when, but also with regard to how, her pregnancy will be terminated.

Just as it has been possible to enact liberal abortion laws in conjunction with laws restricting fetal experimentation, it is also possible to oppose abortion on moral grounds, and still approve the use of fetal tissue for research and/or therapy. It is only possible, however, if the procedures of abortion and transplantation are practically and intentionally distinct, rather than integrally related as means and end.

Theoretically, abortion may be undertaken as a means of facilitating research or clinical applications for others; in fact, however, abortions are typically chosen by individuals as ends for themselves. The end of transplantation is achieved by the means of retrieving tissue from an already nonviable fetus. The physician who performs an abortion, whether therapeutic or elective, is doing something for the pregnant woman; the physician who transplants fetal tissue into the body of another patient is doing something for that person. These two individuals ought to be distinct, just as they are in the analogous situation of organ retrieval from living related or cadaver donors. Real or apparent conflicts of interest are thereby avoided.

The physician who performs an abortion may have moral responsibilities to the fetus that are secondary to those toward the pregnant woman. For example, from methods that present an equal risk to the pregnant woman, the physician may be obligated to choose the one least directly destructive, or least painful to the fetus (if the fetus can experience pain). This is comparable to a situation in which capital punishment is viewed as morally justifiable, while torture is clearly an objectionable means of implementation. Or, physicians may be morally obligated (as they are already legally obligated) to treat a viable abortion survivor. In *Planned Parenthood of Kansas v. Missouri*, the majority opinion of the U.S. Supreme Court affirmed the following: "Preserving the life of a viable fetus that is aborted may not often be possible, but the State legitimately may choose to provide safeguards for the comparatively few instances of live birth that occur."[22] But this array of obligations applies to the physician involved in the abortion, not the transplant surgeon. A transplant surgeon who is morally opposed to abortion may morally use the tissue of a nonviable fetus, obtained through an abortion, in order to cure serious diseases in other patients, *so long as both practical and intentional distinctions between the two procedures are clearly maintained*.

Further Limitations and Objections

Whether or not abortion is a morally acceptable option, further moral considerations are applicable to fetal tissue transplantation. Two of these are specific to evolving knowledge regarding the technology: (1) the requirement of consent on the part of the pregnant woman; (2) the avoidance of pain to the fetus (for example, by insuring that the fetus is already dead, or by using anesthesia). Two other conditions apply here, as they would to other transplantation situations and to any experimental use of human subjects: (3) other modes of research or therapy are not available, and (4) the good expected is at least proportionate to the risk and/or harm that is also expected.[23]

History furnishes convincing examples of the moral uses of results that have been obtained by questionable, illegal, or immoral means. In fact, the argument that it is immoral not to use such results for good purposes is more compelling than its counterargument. For example, although many consider the American bombing of Nagasaki immoral, no one seems to question the morality of utilizing the information thereby provided to learn about radiation (a research goal) and to benefit future victims of radiation fallout (a therapeutic goal). Much earlier, dissection of human corpses was an illegal act; yet those who practiced dissection may have justified it as a form of "civil disobedience," essential to the successful treatment of others or to developing an adequate understanding of the human body. Their posterity undoubtedly used the knowledge thus obtained for moral purposes, without incurring the accusation that they were acting immorally.

Admittedly, these examples involve our use of knowledge rather than tissue or organs. They thus address the research goal of fetal tissue transplants, not their therapeutic goal. Yet the therapeutic goal provides the more persuasive case for use of the new transplant technology, based partly on its analogy with use of organs and tissue from cadaver donors or from living donors. Crucial principles that apply to both sides of the analogy are: respect for autonomy (of pregnant woman or donor); beneficence toward both donor and recipient, and justice or fairness (an equitable distribution of harms and benefits among those affected).

Obviously these principles may also be considered in defending the position that transplantation of fetal tissue is morally wrong, even though the procedure might save a life or cure a debilitating illness. Unless we subscribe to a crassly utilitarian (even eugenic) ethic, scientific progress and therapeutic effectiveness are not adequate grounds for *using* people. It may be objected that nonviable fetuses are not persons anyway, at least not legally. If established personhood is a sufficient basis for opposing transplantation, however, organ transplantation from living adults should also be rejected.

The crucial role of informed consent, as Hans Jonas has suggested, is to transform the situation from one in which a donor is used to one in which the donor's or proxy's autonomy is respected.[24] Or, as Richard McCormick has argued with respect to the participation of children in low-risk experimentation, membership in a community may justify the procedure.[25] The situation may be considered "low risk" on the basis of the donor's inability to survive, regardless of whether the transplantation takes place.

A Slippery Slope—
the Need for Wedges

As with many troublesome ethical issues, the slippery slope argument is applicable to transplantation of fetal tissue. For example, we may initially permit only the transplantation of tissue from dead fetuses. If this does not prove successful or adequate, we may then transplant tissue from nonviable (living) fetuses or abortuses. Routinization of the practice could lead to transplantation of larger and larger portions of the brain, to transplantation of entire brains from viable fetuses, or to harvesting organs from other donors who are not dead, but are dying or chronically ill. In those circumstances too we may have the moral benefit of consent, whether direct or proxy, but consent alone is not sufficient warrant for using human organs or tissue. Moreover, while the technology might at first be used purely for convincing therapeutic reasons (to heal or save lives in situations of seriously debilitating disease, for example), morally questionable motives such as profit making could eventually take over. That possibility has of course existed throughout the history of organ and tissue transplantation. Here one could envision a situation in which women would be paid to become pregnant and undergo abortion exclusively for the sake of fetal tissue transplantation.[26] The moral problems thus raised parallel those that may occur in surrogate motherhood.

While arguments of this sort are valid and important, they are no more compelling than arguments about the permissibility of abortion or withdrawal of life-sustaining treatment. The roadway travelled by those who make ethical decisions is unavoidably a slippery slope. To traverse it successfully requires placing wedges at the right places, in order to restrict or stop travel at those points where one is most likely to fall. Accordingly, if transplantation of fetal tissue is permitted, there must be reliable checks against extending the technique to living, viable individuals, and against commercialization, which would trivialize human life in its nonviable stage. Such checks are neither new nor ineffective; they have been successfully applied to organ and tissue retrieval from cadaver donors.

There is no doubt that fetal tissue transplantation evokes ghoulish images of the procedure itself as an assault and a mutilation of immature human beings. Similar images arise with regard to organ retrieval from cadaver donors. However, recent suggestions for alleviating psychosocial problems associated with organ retrieval are applicable here also. These include educating the staff regarding the procedure, its therapeutic possibilities, and applicable moral guidelines; showing consideration for families, and allowing for refusal to participate in the procedure; recognizing the legitimacy of "emotional discomfort and cognitive dissonance" regarding the issue.[27] While these steps may facilitate the use of fetal tissue where it is morally defensible, they need not and should not obviate the need for continuing scrutiny of its moral basis in particular cases. A degree of aversion will serve as a wedge, helping to maintain our moral balance along the slippery slope.

Acknowledgment

We wish to thank John Sladek, Jeff Rosenstein, Stuart Youngner, and Barbara Juknialis for helpful comments in preparing this article.

References

1. D. Eugene Redmond, et al., "Fetal Neuronal Grafts in Monkeys Given Methylphenyltetrahydropyridine," *The Lancet* (May 17, 1986), pp. 1125–27.

2. William James, *The Will to Believe* (New York: Dover Publications, 1956), p. 3.

3. Fred H. Gage and Anders Bjorklund, "Intracerebral Grafting of Neuronal Cell Suspensions into the Adult Brain," *CNS Trauma* (1984), pp. 47–56.

4. Edwin Kiester, Jr., "Spare Parts for Damaged Brains," *Science 86* 7:2 (March 1986), 34.

5. Steven McLoon and Raymond Lund, "Development of Fetal Retina, Tectum and Cortex Transplanted to the Superior Colliculus of Adult Rats," *Journal of Comparative Neurology* 217 (1983), 376–89.

6. Kiester, pp. 37–38; cf. E.W. Harris and C.W. Cotman, "Brain Tissue Transplantation Research," *Applied Neurophysiology* 47 (1984), 9–15; C.W. Cotman, et al., "Enhancing the Self-Repairing Potential of the CNS after Injury," *CNS Trauma* (1984), pp. 3–14.

7. George M. Smith, Robert H. Miller, and Jerry Silver, "The Changing Role of Forebrain Astrocytes during Development, Regenerative Failure, and Induced Regeneration upon Transplantation," *Journal of Comparative Neurology* 251 (1986), 23–43.

8. Walter Sullivan, "Cell Implants Curb Parkinson's in Two Monkeys," *New York Times*, May 17, 1986, p. 8.

9. Kiester, p. 33.

10. Alan Fine, "Transplantation in the Central Nervous System," *Scientific American* 255 (1986), 52–58b, cf. A.J. Silverman, et al., "Ultrastructure of Gonadotropin-Releasing Hormone Neuronal Structures Derived from Normal Fetal Preoptic Area and Transplanted into Hypogonadal Mutant (HPG) Mice," *Journal of Neuroscience* 6 (1986), 2090–96.

11. "Uniform Anatomical Gift Act," *Table of Jurisdictions Wherein Act Has Been Adopted*, 8A Unif. Laws Annot. 15–16 (1983).

12. Charles H. Baron, "Fetal Research: The Question in the States," *Hastings Center Report* 15:2 (April 1985), 12–16.

13. National Commission for the Protection of Human Subjects of Biomedical and Behavioral Research, *Report and Recommendations: Research on the Fetus* (Washington, 1975).

14. Thomas E. Starzl, "Will Live Organ Donations No Longer be Justified?" *Hastings Center Report* 15:2 (April 1985), 5.

15. Stuart Youngner, et al., "Psychosocial and Ethical Implications of Organ Retrieval," *New England Journal of Medicine* 313 (Aug. 1985), 322–23.

16. Cf. John Perry, ed., *Personal Identity* (Berkeley: University of California Press, 1975); Amelie Rorty, ed., *The Identities of Persons* (Berkeley: University of California Press, 1976); Michael Green and Daniel Wikler, "Brain Death and Personal Identity," *Philosophy and Public Affairs* 9 (1980), 105–33; Walter Quinn, "Abortion: Identity and Loss," *Philosophy and Public Affairs* 13 (1984), 24–54.

17. Michael P. Harrison, "The Anencephalic Newborn as Organ Donor," *Hastings Center Report* 16:2 (April 1986), 21–22.

18. R.D. Wilson, et al., "Spontaneous Abortion and Pregnancy Outcome after Normal First-Trimester Ultrasound Examination," *Obstetrics and Gynecology* 67:3 (March 1986), 352–55.

19. Centers for Disease Control, *Abortion Surveillance* (Public Health Service, Department of Health and Human Services, Atlanta, Georgia, November 1980), p. 48.

20. See Mary B. Mahowald, "Concepts of Abortion and Their Relevance to the Abortion Debate," *Southern Journal of Philosophy* XX:2 (Summer 1986), 195–207.

21. Centers for Disease Control, *Abortion Surveillance*, Table 23, p. 49.

22. Planned Parenthood of Kansas City v. Missouri, *United States Law Week* 51 (June 14, 1983), 4783–85.

23. National Commission for the Protection of Human Subjects, *Report and Recommendations: Institutional Review Boards*, and *Appendix* (Washington: Department of Health and Human Services Publication Nos. OS 78-0008 and OS 78-0009, 1978).

24. Hans Jonas, "Philosophical Reflections on Experimenting with Human Subjects," *Philosophical Essays: From Current Creed to Technological Man* (Chicago: University of Chicago Press, 1980), pp. 105–31.

25. Richard A. McCormick, "Experimentation in Children: Sharing in Sociality," *Hastings Center Report* 6:6 (December 1976), 42.

26. Mary Anne Warren, Daniel Maguire, and Carol Levine, "Can the Fetus Be an Organ Farm?" *Hastings Center Report* 8:5 (October 1978), 23–25.

27. Youngner, et al., p. 323.